Successful Local Anesthesia for Rest(

*Second E*

MW00836994

# Successful
# Local Anesthesia

## FOR RESTORATIVE DENTISTRY AND ENDODONTICS

### *Second Edition*

**Al Reader,** DDS, MS
Emeritus Professor and Past Director of the
Advanced Endodontic Program
College of Dentistry
The Ohio State University
Columbus, Ohio

**John Nusstein,** DDS, MS
Professor and Chair of the Division of Endodontics
College of Dentistry
The Ohio State University
Columbus, Ohio

**Melissa Drum,** DDS, MS
Associate Professor and Director of the
Advanced Endodontic Program
College of Dentistry
The Ohio State University
Columbus, Ohio

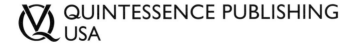

**QUINTESSENCE PUBLISHING**
USA

Chicago, Berlin, Tokyo, London, Paris, Milan, Barcelona,
Istanbul, Moscow, New Delhi, Prague, São Paulo, Seoul, and Warsaw

# Dedication

*This book is dedicated to the current and former endodontic graduate students who shared our goal of profound pulpal anesthesia.*

**Library of Congress Cataloging-in-Publication Data**

Names: Reader, Al, author. | Nusstein, John, author. | Drum, Melissa, author.
Title: Successful local anesthesia for restorative dentistry and endodontics
  / Alfred Reader, John Nusstein, Melissa Drum.
Description: Second edition. | Hanover Park, IL : Quintessence Publishing Co
  Inc, [2017] | Includes bibliographical references and index.
Identifiers: LCCN 2016045951 (print) | LCCN 2016046585 (ebook) | ISBN
  9780867157437 (softcover) | ISBN 9780867157505 ()
Subjects: | MESH: Anesthesia, Dental | Anesthesia, Local--methods | Dental
  Restoration, Permanent | Root Canal Therapy
Classification: LCC RK510 (print) | LCC RK510 (ebook) | NLM WO 460 | DDC
  617.9/676--dc23
LC record available at https://lccn.loc.gov/2016045951

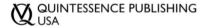

**QUINTESSENCE PUBLISHING**
USA

©2017 Quintessence Publishing Co, Inc

Quintessence Publishing Co Inc
4350 Chandler Drive
Hanover Park, IL 60133
www.quintpub.com

5  4  3  2  1

Editor: Leah Huffman
Design: Erica Neumann
Production: Angelina Schmelter
Printed in the USA

# Contents

# Preface

Why do patients avoid going to the dentist? According to a survey by the American Dental Association,[1] fear of pain is the greatest factor that prevents patients from visiting their dentist. Additional surveys[2,3] have found that 90% of dentists have some anesthetic difficulties during restorative dentistry procedures. Because adequate pulpal anesthesia is a clinical problem, we and other authors have performed a number of research studies on local anesthesia over the last 30 years. We are excited to present some of these findings in this book.

From the Latin word *patiens*, the word *patient* in English originally meant "one who suffers." Unfortunately, some patients may still "suffer" when visiting the dentist. Our goal is to reduce pain and manage it successfully. That being said, profound pulpal anesthesia is a cornerstone to the delivery of dental care. Administration of local anesthesia is one of the most common procedures in clinical practice. It is invariably the first procedure we perform, and it affects almost everything we do during that appointment. If the patient is not adequately anesthetized and you have some extensive restorative work planned, difficulties arise. The information in this book explains why problems occur and offers clinical solutions to help clinicians stay on schedule.

Fortunately, local anesthesia has evolved tremendously over the last 25 years just as the materials and techniques have evolved in restorative dentistry and endodontics. The current technology and drug formulations used for local anesthesia have made it so much easier to treat patients successfully. We now have the ability to anesthetize patients initially, provide anesthesia for the full appointment, and reverse some of the effects of soft tissue anesthesia if desired. Priceless!

This book covers the research-based rationale, advantages, and limitations of the various anesthetic agents and routes of administration. A special emphasis is placed on supplemental anesthetic techniques that are vital to the practice of dentistry. However, this book does not cover the basic techniques utilized for the delivery of local anesthetics because that information is readily available elsewhere in textbooks and other publications.

In addition, this book emphasizes information for the restorative dentist and endodontist because the requirements for pulpal anesthesia are different than those for oral surgery, implant dentistry, periodontics, and pediatric dentistry. Eighty-five percent of local anesthesia teaching in dental school is done by oral and maxillofacial surgery departments,[4] and while they do an excellent job, it is sometimes difficult for oral surgeons to appreciate the requirements for pulpal anesthesia in restorative dentistry and endodontic therapy. Furthermore, we should value our experience. Whereas education is what you get during your training, experience is what you get afterward. A young practitioner knows the rules, but an older practitioner knows the exceptions. Experience is a wonderful thing that enables us to recognize a mistake when we make it.

Throughout the book, the information has been divided into specific topics so it is understandable and easy to reference. When indicated, summary information has been provided. References to published literature are included in the chapters because clinicians within the specialty of endodontics (of which we are members) communicate with each other by quoting authors and studies. We also think it is important to credit the authors for their contributions to the literature on local anesthesia.

This book is a clinical adjunct to help you successfully anesthetize patients using the newest technology and drugs available. Indeed, the information presented here will help you to provide painless treatment. Pulpal anesthesia is emphasized throughout this book. That is, pulpal anesthesia is required by the restorative dentist and endodontist in order to perform painless treatment. We think that is a worthy goal for the dental profession. However, as Will Rogers once said, to be successful, you must *know* what you are doing, *like* what you are doing, and *believe in* what you are doing.

## References

1. ADA survey. Influences on dental visits. ADA News 1998;11(2):4.
2. Kaufman E, Weinstein P, Milgrom P. Difficulties in achieving local anesthesia. J Am Dent Assoc 1984;108:205–208.
3. Weinstein P, Milgrom P, Kaufman E, Fiset L, Ramsay D. Patient perceptions of failure to achieve optimal local anesthesia. Gen Dent 1985;33:218–220.
4. Dower JS. A survey of local anesthesia course directors. Anesth Prog 1998;45:91–95.

# Acknowledgments

We want to acknowledge the time spent away from our spouses (Dixie Reader, Tammie Nusstein, and Jason Drum) in completing this work. We are so grateful they were willing to help us produce a thoughtful addition to local anesthesia.

As the senior author, Al Reader would like to thank his coauthors for all their help: "My associates and I always compromise. I admit I'm wrong and they agree with me."

All royalties from the sale of this book will be equally divided between the American Association of Endodontists' Foundation and The Ohio State University Endodontic Graduate Student Research Fund to support further research on anesthesia and pain control.

# 1

# Clinical Factors Related to Local Anesthesia

**After reading this chapter, the practitioner should be able to:**

- Discuss the clinical factors related to local anesthesia.
- Provide ways of confirming clinical anesthesia.
- Describe issues related to local anesthesia.
- Explain the effects anxiety has on local anesthesia.
- Discuss the use of vasoconstrictors.
- Characterize injection pain.
- Evaluate the use of topical anesthetics.
- Discuss alternative modes of reducing pain during injections.

Clinical pulpal anesthesia is dependent on the interaction of three major factors: *(1)* the dentist, *(2)* the patient, and *(3)* local anesthesia (Fig 1-1). The dentist is dependent on the local anesthesia agents as well as his or her technique. In addition, the dentist is dependent on the interaction with the patient (rapport/confidence). How the patient interacts with the administration of local anesthesia is determined by a number of clinical factors.

# Confirming Pulpal Anesthesia in Nonpainful Vital Teeth

## Lip numbness

A traditional method to confirm anesthesia usually involves questioning patients by asking if their lip is numb (Fig 1-2). Although lip numbness can be obtained 100% of the time, pulpal anesthesia may fail in the mandibular first molar in 23% of patients.[1–16] Therefore, lip numbness does not always indicate pulpal anesthesia. However, lack of lip numbness for an inferior alveolar nerve block (IANB) does indicate that the injection was "missed," and pulpal anesthesia will not be present.

    **IN CONCLUSION,** *lip numbness does not always indicate pulpal anesthesia.*

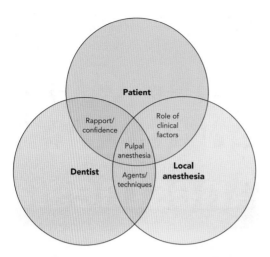

**Fig 1-1** The relationship of pulpal anesthesia to the patient, dentist, and local anesthesia.

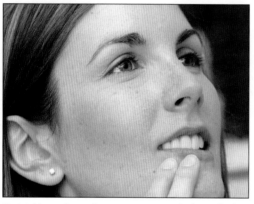

Fig 1-2 Lip numbness does not guarantee pulpal anesthesia.

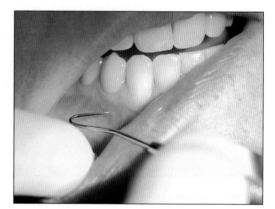

**Fig 1-3** A lack of patient response to mucosal or gingival "sticks" is a poor indicator of pulpal anesthesia.

## Soft tissue testing

Using a sharp explorer to "stick" the soft tissue (gingiva, mucosa, lip, tongue) in the area of nerve distribution (Fig 1-3) has a 90% to 100% incidence of success.[2–5] Regardless, pulpal anesthesia may still not be present for the mandibular first molar in 23% of patients.[1–16] Negative mucosal sticks usually indicate that the mucosal tissue is anesthetized.

**IN CONCLUSION,** *the lack of patient response to sharp explorer sticks is a poor indicator of pulpal anesthesia.*

## Commencing with treatment

The problem with commencing treatment without confirming anesthesia is that there is no way to know if the patient is numb until we start to drill on the tooth. This may create anxiety for both the patient and the dentist. A typical scenario involving a crown preparation on a mandibular molar can become problematic if the patient feels pain when the mesiobuccal dentin is reached with the bur. If the patient reacts to the pain, the dentist may say, "Oh, did you feel that?" and then may try to continue with treatment. If the patient reacts again when the mesiobuccal dentin is touched with the bur,

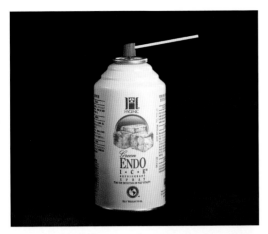

Fig 1-4 A cold refrigerant may be used to test for pulpal anesthesia before the start of a clinical procedure. (Courtesy of Coltène/Whaledent.)

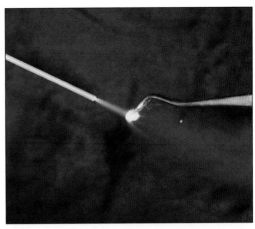

Fig 1-5 The cold refrigerant is sprayed on a large cotton pellet.

the dentist may try to work around the pain the patient is feeling by saying, "I'll be done in a minute." Such a situation would not make a good day for the dentist or the patient.

**IN CONCLUSION,** *commencing with treatment without confirming anesthesia may add apprehension for the dentist and patient because neither one knows if the tooth is anesthetized.*

## Cold refrigerant or electric pulp testing

A more objective measurement of anesthesia in nonpainful vital teeth is obtained with an application of a cold refrigerant of 1,1,1,2-tetrafluoroethane or by using an electric pulp tester (EPT). Cold refrigerant or the EPT can be used to test the tooth under treatment for pulpal anesthesia prior to beginning a clinical procedure.[17–20] A dental assistant could test the tooth to determine when pulpal anesthesia is obtained and then inform the dentist that treatment can be started.

In a very anxious patient, the use of pulp testing may cause a very painful reaction. Apprehensive patients can become sufficiently keyed up to react to even minimal stimulation. They may say, "Of course I jumped, it hurts!" or "It's only normal to jump when you know it is going to hurt."

**IN CONCLUSION,** *pulp testing with a cold refrigerant or an EPT will indicate if the patient has pulpal anesthesia. For anxious patients, pulp testing may need to be postponed until the patient can be conditioned to accept noninvasive diagnostic procedures.*

### Cold testing

A cold refrigerant tetrafluoroethylene (Hygenic Endo-Ice, Coltène/Whaledent) (Fig 1-4) can be used to test for pulpal anesthesia before commencing drilling on the tooth. The technique for cold testing is quick and easy; it takes only seconds to complete and does not require special equipment. Once the patient is experiencing profound lip numbness, the cold refrigerant is sprayed on a large cotton pellet held with cotton tweezers[21] (Fig 1-5). The cold pellet is then placed on the tooth (Fig 1-6). If clinical anesthesia has been successful, applications of cold refrigerant should not be felt. If the patient feels pain with application of the cold, supplemental injections should be given. If no pain is felt with the cold, it is likely that pulpal anesthesia has been obtained. Testing with a cold refrigerant is more convenient than with an EPT and gives a good indication of clinical anesthesia.

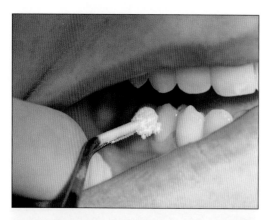

**Fig 1-6** The pellet with the cold refrigerant is applied to the surface of the tooth.

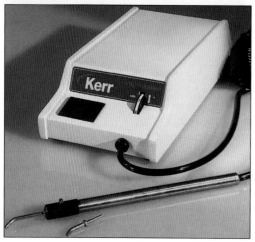

**Fig 1-7** An EPT may also be used to test for pulpal anesthesia before a clinical procedure is started. (Courtesy of SybronEndo.)

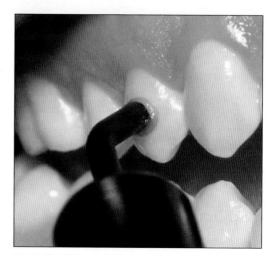

**Fig 1-8** The EPT probe is placed on the surface of the tooth.

Pulp testing with a cold refrigerant can be performed effectively on gold crowns and porcelain-fused-to-metal crowns. In fact, pulp testing is fairly easy to use in these situations because the metal conducts the cold very nicely. Miller and coauthors[21] also showed that pulp testing with a cold refrigerant is effective for all-ceramic crowns.

**IN CONCLUSION,** *pulp testing with a cold refrigerant is a reliable way to confirm clinical pulpal anesthesia, even in teeth with gold, porcelain-fused-to-metal, and all-ceramic crowns.*

### Electric pulp testing

In order to use the EPT (Kerr Vitality Scanner, SybronEndo) (Fig 1-7), the tooth should be dried with a gauze pad or cotton roll. Toothpaste is applied to the probe tip of the pulp tester before placing the tip on the middle of the labial surface (for anterior teeth) or buccal surface (for posterior teeth) of the tooth to be anesthetized (Fig 1-8). The Kerr EPT automatically starts on contact with the tooth and continues to apply current until the maximum output of a reading of 80 is reached. On removal from the tooth, the EPT automatically resets to 0. Contemporary EPTs are easy to use and no longer rely on the dentist to increase the current rate manually via a dial or to reset the unit manually.

Kitamura and coauthors[22] reported that the EPT was 99% accurate when testing teeth determined to be vital. Dreven and colleagues[17] and Certosimo and Archer[18] showed that a lack of patient response to an 80 reading with the EPT was an assurance of pulpal anesthesia in nonpainful vital teeth.

Certosimo and Archer[18] demonstrated that patients who responded to EPT readings of less than 80 experienced pain during operative procedures in normal teeth. Therefore, using the EPT prior to beginning dental procedures on nonpainful vital teeth will provide the clinician with a reliable indicator of pulpal anesthesia. We have used the EPT experimentally in many of the studies outlined in this book because it is easier to use for constant pulp testing over a period of 60 minutes.

**IN CONCLUSION,** *the EPT is very reliable in determining pulpal anesthesia in nonpainful vital teeth. Patient response to EPT readings less than the maximum output reading (80) indicate a lack of pulpal anesthesia.*

### EPT and cold testing in clinical practice

Almost all of the studies outlined in this book can be duplicated in your office. That is, by pulp testing teeth after giving different local anesthetic formulations and techniques, you can perform the same tests in your office to evaluate pulpal anesthesia. Wow!

Some may say that a negative response to pulp testing is not needed to perform restorative dentistry. This is true if you don't mind the patient often experiencing pain during treatment.[18] However, our goal is to have the patient experience no pulpal pain. While patients may tolerate being hurt during dental procedures, we think this is unnecessary in today's modern dental practice.

**IN CONCLUSION,** *pulp testing is a very valuable tool to determine pulpal anesthesia in clinical practice.*

# Clinical Local Anesthesia–Related Issues

## Patient considerations

### Pain versus pressure during treatment

The senior author remembers that when extracting painful teeth, I used to explain to patients that they were only feeling pressure during treatment—not pain. The explanation was that, although the local anesthetic was very effective at inhibiting the nerve fibers that transmit pain sensations, it did not have much of an effect on the nerves that transmit pressure sensations. While this theory may have some merit, it has never been proven, and the reason patients feel pain during treatment is much more complicated (see chapters 2 and 4). For example, voltage-gated sodium channels (VGSCs) exist on nerve membranes and differ in their roles in mediating peripheral pain.[23–25] They are divided into channels that are blocked by the toxin tetrodotoxin (TTX) and the channels that are resistant to the toxin (TTX-R).[26] A number of TTX-R channels are found on pain receptors NaV 1.8 and NaV 1.9,[26] and these channels are somewhat resistant to local anesthetics.[27]

**IN CONCLUSION,** *pressure transmission is an incomplete explanation of why patients react to dental treatment, and TTX-R channels are involved in resistance to local anesthetic action on nerves.*

## Patient reaction to local anesthetic injection

Brand and coauthors[28] found that feeling tense (42%), clenching fists (14%), and moaning (13%) were the most common reactions to an IANB. Vika and coauthors[29] reported that about 17% of patients indicated high fear to an injection during their last dental appointment, which may lead to avoidance of necessary treatment in the future.

**IN CONCLUSION,** *some patients react negatively to receiving an IANB.*

*Patients who report previous difficulty with local anesthesia*

In addition, patients who report having had difficulty with local anesthesia in the past are more likely to experience unsuccessful anesthesia.[30] These patients will generally identify themselves with comments such as, "Novocaine doesn't work on me" or "a lot of shots are needed to get my teeth numb." A good clinical practice is to ask the patient if he or she has had previous difficulty achieving clinical anesthesia. If so, supplemental injections should be considered.

**IN CONCLUSION,** *patients who report previous difficulty with anesthesia are more likely to experience unsuccessful anesthesia.*

## Dentist considerations

*Dentist reaction to injections of local anesthetic*

Simon and coauthors[31] found that 19% of dentists reported that the administration of local anesthetic injections caused enough distress that they had at some point reconsidered dentistry as a career. And 6% considered it a serious problem. This study indicates that the administration of local anesthetic injections might contribute to overall professional stress for some dentists.

Anxious patients may not be the only ones anxious about local anesthetic injections. Dower and coauthors[32] found that two-thirds of dentists described anxious patients as the main source of their anxiety, and 16% identified children as the main source of anxiety.

**IN CONCLUSION,** *some dentists are stressed by giving a local anesthetic injection, and anxious patients and children can be sources of anxiety for the dentist.*

*Compassion fatigue*

Moreover, a type of emotional burnout called compassion fatigue may affect many health care workers.[33,34] Although we become doctors because we want to help people, controlling pain on a daily basis and performing treatment at a very high level of precision may take its toll. In fact, if patients feel pain during restorative treatment, we sometimes internalize the feeling as failure.

As dentists and professionals, we provide an extraordinary service to our patients. Our ability to provide exceptional treatment with a caring attitude is a most rewarding art. However, we also have the ability to not accept failure because we have the means to prevent it. Dentists have been maligned for many years because of pain. Unfortunately, some of the information that we have today that allows us to prevent patient pain was not available in the past. This is particularly true with the IANB; this injection fails often enough to present meaningful clinical problems. This book will outline the steps you need to take to overcome failure with this block.

**IN CONCLUSION,** *we should not accept clinical failure of pulpal anesthesia when we have the means to prevent it from happening.*

## Anesthetic agents and dosages

Table 1-1 outlines the local anesthetic formulations available in the United States. The American Dental Association has specified a uniform color code to prevent confusion among brands. The maximum allowable dosage applies to complex oral and maxillofacial surgery procedures. The typical maximum dosage is for adults (weighing 150 pounds) who are undergoing typical restorative and endodontic procedures. Local anesthetic agents, common names, and milligrams per cartridge are presented in Table 1-2.

| Table 1-1 | Local anesthetics available in the United States[a] | | | |
|---|---|---|---|---|
| Anesthetic | Vasoconstrictor | Dental cartridge color code[b] | MAD[c] | TMD[c] |
| 2% lidocaine | 1:100,000 epinephrine | Red | 13 | 8 |
| 2% lidocaine | 1:50,000 epinephrine | Green | 13 | 8 |
| 2% lidocaine plain | No vasoconstrictor | Light blue | 8 | 8 |
| 2% mepivacaine | 1:20,000 levonordefrin | Brown | 11 | 8 |
| 3% mepivacaine plain | No vasoconstrictor | Tan | 7 | 5½ |
| 4% prilocaine | 1:200,000 epinephrine | Yellow | 5½ | 5½ |
| 4% prilocaine plain | No vasoconstrictor | Black | 5½ | 5½ |
| 0.5% bupivacaine | 1:200,000 epinephrine | Blue | 10 | 10 |
| 4% articaine | 1:100,000 epinephrine | Gold | 7 | 7 |
| 4% articaine | 1:200,000 epinephrine | Silver | 7 | 7 |

[a]The dosages were adapted from Malamed.[35]
[b]Uniform dental cartridge color codes.
[c]This table provides the maximum dosage in two formats. The maximum allowable dose (MAD) generally is approached only with complex oral and maxillofacial surgical procedures. The typical maximum dose (TMD) is the usual upper limit of drug dosage for most restorative and endodontic dental procedures. Both columns show the number of cartridges that would be required for an adult weighing 150 pounds (67.5 kg).

| Table 1-2 | Local anesthetics, common names, and milligrams per cartridge | |
|---|---|---|
| Local anesthetic agent | Common name(s) | Cartridge (mg) |
| 2% lidocaine with 1:100,000 epinephrine | Xylocaine (Dentsply) Lidocaine | 36 |
| 2% lidocaine with 1:50,000 epinephrine | Xylocaine Lidocaine | 36 |
| 2% mepivacaine with 1:20,000 levonordefrin | Carbocaine (Cook-Waite) Polocaine (Dentsply) | 36 |
| 3% mepivacaine plain (no vasoconstrictor) | Carbocaine Polocaine | 54 |
| 4% prilocaine with 1:200,000 epinephrine | Citanest Forte (Dentsply) | 72 |
| 4% prilocaine plain (no vasoconstrictor) | Citanest Plain (Dentsply) | 72 |
| 0.5% bupivacaine with 1:200,000 epinephrine | Marcaine (Cook-Waite) | 9 |
| 4% articaine with 1:100,000 epinephrine | Septocaine (Septodont) Zorcaine (Cook-Waite) Articadent (Dentsply) | 72 |
| 4% articaine with 1:200,000 epinephrine | Septocaine | 72 |

## Gray rubber stoppers

Most of the rubber stoppers of cartridges are colored gray (Fig 1-9). These rubber stoppers are not color coded and are not indicative of the drug the cartridge contains.

## Orabloc articaine formulation

Orabloc (Patterson Dental) is an articaine local anesthetic containing a vasoconstrictor and is available in two epinephrine formulations—1:200,000 and 1:100,000. Supposedly, it is a "purer" form of articaine that has a 24-month shelf life at room temperature and very low manufacture-related degradation

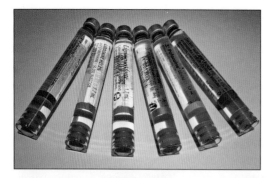

**Fig 1-9** Gray anesthetic cartridge stoppers.

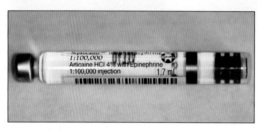

**Fig 1-10** Articaine cartridge showing 1.7 mL of anesthetic solution.

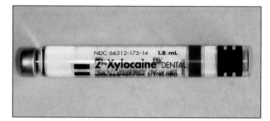

**Fig 1-11** Lidocaine cartridge showing 1.8 mL of anesthetic solution.

products, including articaine acid and epinephrine sulfonic acid, and it is sodium edetate free, methylparaben free, and latex free. As far as we are aware, no research has been performed on Orabloc in comparison with other commercially available products.

**IN CONCLUSION,** *the articaine formulation of Orabloc needs to be evaluated for clinical efficacy.*

## Media hype: "Local anesthetics cause tooth cell death"

Zhuang and coauthors,[36] using pig teeth and young permanent tooth pulp cells, found that prolonged exposure to high doses of local anesthetics interfered with the mitochondria of tooth cells and led to cell death. The researchers noted that further clinical studies are required before there is enough data to change clinical guidelines. They also urged parents not to be alarmed or withdraw their children from treatment if they need it.

**IN CONCLUSION,** *exposing pig teeth and pulp cells to high doses of local anesthetics does not prove a correlation with clinical outcomes.*

## Cartridge volume—1.7 mL versus 1.8 mL

Robertson and coauthors[37] measured the amount of anesthetic solution delivered with an aspirating syringe, a standard syringe with a 27-gauge needle, and the contents of 50 articaine cartridges and 50 lidocaine cartridges into a graduated syringe with 0.01 milliliter–increment divisions. Even though the articaine cartridge was marked externally as containing 1.7 mL (Fig 1-10), on average the anesthetic solution expressed was 1.76 mL. For the lidocaine cartridge, the amount was marked as 1.8 mL (Fig 1-11), but on average the anesthetic solution expressed was 1.76 mL. In general, a small amount of anesthetic solution remained in both cartridges after delivery of the solution with an aspirating syringe. The amount of anesthetic solution expressed was basically the same for both articaine and lidocaine. Some manufacturers are now labeling cartridges as 1.7 mL even though the anesthetic solution expressed is 1.76 mL.

**IN CONCLUSION,** *cartridges marked 1.7 mL and 1.8 mL express the same amount of anesthetic solution.*

Fig 1-12 Will this woman with red hair be more difficult to anesthetize?

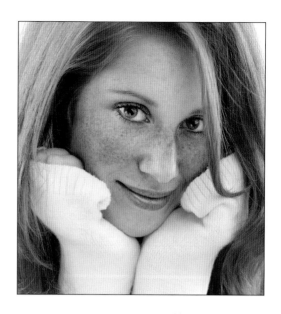

## Classification of local anesthetics and clinical implications

Generally, local anesthetic agents are classified as short, intermediate, or long-acting based on their pKa, lipid solubility, and protein binding.[35] Short-duration drugs include 3% mepivacaine and 4% prilocaine. A long-acting drug is 0.5% bupivacaine with 1:200,000 epinephrine. Lidocaine, articaine, mepivacaine, and prilocaine, all with vasoconstrictors, are considered intermediate in action. However, Pateromichelakis and Prokopiou[38] found that studies on isolated nerves can be poor guides to the clinical comparisons of local anesthetics. For example, clinical studies indicate that the duration of these drugs is different when used in nerve blocks versus infiltration or intraosseous injections. A good example is anesthetic agents like bupivacaine and etidocaine. While classified as long-acting agents, this duration only holds true for nerve blocks—not for maxillary infiltration, intraligamentary, or intraosseous anesthesia.[11,39–41] Short-duration drugs like 3% mepivacaine and 4% prilocaine are effective for IANBs of at least 50 minutes[4] but have a short duration for infiltration anesthesia in the maxilla.[42,43]

IN CONCLUSION, the overall classification of local anesthetics does not always correlate with clinical effectiveness.

## Factors influencing local anesthetic effectiveness

### Genetics

Some patients may not respond adequately to local anesthetic administration. Various studies[44–47] have related pain or ineffectiveness of local anesthetic to genetic factors. Perhaps, one day in the future, we may be able to use genomic testing to improve the efficacy of local anesthetics by selecting drugs that offer the most appropriate pharmacologic usefulness. However, the problem with the gene pool is that there is no lifeguard.

IN CONCLUSION, genetics may play a role in anesthetic failure.

### Red hair phenotype

Natural red hair color results from distinct mutations of the melanocortin-1 receptor (MC1R), which may modulate pain pathways.[48–50] Red hair color is the phenotype for MC1R gene, which is associated with red hair, fair skin, and freckles in humans (Fig 1-12). Women with red hair have been reported to be more sensitive to some types of pain and may be resistant to subcutaneous lidocaine.[48] Liem and

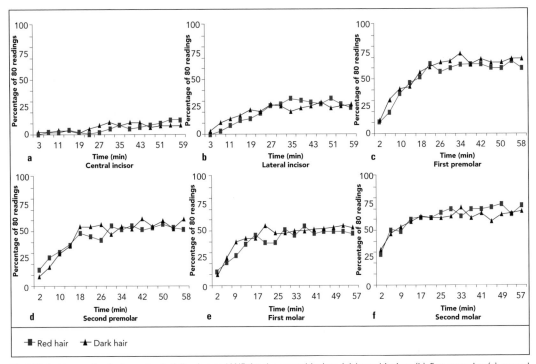

**Fig 1-13** Incidence of pulpal anesthesia following an IANB for the central incisor *(a)*, lateral incisor *(b)*, first premolar *(c)*, second premolar *(d)*, first molar *(e)*, and second molar *(f)* as determined by lack of response to an EPT at maximum reading (percentage of 80 readings), at each postinjection time interval, for red-haired and dark-haired women. There were no significant differences in anesthetic success for any of the teeth. Red hair was significantly linked to higher levels of dental anxiety but was unrelated to success rates of the IANB in women with healthy pulps. (Reprinted from Droll et al[52] with permission.)

coauthors[49] reported that the anesthetic requirement for desflurane was increased in redheads. In a follow-up study, Binkley and coauthors[50] found that genetic variations associated with red hair color were also associated with fear of dental pain and anxiety. However, Myles and coauthors[51] found no evidence that patient hair color affects requirements or recovery characteristics in a broad range of surgical procedures.

Droll and coauthors[52] investigated a possible link between certain variant alleles of the *MC1R* or its phenotypic expression (red hair) and anesthetic efficacy of the IANB in women. They found that neither red hair nor *MC1R* was significantly linked to success rates of the IANB in women with healthy pulps (Fig 1-13). Importantly, women with red hair and women with two red hair color alleles reported significantly higher levels of dental anxiety compared with women with dark hair or women with no red hair color alleles. Women with red hair also reported greater pain on needle insertion during the injection. It may be that the clinical impression of failed anesthesia in red-haired individuals is owed to the higher anxiety levels perceived in this population. During dental treatment, this population may be more likely to report nonpainful sensations (pressure, vibration, etc) as painful.

**IN CONCLUSION,** *red-haired women do not have more failure with the IANB. However, red-haired women report significantly higher dental anxiety.*

## Gender differences

Authors have found that women try to avoid pain more than men, accept it less, and fear it more.[53–55] Morin and coauthors[56] found that women find postsurgical pain more intense than men, but men are more disturbed than women by low levels of pain that last several days. Anxiety may also modulate differences in pain response between men and women.[54] Thus, we should be aware that women might react differently to pain than men. Tofoli and coauthors[57] found that injection discomfort and effectiveness of local anesthetics were not related to phases of the menstrual cycle or use of oral contraceptives. However, Loyd and coauthors[58] reported that a sexually dimorphic peripheral mechanism may modulate trigeminal pain processing and may be related to the luteal phase of the menstrual cycle.

**IN CONCLUSION,** *women try to avoid pain more than men, accept it less, and fear it more.*

## Catastrophizing

Some patients may have an exaggerated negative mental set that occurs during an actual or anticipated painful experience.[59] This is called catastrophizing. That is, these patients are already predisposed to have a painful experience during dental treatment.

**IN CONCLUSION,** *clinicians may need to probe patients' pain experiences and help them reappraise threats.*

## Pathways of dental fear

Five pathways related to dental fear have been recognized[60]: *(1)* The conditioning pathway occurs as a result of direct traumatic experiences. *(2)* The parental pathway relates to dental fear learned from parents or guardians. *(3)* The informative pathway is related to fearful experiences learned or heard about from others. *(4)* The verbal threat pathway comes from parents using the dental environment as punishment for bad behavior in children. *(5)* The visual vicarious pathway is caused by fear-inducing dental situations seen in the media. A recent study[60] found that less fear was shown in older patients, men were more likely to cancel dental appointments because of fear, and different ethnic backgrounds adopt different pathways of fear.

**IN CONCLUSION,** *there are different pathways of dental fear, and each has an influence on fear of dentistry.*

## Pregnancy and breastfeeding

For pregnant patients, elective treatment should be deferred, particularly in the first trimester. However, if treatment involving a painful procedure is required, many of the commonly available local anesthetic agents are safe to use.[61] The United States Food and Drug Administration classifies articaine, mepivacaine, and bupivacaine as category C drugs.[35] A category C classification means that "Either animal-reproduction studies have revealed adverse effects and there are no controlled studies in women or studies in women and animals are not available. Drugs should be given only if the potential benefit justifies the potential risk to the fetus."[35,61] Lidocaine and prilocaine are classified as category B drugs. A category B classification means that "Either animal-reproduction studies have not demonstrated a fetal risk but there are no controlled studies in pregnant women or animal-reproduction studies have shown an adverse effect that was not confirmed in controlled studies in women in the first trimester (and there is no evidence of a risk in later trimesters)."[35]

The manufacturer drug monographs that accompany local anesthetic agents place warning statements that these agents should not be used during pregnancy. These statements are placed for medicolegal reasons because the anesthetics have not been tested during pregnancy. To put things in perspective, congenital anomalies occur in 3% of the general population, yet the causes can be determined in less than 50% of these cases.[61] Hagai and coauthors[62] evaluated the rate of major anomalies after exposure to local anesthetics as part of dental care during pregnancy. They found that the use of local anesthetics, as well as dental treatment during pregnancy, did not present a major risk for anomalies.

In patients who are lactating, drugs do pass into the breast milk in very small quantities.[63] If there is concern, the patient may be comforted by electing to use a breast pump, discarding the milk, and then providing the infant with formula or previously expressed milk for a day. If the practitioner is unsure about the safety of a drug, he or she could consult the National Institutes of Health LactMed database. This resource provides information on drug transference to breast milk, drug safety, and safe alternative drugs.

The most important aspect of care in the pregnant patient in pain is elimination of the source of pain by performing the indicated treatment. This approach will reduce the need for systemic medications.[61]

**IN CONCLUSION,** *defer elective treatment for pregnant patients, particularly in the first trimester. However, if treatment involving a painful procedure is required for the pregnant or lactating patient, many of the commonly available local anesthetic agents are safe to use.*

### Elderly patients

Nordenram and Danielsson[64] found that elderly patients had significantly shorter onset times of anesthesia when compared with younger patients. In general, older patients may also be more tolerant of pain than younger patients.[65,66]

**IN CONCLUSION,** *older patients may tolerate pain better than younger patients.*

### Alcohol addiction

Patients with alcoholism have been found to be more sensitive to painful stimulation, and those with a history of depression/unhappiness may also have shallower pulpal anesthesia.[67,68] In contrast, patients in recovery for alcohol addiction may not be at increased risk for inadequate pain control with local anesthesia.[68]

**IN CONCLUSION,** *patients with alcoholism who are not in recovery may be more difficult to anesthetize.*

## Allergies and local anesthetics

### Local anesthetics

Generally, amide local anesthetics have a very low chance of allergic reactions.[69] Batinac and coauthors[70] found that the most common symptoms related to administration of local anesthetics were cardiovascular reactions (18%). True allergic reactions were rare (less than 1%). In patients who have reported adverse reactions to local anesthetics, none had hypersensitivity reactions to the intradermal injection of local anesthetics.[69] However, there have been case reports of hypersensitivity reactions to local anesthetics.[69–78] Patients who have had anaphylactic reactions or serious idiosyncratic reactions to administration of local anesthetics should be referred to a dental anesthesiologist or oral surgeon for deep sedation or general anesthesia prior to restorative procedures.

**IN CONCLUSION,** *patients who have had serious reactions to local anesthetics should be treated in conjunction with a dental anesthesiologist or oral surgeon.*

### Latex in dental cartridges

Shojaei and Haas[76] performed a literature review on latex allergies. They concluded that the medical literature provides some evidence that latex allergen can be released into solutions by direct contact with natural latex stoppers within the cartridges. However, they stated that there are no cases of documented allergy for dental local anesthetics. Recently, some manufacturers have introduced latex-free dental cartridges for all of their product lines.

**IN CONCLUSION,** *dental cartridges present little risk in latex allergy patients.*

### Sulfites

Sulfites are common additives to many food products and are present in small amounts in local anesthetic cartridges. The sulfites prevent the oxidation of the vasoconstrictor in dental formulations. Smolinske[77] felt that anaphylactic or asthmatic reactions caused by parenteral administration of sulfite

**Fig 1-14** OraVerse is a safe product to help reverse soft tissue anesthesia.

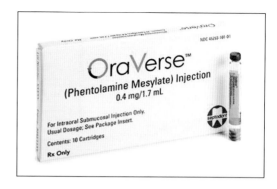

agents were different than reactions caused by foods. The reactions were rapid and had no predilection for steroid-dependent asthmatics. As stated by Naftalin and Yagiela,[78] the best way to avoid a reaction in a patient with a true sulfite allergy would be to use a local anesthetic without a vasoconstrictor.

**IN CONCLUSION,** *if a patient has a severe sulfite allergy, use an anesthetic solution without a vasoconstrictor.*

## Reversing soft tissue numbness

Patients may feel that residual soft tissue numbness interferes with their normal daily activities in three specific areas—perceptual (perception of altered physical appearance), sensory (lack of sensation), and functional (diminished ability to speak, smile, drink, and control drooling). Patients may complain that they are unable to eat a meal or talk normally after their dental visit. Patients often do not want to have lip and tongue numbness for hours after the appointment. Phentolamine mesylate (0.4 mg in a 1.7-mL cartridge; OraVerse, Septodont) is an agent that shortens the duration of soft tissue anesthesia (Fig 1-14). The duration of soft tissue anesthesia is longer than pulpal anesthesia and is often associated with difficulty eating, drinking, and speaking.[79-81] The greatest value of using OraVerse is in the majority of dental procedures in which postoperative pain is not of concern. Clinical trials have evaluated the use of phentolamine in patients undergoing routine nonsurgical operative or periodontal procedures or implant placement and in asymptomatic endodontic patients.[79-87] These studies have shown that phentolamine statistically reduces the time of soft tissue numbness when compared with a sham injection. Saunders and coauthors[86] found that patients who experienced OraVerse reported a reduced duration of numbness (92%) and an improved dental experience (84%), 83% of the patients would recommend OraVerse to others, and 79% would have OraVerse used in future dental visits.

Fowler and coauthors[85] studied the use of OraVerse for reversal of soft tissue anesthesia in asymptomatic endodontic patients. They found that patients experienced an 88-minute decrease in time to return to normal maxillary soft tissue sensation, and a 47-minute decrease in time to return to normal in mandibular lip sensation. Postoperative pain and complications were minimal. Many patients may benefit from the use of a reversal agent when they have speaking engagements or important meetings or perform in musical or theatrical events.

Elmore and coauthors[88] found that phentolamine significantly reduced duration of both pulpal and soft tissue anesthesia when administered either at 30 or 60 minutes after an IANB (Fig 1-15). Therefore, because pulpal anesthesia is also reversed fairly rapidly, phentolamine should be administered at the end of the dental appointment.

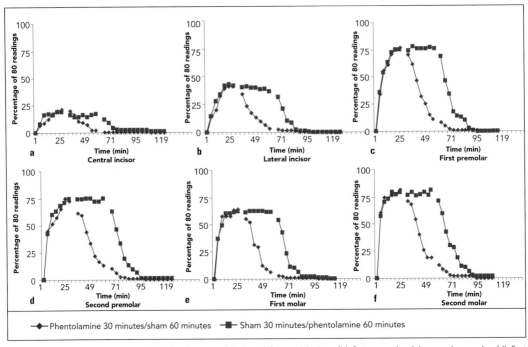

**Fig 1-15** Incidence of pulpal anesthesia for the central incisor *(a)*, lateral incisor *(b)*, first premolar *(c)*, second premolar *(d)*, first molar *(e)*, and second molar *(f)* as determined by lack of response to an EPT at maximum reading (percentage of 80 readings), at each postinjection time interval, for phentolamine/sham and sham/phentolamine injections. The injection of phentolamine at 30 minutes reversed pulpal anesthesia fairly rapidly. Phentolamine would be beneficial for patients who would like to experience a faster return to normal soft tissue function and sensation after the administration of local anesthesia. However, pulpal anesthesia is also reversed fairly rapidly. (Reprinted from Elmore et al[88] with permission.)

OraVerse is administered with a standard syringe using the same location and same technique (infiltration or nerve block) and in the same proportion (1 to 1) as was used initially for the local anesthetic injection.

**IN CONCLUSION,** *OraVerse is a safe product and would be beneficial for patients who would like to experience a faster return to normal soft tissue function after the administration of local anesthesia.*

# Anxiety and Pain

Anxious patients may be harder to anesthetize. Although dental injections are an important aspect of treatment for patients, injections can induce anxiety or fear and may be a reason for patients to avoid dental treatment.[89] Van Wijk and Hoogstraten[90] found that anxious patients felt more pain than that reported by less anxious patients. Anxious patients also have a tendency to overestimate anticipated pain.[91] Vika and coauthors[92] reported that about 17% of patients indicated high fear during their last dental appointment.

Patients who are anxious have reduced pain tolerances.[93] Therefore, anxious patients may be harder to anesthetize and may require supplemental techniques (articaine infiltration of mandibular teeth or intraosseous or intraligamentary injections).

In addition, dental anxiety is less prevalent among older adults (over 50 years of age) than in younger patients.[94]

Especially for dental students transitioning to the clinical years, one of the highest levels of anxiety was associated with hurting patients.[95] When faced with specific clinical situations, students were stressed by failed local anesthesia.[95]

However, Corah and coauthors[96] found that the dentist's explicit dedication to prevent pain was the most important dentist behavior to the patient to reduce patient anxiety and increase satisfaction. Friendliness, working quickly, being calm, and giving moral support were important auxiliary behaviors.

**IN CONCLUSION,** *anxious patients may be harder to anesthetize. However, dentist dedication to preventing pain is the most important behavior to patients.*

## Oral conscious sedation

Patients in pain are often anxious and fearful of dental treatment.[97] Patients reporting for emergency treatment with pain are even more fearful. Therefore, in situations with anxious and fearful patients, will the IANB be more successful if the patient is consciously sedated? Lindemann and coauthors[98] determined the effect of the administration of a 0.25-mg sublingual does of triazolam (Halcion, Pfizer) on the efficacy of the IANB in patients experiencing irreversible pulpitis. Success was defined as no or mild pain upon endodontic access or initial instrumentation. The success rate for the IANB was 43% with triazolam and 57% with the placebo. There was no significant difference between the two groups. Likewise, Khademi and coauthors[99] found that the preoperative oral administration of 0.5 mg of alprazolam did not improve the success of the IANB in mandibular molars in patients presenting with irreversible pulpitis. Success (no or mild pain upon access or initial instrumentation) was 53% with alprazolam and 40% with the placebo, with no significant difference between the two groups. In conclusion, for mandibular posterior teeth, preoperative triazolam or alprazolam will not result in an increase in success of the IANB in patients with irreversible pulpitis.

Thus, if a painful procedure is anticipated, conscious sedation with triazolam or alprazolam will not reduce pain during dental treatment. Profound local anesthesia is still required. That is, conscious sedation should not be used as a way to reduce pain during dental treatment! The results of these studies should not be interpreted to mean that triazolam or alprazolam sedation should not be used to reduce patients' anxiety. Anxiety reduction may make the process of dental treatment more acceptable to the patient.

**IN CONCLUSION,** *oral conscious sedation with triazolam (Halcion) or alprazolam (Xanax, Pfizer) will not reduce pain during dental treatment. Profound local anesthesia is still required.*

### Patient satisfaction with painful treatment

A dentist's caring manner relates to patient satisfaction even though painful treatment may be involved. A number of studies in endodontics[98,100–104] have found high satisfaction ratings (96% to 100%) despite the findings that most patients experienced moderate-to-severe pain during endodontic treatment. Gale and coauthors,[105] Davidhizar and Shearer,[106] Schouten and coauthors,[107] and Fletcher and coauthors[108] found that patient satisfaction is related to maintaining a positive and professional attitude, practicing encouragement, exhibiting a caring manner, and avoiding defensiveness. Communicative behavior of the dentist (rapport or "bedside manner") is positively related to patient satisfaction and explains why patients are satisfied with dental treatment even though pain may be involved. In endodontics, high satisfaction ratings may also be related to the expectation that the patient's pain will be relieved.

**IN CONCLUSION,** *a dentist's caring manner relates to patient satisfaction even though painful treatment may be involved. In endodontics, high satisfaction ratings may be related to the expectation that the patient's pain will be relieved.*

## Nitrous oxide

Nitrous oxide has an impressive safety record and is excellent for minimal conscious sedation for apprehensive patients.[109] Nitrous oxide produces an analgesic effect[110–112] and has been used to decrease the pain of venipuncture[113] and minor pediatric surgical procedures[114] as well as the injection pain of the initial IANB[115] using a standard block, Gow-Gates, or Vazirani-Akinosi technique. It has also been used to reduce the pain of IANB injections in children, resulting in improvement in behavior.[116]

Stanley and coauthors[100] determined the effect of nitrous oxide on the anesthetic success of the IANB in patients experiencing symptomatic irreversible pulpitis. They found that nitrous oxide sedation did increase the success of an IANB and was a useful technique in the treatment of painful teeth. Furthermore, if a patient were to present with anxiety and request sedation, nitrous oxide sedation may be preferable to oral sedation. Nitrous oxide sedation allows a titratable dosage, and the patient is not sedated beyond the length of the treatment appointment, meaning the patient would not require someone else to drive after the appointment.

**IN CONCLUSION,** *nitrous oxide is very useful for minimal conscious sedation in apprehensive and emergency patients because it has both analgesic and antianxiety effects.*

## Aromatherapy

Kiecolt-Glaser and coauthors[117] studied aromatherapy and found that it failed to show any improvement in pain control. However, lemon aroma did enhance positive moods, while lavender had no effect on mood. Maybe we should dust with lemon-scented Pledge to enhance the mood of our patients, assistants, and ourselves. Just kidding.

**IN CONCLUSION,** *aromatherapy does not improve pain control in anxious patients.*

# Vasoconstrictors

## Cardiovascular reactions

Several authors[118–122] have reported increases in heart rate with infiltration injections and nerve blocks using 2% lidocaine with 1:100,000 epinephrine, while others[123–128] have reported no significant changes in heart rate or reported that the changes were clinically insignificant. When specific information was given on dosing and heart rate increases, five studies[118–122] found mean heart rate increases. Two studies found increases of 4 beats per minute using approximately 20 μg of epinephrine (one cartridge of 1:100,000 epinephrine contains 18 μg),[119,120] three studies recorded increases from 10 to 15 beats per minute using 45 to 80 μg of epinephrine (approximately 2½ to over 4 cartridges of 1:100,000 epinephrine),[118,120,121] and one study found increases of approximately 21 beats per minute using 144 μg of epinephrine (eight cartridges of 1:100,000 epinephrine).[122]

Moore and coauthors[123] found no differences in the cardiovascular profiles of 4% articaine with 1:100,000 or 1:200,000 epinephrine when using a one-cartridge volume. However, when using large volumes (almost seven cartridges, which is the maximum allowable dose of 4% articaine), Hersh and coauthors[124] reported that the 1:100,000 epinephrine produced significantly higher heart rates and systolic blood pressure 10 minutes following injection. The increase in heart rate is caused by the stimulation of the beta1 receptors. Therefore, increasing the amount of epinephrine in an infiltration or block injection increases the likelihood of an increase in heart rate.

Intraosseous injections, but not intraligamentary injections, will increase heart rate when local anesthetics with vasoconstrictors are used[11,13,129–131] (see chapter 4 for a complete discussion).

**IN CONCLUSION,** *using 1.8 mL of local anesthetic with vasoconstrictors for infiltrations and nerve blocks generally will not increase heart rate. Increasing the volume will increase heart rate. Intraosseous injections using local anesthetic agents with vasoconstrictors will almost always increase heart rate.*

## Considerations in patients with cardiovascular disease

Treatment should be individualized based on a comprehensive assessment of the patient and medical consultation. Niwa and coauthors[132] concluded that 1.8 mL of 2% lidocaine with 1:80,000 epinephrine was safe and had few, if any, hemodynamic consequences in patients with cardiovascular disease. Likewise, Elad and coauthors[133] found that dental treatment using 1.8 mL of 4% articaine with 1:200,000 epinephrine or 2% lidocaine with 1:100,000 epinephrine was safe in medically compromised cardiac patients. Niwa and coauthors[134] reported that many patients with unstable angina pectoris or acute myocardial infarction (within 6 months) tolerated tooth extraction and pulpectomy under local anesthesia when appropriate stress-control measures were used.

**IN CONCLUSION,** *medical consultation is advised before treating patients with cardiovascular disease.*

## Contraindications

Epinephrine is contraindicated in patients with untreated hyperthyroidism and pheochromocytoma.[35]

Pheochromocytoma is a rare neuroendocrine tumor of the medulla of the adrenal glands causing secretion of excessive amounts of catecholamines.[135] Patients should be well aware that they have this condition, and medical consultation is required. Because of the excessive secretion of catecholamines, they should not be given vasoconstrictors.

Hyperthyroidism is an increase in thyroid hormone production and may cause irregular heart rhythms.[135] In its most severe form, untreated hyperthyroidism may result in thyroid storm, a condition involving high blood pressure, fever, and heart failure. Usually the symptoms of hyperthyroidism are so gradual in their onset that patients do not realize the symptoms until they become more severe. This means the symptoms may continue for weeks or months before patients fully realize that they are sick. In older people, some or all of the typical symptoms of hyperthyroidism may be absent, and the patient may just lose weight or become depressed. Therefore, patients may come into the dental office with undiagnosed hyperthyroidism. Symptoms include patients often feeling hotter than those around them because the body's metabolism is increased and slowly losing weight even though they may be eating more.[135] Patients with hyperthyroidism usually experience fatigue at the end of the day but have trouble sleeping. Trembling of the hands and heart palpitations may develop. These individuals may become irritable and easily upset. When hyperthyroidism is severe, patients can suffer shortness of breath, chest pain, and muscle weakness.[135]

Moreover, Malamed[35] stated that vasoconstrictors should be avoided in patients with high blood pressure (higher than 200 mmHg systolic or 115 mmHg diastolic), cardiac dysrhythmias, unstable angina, severe cardiovascular disease, or patients who have experienced a myocardial infarction or cerebrovascular accident within the last 6 months. It must be stated that these conditions are contraindications to even routine dental treatment. Therefore, the contraindication to epinephrine, or levonordefrin, is not the crucial issue in these patients; rather it is the safety of performing in-office dental treatment at all.

In addition, it is possible that patients may be allergic to the epinephrine in an anesthetic cartridge, but this must be considered an extremely rare occurrence. Kohase and Umino[136] reported two cases of confirmed hypersensitivity to epinephrine (hydrochloride or bitartrate) in a 2% lidocaine formulation. Although some patients may actually be allergic to exogenous epinephrine preparations, patients who say they are allergic to epinephrine because of an increased heart rate or palpitations are only reacting to the epinephrine released into their blood stream.

**IN CONCLUSION,** *serious medical conditions are contraindications to routine dental treatment. It is possible that patients may be allergic to the epinephrine in an anesthetic cartridge, but this must be considered an extremely rare occurrence.*

## Consultation with the patient's physician

It is often best to contact the patient's physician directly to discuss the proposed treatment. By doing this, the physician can appreciate our concern for the patient and our rationale for treatment. We also want to discuss that all injections are given only after repeated aspirations and are given slowly over a 1-minute time period. It is best not to ask if it is safe to use epinephrine because many physicians have been taught to use high doses of epinephrine to treat allergic reactions—giving 0.3 to 0.5 mg of a 1:1,000 epinephrine solution. They are less familiar with the doses used in dental cartridges.

For IANBs, 3% mepivacaine is similar to 2% lidocaine with 1:100,000 epinephrine in efficacy and duration of approximately 50 minutes. Supplemental intraosseous injections, but not intraligamentary injections, will be successful with 3% mepivacaine. Therefore, 3% mepivacaine can be used in these situations.

**IN CONCLUSION,** *emphasize our anticipated treatment and the rationale for local anesthesia.*

## Plain anesthetic formulations

Historically, emphasis has been placed on the dangers of using vasoconstrictors with certain medical conditions or drug interactions. While this is important, the clinician must also realize that local anesthetic solutions without vasoconstrictors contain more drug because of higher concentrations (3% mepivacaine and 4% prilocaine). In thinking these drugs are safer than solutions without vasoconstrictors, clinicians may give larger amounts of these anesthetics, which can lead to toxicity and central nervous system depression.[137] We have to remember that without the vasoconstrictor, the anesthetic solution will be removed more rapidly from the injection site into the systemic circulation—causing higher blood levels of the anesthetic.

**IN CONCLUSION,** *anesthetic solutions without vasoconstrictors are not safer than anesthetic solutions with vasoconstrictors and should not be given in large amounts.*

## Drug interactions

We should be cautious about administering a vasoconstrictor, or at least limit the amount of vasoconstrictor, in certain patients taking systemic drugs, including antidepressants, beta-blocking agents, medicines that treat Parkinson disease, and cocaine. For patients taking the majority of these drugs, 3% mepivacaine can be used for an IANB. For supplemental intraosseous injections, only 3% mepivacaine should be used; intraligamentary injections with 3% mepivacaine are not effective.

### Monoamine oxidase inhibitors

Epinephrine and levonordefrin are catecholamines metabolized by catechol-o-methyltransferase and not monoamine oxidase (MAO).[138] Therefore, patients on MAO inhibitors can receive either of these vasoconstrictors.

### Antidepressants

Fluoxetine (Prozac, Eli Lilly) selectively inhibits serotonin uptake and does not present a problem.[138] However, patients on tricyclic antidepressants may have cardiac arrhythmias that could be potentiated by vasoconstictors.[139] The number of cartridges containing epinephrine or levonordefrin should be limited to one or two.

## Beta-blocking agents

Patients taking nonselective beta-blocking agents (eg, propranolol, nadolol) may have a sensitivity to vasopressors, causing increases in blood pressure and reflex bradycardia.[138] Caution in the use of vasoconstrictors is prudent. Patients on selective beta1 blockers (atenolol, metroprolol) at normal doses do not demonstrate the sensitivity to vasopressors.[138] However, the amount of vasoconstrictors administered should not be excessive.

## Medicines treating Parkinson disease

Because of an exaggerated effect on blood pressure and heart rate due to drug interactions with medicines to treat Parkinson disease (levodopa and entacapone), we should limit 2% lidocaine with 1:100,000 epinephrine to three cartridges per half hour.[140] If the patient is receiving selegiline, no epinephrine or levonordefrin should be used.[140]

## Cocaine

Cocaine produces a state of catecholamine hypersensitivity, causing dysrhythmias and other serious cardiac problems.[35] Local anesthetic with vasoconstrictors should never be administered to patients who have used cocaine within the last 24 hours.[35] Unfortunately, cocaine users may not be honest when reporting their habit. We must be frank in asking patients if they have used cocaine, particularly if we see physical signs of abuse: red bloodshot eyes, runny nose or frequent sniffing without allergies or cold symptoms, increased blood pressure, dilated pupils, increased heart rate, or nosebleeds.

Additionally, Saraghi and Hersh[141] cautioned practitioners to keep track of their lidocaine supplies because of the potential that local anesthetics are being diverted from dental offices to be used as cocaine adulterants (they augment the nasal numbness produced by inhaling cocaine).

# Injection Pain

Like dental injections, medical injections also have the potential to be painful. One only has to watch children receiving immunization injections; the reaction is usually painful. Perhaps medical injections are sensitizing individuals to injection pain at an early age. Additionally, vaccines have no local anesthetic properties during the injection. Taddio and coauthors[142] stated that pain interventions are not commonly used during childhood vaccination, despite the fact that two-thirds of children are afraid of needles and one-tenth are noncompliant with immunizations. The reason is cost and inconvenience.[143] The authors reported that managing vaccination pain is important and that analgesic interventions (distraction techniques, topical anesthetics, and injection techniques) should be used routinely, thereby promoting more positive attitudes and behaviors.

Taddio and coauthors[143] compared the effectiveness of topical liposomal bupivacaine to vapocoolant spray, nurse-administered tactile stimulation, or self-directed distraction (reading a magazine). The authors found that liposomal bupivacaine was more effective than distraction but did not differ from either vapocoolant spray or tactile sensation. They concluded that vaccinators should routinely offer to mitigate pain during immunizations. Other medical injections, including venipuncture and cosmetic and plastic surgery procedures, also have the potential to be painful.

Versloot and coauthors[144] assessed the pain and distress by a pediatric patient, a dentist, and independent observers during a dental injection. A correlation was found between the child's self-reported pain and the pain assessed by independent observers. The dentists' pain assessment was the lowest. Therefore, a dentist's assessment of a patient's pain may not always be accurate.

We think we administer a relatively painless injection to the majority of patients. However, it is rare that we actually have patients objectively rate the pain they experienced.

## Effect of operator and patient gender on injection pain

Experimental studies have shown that women have a lower acceptance of pain, fear pain more, and avoid pain more than men.[55] Perry and coauthors[145] studied the effect of the gender of the operator giving the injection on the pain of asymptomatic men and women receiving the injection. That is, they evaluated operator gender and its influence on maxillary lateral incisor injection pain in males versus females. The authors found that females reported higher pain ratings when a male operator administered the anesthetic solution. Other pain interactions of male operator/male patients, female operator/female patients, and female operator/male patients were not significant. One explanation as to why a discrepancy in pain exists between men and women is a result of social expectations suggesting that men are expected to behave in a more stoic manner. We have all known men who do not know the meaning of pain, but then again, some of them do not know the meaning of most words. I think "macho law" prohibits some men from admitting things hurt in a public setting.

IN CONCLUSION, *higher pain ratings may occur when a male operator gives an injection to a female patient.*

## Phases of a dental injection and pain

Each dental injection has three phases: *(1)* initial needle placement through the alveolar mucosa, *(2)* needle placement to the target site, and *(3)* deposition of the anesthetic solution at the target site. Each phase has different requirements for controlling pain.

### IANB injection pain

The IANB has been associated with pain in asymptomatic patients. For the needle insertion phase, Nusstein and Beck[146] reported an incidence of moderate-to-severe pain ranging from 14% to 22% in a retrospective study of 1,635 IANBs. For needle placement to the target site, Nusstein and coauthors[147] found that 39% to 54% of the subjects reported moderate-to-severe pain. For the deposition of the anesthetic solution at the target site, various authors[2,7,15,16,148] have reported the incidence of moderate-to-severe pain ranging from 20% to 40%. The pain occurred despite the fact that anesthetic solution was deposited over a 1-minute time period. Nusstein and coauthors[147] found that needle placement to the target site was more painful than needle insertion pain or anesthetic solution deposition pain for the IANB. Therefore, we need to develop methods to decrease the pain of the IANB.

IN CONCLUSION, *the IANB has the potential to be a painful injection.*

## Injection pain in the maxilla and mandible

Kaufman and coauthors[149] found that the IANB resulted in more discomfort than infiltration, intraligamentary injection, and mental nerve block. However, local infiltration in the maxillary anterior region yielded the highest discomfort scores. Aminabadi and coauthors[150] also found that maxillary anterior infiltration had higher pain scores than IANB or mandibular infiltrations in children. Wahl and coauthors[151] found that palatal injections caused significantly more pain than anterior or posterior maxillary infiltrations or IANBs. Meechan and coauthors[152] compared needle penetration in the anterior and posterior palate and found that infiltration was more uncomfortable in the anterior palate than posterior palate.

Maxillary infiltration anesthesia has the potential to be a painful injection. For the needle insertion phase, Nusstein and Beck[146] reported an incidence of moderate-to-severe pain ranging from 18% to 21% in a retrospective study of 422 maxillary infiltrations in anterior teeth. Perry and coauthors[145] found that needle insertion resulted in moderate-to-severe pain 32% to 44% of the time. For maxillary infiltrations in posterior teeth, Nusstein and Beck[146] reported an incidence of moderate-to-severe pain

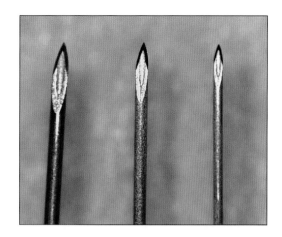

**Fig 1-16** Tribeveled 25-, 27-, and 30-gauge needles. Needle gauge does not seem to matter in perception of pain in the oral cavity.

ranging from 12% to 17% in a retrospective study of 279 injections. Topical anesthesia significantly increased the odds of patients experiencing no pain upon needle insertion during maxillary anterior infiltrations but not during maxillary posterior infiltrations.

For needle placement over the lateral incisor, Scott and coauthors[153] reported that 20% to 28% of the patients had moderate pain while 3% had severe pain. Perry and coauthors[145] reported that needle placement resulted in moderate-to-severe pain 25% to 46% of the time.

For deposition of 1.8 mL of 2% lidocaine with 1:100,000 epinephrine over the lateral incisor, Mikesell and coauthors[154] and Scott and coauthors[153] reported that 23% to 34% of the patients had moderate pain while 3% had severe pain. Perry and coauthors[145] reported that solution deposition resulted in moderate pain 35% to 53% of the time, with an incidence of 4% to 14% for severe pain. Mikesell and coauthors[154] reported that 9% of the patients had moderate pain over the first premolar site, and 6% had moderate pain over the first molar site. The pain occurred despite the fact that anesthetic solution was deposited over a 1-minute time period.

**IN CONCLUSION,** *maxillary infiltration anesthesia has the potential to be a painful injection.*

## Needle size

Dentists may use smaller needles because they think they hurt less (Fig 1-16). However, Fuller and coauthors[155] found no significant differences in the perception of pain produced by 25-, 27-, and 30-gauge needles in the retromolar fossa. Flanagan and coauthors[156] found no significant difference for injection pain between 25-, 27-, and 30-gauge needles, in 930 injections, for IANBs, maxillary buccal infiltrations, and palatal injections. They coined the phrase "size doesn't matter," at least for dental injections.

McPherson and coauthors[157] investigated whether a larger internal bore needle reduced pain during an IANB and long buccal nerve block. The enlarged bore (43% wider than a standard needle) supposedly reduces the level of pressure during injection, thus reducing pain. However, the authors found that the larger-bore 27-gauge needle did not reduce injection pain compared with the standard-bore 27-gauge needle.

Meechan and coauthors[152] found that a needle used for a previous needle penetration for a palatal injection in the same patient caused more discomfort in female patients. Perhaps it would be best to use a fresh needle for additional injections in the palate.

**IN CONCLUSION,** *needle gauge (25-, 27-, and 30-gauge) does not seem to matter in perception of pain in the oral cavity.*

## Injection discomfort with plain and epinephrine-containing solutions

Some authors have found that there is a reduction in injection pain when using plain anesthetic solutions.[158] The higher pH of the plain solutions is believed to contribute to this effect. However, Meechan and Day[159] did not find a difference between a plain solution and one containing epinephrine for a palatal injection. Wahl and coauthors[160] were unable to find a difference in the pain of injection when using a plain or an epinephrine-containing solution for maxillary buccal infiltrations or IANB. In a later study, Wahl and coauthors[161] found that injection of prilocaine plain (Citanest Plain, Dentsply) produced significantly lower pain scores than lidocaine with epinephrine, mepivacaine plain, or articaine with epinephrine for maxillary buccal infiltration, palatal infiltration, or IANBs. However, needle insertion, and to some extent needle placement, would not be affected by the anesthetic solution. While 4% prilocaine plain may decrease solution deposition pain, it is not a painless injection.

Some clinicians initially administer 3% mepivacaine plain and then add 2% lidocaine with 1:100,000 epinephrine for IANBs. The rationale is that 3% mepivacaine has a higher pH because it does not contain epinephrine. In theory, using 3% mepivacaine initially would decrease the pain of injection. Lammers and coauthors[162] found that injection pain with the initial administration of 3% mepivacaine plain (Carbocaine) followed by 2% lidocaine with 1:100,000 epinephrine was not significantly different than that with the initial administration of 2% lidocaine with 1:100,000 epinephrine followed by 2% lidocaine with 1:100,000 epinephrine for an IANB.

In the maxilla, infiltration of plain solutions without vasoconstrictors will only provide pulpal anesthesia for 10 to 15 minutes. So an additional infiltration would be needed if anesthesia past 15 minutes were required. In the IANB, plain solutions will provide at least 50 minutes of pulpal anesthesia for the patients who achieve pulpal anesthesia.

Another consideration is whether 4% prilocaine or 3% mepivacaine decreases the pain of injection with a standard syringe better than use of the computer-controlled local anesthetic delivery (CCLAD) system.

**IN CONCLUSION,** *injection pain of the IANB with 3% mepivacaine plain is the same as using 2% lidocaine with 1:100,000 epinephrine. A 4% prilocaine plain solution may decrease the pain of the IANB, but further study is needed. Factors other than pain, such as the efficacy of 4% prilocaine and 3% mepivacaine in the maxilla, need to be considered for their clinical use.*

## Articaine injection pain

Mikesell and coauthors,[154] Evans and coauthors,[163] Haase and coauthors,[164] and Robertson and coauthors[37] found no significant differences between a 4% articaine formulation with 1:100,000 epinephrine and a 2% lidocaine formulation with 1:100,000 epinephrine for the three phases of the injection. Sumer and coauthors[165] studied 497 maxillary infiltrations or IANBs using an articaine formulation or lidocaine formulation. They also found similar pain for both formulations.

**IN CONCLUSION,** *injection pain is the same for an articaine formulation when compared with a lidocaine formulation.*

## Injection techniques

### Slow injection
Hochman and coauthors[166] and Kudo[167] measured injection pressures of dental injections. Injecting with low pressures (slow injection) significantly reduced pain and anxiety.[167] Therefore, a slow injection (deposition of anesthetic solution) decreases pressure and patient discomfort during injection. Kanaa and coauthors[168] found that a slow IANB injection (60 seconds) was more comfortable than a rapid injection (15 seconds).

Fig 1-17 Older CompuDent unit, formerly referred to as the *Wand*. The handpiece assembly and microtubing are also shown. (Courtesy of Milestone Scientific.)

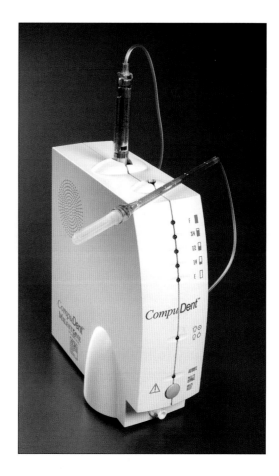

One way to give a slow injection is to use the CompuDent (Milestone Scientific) CCLAD system—formerly referred to as the *Wand* (Fig 1-17). The CompuDent CCLAD system delivers 1.4 mL of anesthetic solution over a time period of 4 minutes and 45 seconds (slow rate). There are also faster rates available with the CompuDent. The majority of the literature on CCLAD systems has dealt with the pain of injection with the delivery system compared with standard injections using a syringe.[169–194] From 20 studies, there is very good evidence that the CompuDent CCLAD unit decreases the pain of injections and reduces disruptive behavior in children.[169–189] Four studies show no difference in pain,[190–193] and one study shows higher pain ratings[194] with the CCLAD unit. While the CCLAD unit decreases pain of the injection, the system does not produce a painless injection.[169–194]

**IN CONCLUSION,** *a slow injection is more comfortable than a rapid injection, and the CCLAD system decreases the pain of injection.*

## Two-stage injection

A two-stage injection consists of an initial very slow administration of approximately a quarter cartridge of anesthetic solution just under the mucosal surface. Once regional numbness occurs, the remaining anesthetic solution is given to the full depth at the target site. Nusstein and coauthors[147] found that the two-stage injection, using a standard syringe, decreased the pain of needle placement for the IANB but was only significant for female patients. This injection technique is indicated for

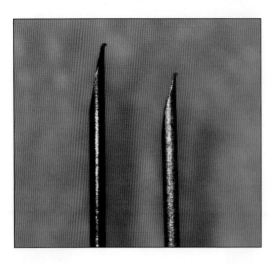

**Fig 1-18** Needles become barbed when they contact the mandibular bone during an IANB.

apprehensive and anxious patients or pediatric patients but may be used on anyone. Sandeep and coauthors[195] found that the two-stage injection technique reduced the pain of nerve blocks in children.

**IN CONCLUSION,** *a two-stage injection may be helpful in reducing the pain of injection.*

## Nerve injury following an IANB

Permanent nerve damage to the lingual and inferior alveolar nerve is a very rare occurrence. Pogrel and Thamby[196] reported the incidence at between 1 in 26,762 and 1 in 160,571. The lingual nerve is affected in 70% to 79% of patients and the inferior alveolar nerve in 21% to 30%.[197,198] A possible cause for the predominance of injury to the lingual nerve may be the smaller number of fascicles, when compared with the inferior alveolar nerve, at the site of the injection.[197] Krafft and Hickel[198] reported sensory disturbances to the lingual nerve in 18 out of 12,104 patients. In 17 of the 18 patients, sensation recovered after 6 months.

Rout and coauthors[199] and Stacy and Hajjar[200] found an incidence of 60% to 97% barbed needle tip damage when needles were examined following an IANB (Fig 1-18). The tips were damaged when the medial surface of the mandibular bone was contacted during the injection. Stacy and Hajjar[200] speculated that the withdrawal of barbed needles might cause nerve damage to the lingual or inferior alveolar nerve. It may be prudent to not contact bone when administering the IANB.

**IN CONCLUSION,** *lingual nerve injury occurs more often than injury to the inferior alveolar nerve. However, permanent damage is rare. Furthermore, needles become barbed when they contact the mandibular bone.*

## Broken needles

According to Pogrel,[201] most needle fractures occur when giving the IANB, often with a 30-gauge needle, and in children who have moved suddenly during the injection. His recommendations are as follows: *(1)* do not bury the needle to the hub, *(2)* avoid using 30-gauge needles for IANBs, and *(3)* avoid bending the needles at the hub before insertion. (This last recommendation does not apply to intraosseous anesthesia because the ultrashort needle is commonly bent to gain access in posterior teeth.) While needle breakage is a rare occurrence with new disposable needles, the dentist should be aware of these recommendations. It is always better to be safe than sorry.

**IN CONCLUSION,** *to prevent broken needles for IANBs, do not use 30-gauge needles, bury the needle to the hub, or bend needles at the hub.*

# Topical Anesthetics

Fear of the needle is one of the major causes of apprehension in dental patients.[202–204] Although some authors[205–208] have demonstrated the effectiveness of topical anesthetics, others[209–211] have reported no significant pain reduction with the use of topical anesthetic. However, a particularly important area of the mouth where topical anesthesia has been shown to be helpful is in the maxillary anterior region.[146] Nusstein and Beck[146] reported that topical anesthesia significantly increased the odds of patients experiencing no needle insertion pain during maxillary anterior infiltration.

Nusstein and Beck,[146] along with other authors,[205,207,208,212–214] found that 20% benzocaine (Hurricaine, Beutlich) requires at least a 1-minute application to be effective in the maxilla, but that increased duration of application may still not be effective with an IANB. Lidocaine has been reported to be effective at concentrations of 5%,[205,215–217] 10%, and 20% (via a patch).[206,218,219] Ineffectiveness of 5% lidocaine has been reported for 30-second applications.[208] A eutectic mixture of local anesthetic (EMLA) containing lidocaine and prilocaine has been found to be successful after 2- and 5-minute applications.[215,216,220,221] de Freiras and coauthors[222] compared the pain of injection of lidocaine using topical benzocaine versus a placebo for the posterior superior alveolar nerve and greater palatine nerve. The authors found the placebo and benzocaine to have similar effects. There was no statistical difference in sex. Ghaderi and coauthors[223] used topical anesthetic (benzocaine) or topical anesthetic plus 1 minute of ice application to the buccal mucosa before injection in pediatric patients. While they found a significant reduction in pain with the topical anesthetic plus ice (42 mm out of 100 mm on a visual analog scale [VAS]) when compared with the topical anesthetic alone (58 mm out of 100 mm), pain was still present during injection.

Franz-Montan and coauthors[224] compared the effectiveness of liposome-encapsulated ropivacaine with EMLA (2.5% lidocaine/2.5% prilocaine) and 20% benzocaine gel for topical anesthesia of the maxillary canine region. The authors found the liposome-encapsulated ropivacaine to be equivalent to EMLA for reducing pain during needle insertion. None of the topical anesthetics were effective for pulpal anesthesia.

Al-Melh and coauthors[225–227] found that EMLA cream was better than benzocaine gel for palatal canine infiltration and maxillary vestibular canine infiltration.

Martin and coauthors[210] found that if patients thought they were receiving topical anesthetic, whether they did or not, they anticipated less pain. Therefore, the most important aspect of using topical anesthetic may not be its clinical effectiveness but rather the psychologic effect on the patient, who feels the practitioner is doing everything possible to prevent pain.

**IN CONCLUSION,** *topical anesthetic is most effective in the maxillary anterior region. Topical anesthetic should be applied for at least 1 minute and before each injection to demonstrate that we are doing everything possible to prevent pain.*

## Safety of compound topical anesthetics

Kravitz[228] reviewed five compound topical anesthetics containing tetracaine, cocaine, prilocaine, and lidocaine, with and without vasoconstrictors. He concluded that legitimate concerns exist regarding their safety because they are unapproved drugs. He went on to say that until compound topical anesthetics become federally regulated, any benefits for topical anesthesia may not outweigh their risks to dental patients. Additionally, the amount of each topical agent may vary greatly in compound anesthetics. Macdonnel[229] also questioned the use of these compound topical anesthetics. While the amount we administer orally would be small, the effectiveness of various compound anesthetics is not well known.

**IN CONCLUSION,** *compound topical anesthetics may contain varied amounts of drugs and are not well studied.*

# Palatal Anesthesia

Bhalia and coauthors[230] found that topical 5% lidocaine reduced the pain of needle insertion if left on the palatal mucosa for 2, 5, or 10 minutes, but it had no effect on clinical pain relief for local anesthetic solution deposition. For palatal injections using a CCLAD system, Johnson and Primosch[211] compared infiltration pain using a topical anesthetic, pressure anesthesia using a cotton tip applicator, a combination of both methods, and use of neither method in the palate. They found no difference among the various site preparation methods used and reported the pain as minimal, probably because of the use of the CCLAD system at a slow injection rate. However, Jälevik and Klingberg[231] found that the pain of a palatal injection was significantly lower with the CCLAD system than with conventional syringe injection. Nusstein and coauthors[179] found that the anterior middle superior alveolar (AMSA) injection using the CCLAD system resulted in similar pain ratings for needle insertion as the conventional syringe but statistically lower pain ratings for anesthetic solution deposition. However, the AMSA, whether using the CCLAD system or a conventional syringe, has the potential to be a painful injection.

For a palatal injection of lidocaine, no difference in pain was found between the application of low-intensity laser therapy, 20% benzocaine, or pressure.[232]

**IN CONCLUSION,** *palatal anesthesia continues to be painful, and further studies are needed to reduce pain. Use of the CCLAD system reduces pain but does not make the injection pain free.*

# Alternative Modes of Reducing Injection Pain

## Warming anesthetic solution

Three studies found that warming local anesthetic solutions to body temperature, when compared with room-temperature solutions, did not reduce the pain of subcutaneous injection.[233–235] However, other studies found that warming anesthetic solution reduced the pain of local infiltration.[236–238] Oikarinen and coauthors[239] found that most subjects could not differentiate between anesthetic solutions at room temperature (21°C) or body temperature (37°C). Volk and Gargiulo[240] questioned the use of cartridge warmers because by the time the cartridge was removed from the warmer and placed in the metal syringe, and the solution was expressed through the metal needle, the temperature was almost at room temperature.

**IN CONCLUSION,** *further research is needed on warming anesthetic solution.*

## Palatal anesthesia with cooling

In medicine, Hijazi and coauthors[241] found that topical vapocoolant spray reduced pain before venous cannulation. Robinson and coauthors[242] reported that intradermal lidocaine was more effective at pain reduction before venous cannulation than ethyl chloride topical spray. Hartstein and Barry[243] failed to find a topical skin coolant beneficial in venous cannulation.

In pediatric patients, precooling the soft tissues with ice helped to reduce the pain of local anesthetic injection.[244] Harbert[245] also described a technique utilizing topical ice to reduce the pain of palatal injections. Kosaraju and Vandewalle[246] compared injection pain of a 5-second application of a cold refrigerant versus a 2-minute application of 20% benzocaine gel in the posterior palate. While the cold refrigerant was better at reducing the pain of injections, there was no postoperative follow-up to determine if tissue damage occurred from the application of cold.

Wiswall and coauthors[247] found that the pain of a palatal injection over the greater palatine foramen was no different using pressure alone, pressure and 20% benzocaine, and pressure and Endo-Ice (10-second application). The pain of needle insertion was less than that of solution deposition. Howev-

**Fig 1-19** Postoperative palatal lesion caused by the application of Endo-Ice.

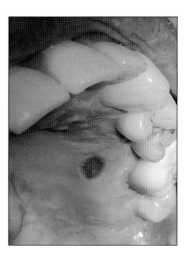

er, over 80% of the subjects reported a sore on their palate (Fig 1-19) occurring 2 to 48 hours after cold application and persisting for 1 to 10 days. The manufacturers of Endo-Ice caution that it should not be applied to mucosal tissues because of freezing of the tissue and soft tissue damage.

**IN CONCLUSION,** *using Endo-Ice or prolonged cold application to the palatal mucosa should not be used clinically to achieve anesthesia.*

## Buffering anesthetic solutions to reduce injection pain

Local anesthetic agents with vasoconstrictors are acidic. A buffered local anesthetic has been proposed to be less painful when injected because the pH of the solution is closer to the physiologic pH. Systematic reviews in medicine have shown reduced injection pain with buffered anesthetics.[248–250] In dentistry, Al-Sultan and coauthors,[251,252] Kashyap and coauthors,[253] Malamed and coauthors,[254] and Bowles and coauthors[255] have shown decreased injection pain with buffered lidocaine. Primosch and Robinson,[256] Whitcomb and coauthors,[257] Balasco and coauthors,[258] Harreld and coauthors,[259] Saatchi and coauthors,[260] Schellenberg and coauthors,[101] Hobeich and coauthors,[261] Shurtz and coauthors,[262] and Comerci and coauthors[263] failed to establish a significant reduction in pain scores for buffered lidocaine and articaine solutions. Buffering the formulation increased the pH of the anesthetic formulation but did not result in less pain during solution deposition. Theoretically, the higher pH should have resulted in decreased pain of injection. However, the body intrinsically has an efficient buffering system that maintains tissues at physiologic pH. The pH conversion buffering process, as reported by Wennberg and coauthors,[264] could occur within several minutes. Punnia-Moorthy[265] reported a freshly prepared 2% lignocaine with adrenaline formulation (pH 5.25) being converted to a pH of 7.17 within 3 minutes following an intradermal injection. This physiologic conversion may help explain why buffering an anesthetic did not demonstrate any benefit in decreasing injection pain.

Another consideration is the initial pain of needle insertion and needle placement. These two aspects of the injection have proven to be painful. In fact, needle insertion pain in an IANB was reported as moderate to severe in 14% to 22% of patients.[146] Needle placement is the most painful part of the injection, and 39% to 54% of patients reported moderate-to-severe pain.[147] Neither of these would be eliminated by buffering!

**IN CONCLUSION,** *buffering local anesthetics does not reduce the pain of dental injections.*

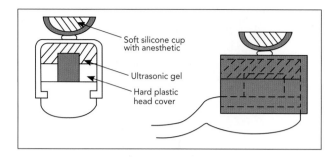

**Fig 1-20** Schematic drawing of a dental anesthesia sonophoresis device head with a silicone cup to hold anesthetic. (Redrawn after Packer et al[266] with permission.)

## Sonophoresis

Sonophoresis produces ultrasonic energy (Fig 1-20) that generates microchannels between the keratinized cells of the stratum corneum—allowing topical anesthetic to penetrate this layer. Packer and coauthors[266] studied the application of sonophoresis and 5% lidocaine in the maxillary canine vestibule of asymptomatic patients. The authors found no significant difference in pain perception using sonophoresis and the control.

**IN CONCLUSION,** *the application of sonophoresis/topical lidocaine does not seem to be effective in reducing injection pain.*

## Jet injection

Intradermal needleless jet injection (J-Tip, National Medical Products) (Fig 1-21) has been shown to be effective in medicine prior to intravenous cannulation.[267–270] It has also been used for needleless vasectomy.[271] Geenen and coauthors[272] reported that the Injex jet injector (Injex Pharma) may have some value in pediatric dentistry. However, patients did not prefer the Injex system over the classical local anesthetic injection with a needle. While Dabarakis and coauthors[273] found good soft tissue anesthesia with Injex, the success rate for pulpal anesthesia of permanent maxillary lateral incisors was poor (13% as judged by electric pulp testing). Arapostathis and coauthors[274] also found the Injex not very effective for infiltration anesthesia; 81% of patients required additional anesthetic for completion of routine dental procedures. They also felt it was difficult to administer the Injex in some areas of the mouth.

Jet injectors may be useful for topical anesthesia but not for pulpal anesthesia. In addition, because jet injectors inject the local anesthetic under pressure using carbon dioxide, their use can sound like opening a pop can. In the mouth, this sound may surprise the patient or result in fear during administration.[273,274]

**IN CONCLUSION,** *jet injection may not be effective orally and does not provide consistent pulpal anesthesia.*

## Counterstimulation and distraction

Counterstimulation (using finger vibration of oral tissue) and distraction (raising the right and left legs) were found to reduce pain reaction in pediatric patients.[275] Nanitsos and coauthors[276] also found that vibration of tissue decreased the pain during local anesthetic administration. Furman and coauthors[277] found that virtual reality distraction was better than a movie for pain control during periodontal scaling and root planing. Dahlquist and coauthors[278] studied the effects of video game and virtual reality distraction for cold pressor pain in children. They found that both methods equally improved pain threshold and pain tolerance.

Fig 1-21 J-Tip jet injectors inject the local anesthetic under pressure after being loaded with local anesthetic solution.

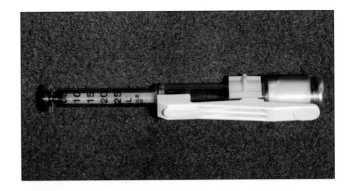

Fig 1-22 Patient using audio sedation. (Courtesy of b-Calm.)

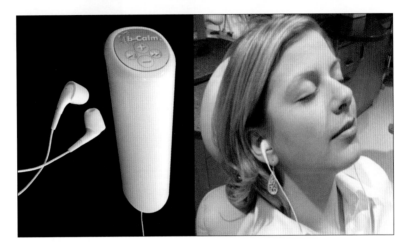

Noise-canceling devices such as b-Calm may help to soothe patients during treatment (Fig 1-22), especially children with sensory challenges or autism. Studies are needed to evaluate the efficacy of these devices.

**IN CONCLUSION,** *counterstimulation and distraction methods may be effective, but further studies are needed.*

## Vibrating devices and their effect on pain

A study by Saijo and coauthors[279] used a vibrating local anesthetic attachment (VibraJect, Vibraject) to potentially reduce injection pain. The concept is similar to the vibrating razors used in the shaving industry. The small VibraJect battery-operated unit is clipped onto the barrel of a conventional syringe and can be used for any injection technique (Fig 1-23). The device was not found to be clinically effective in decreasing pain scores on needle insertion or solution deposition.[279] Roeber and coauthors[280] studied the effectiveness of using VibraJect in reducing pain from dental injections in children. They found that the use of vibration did not significantly reduce pain, pain-related disruptive behavior, or subjective dentist ratings.

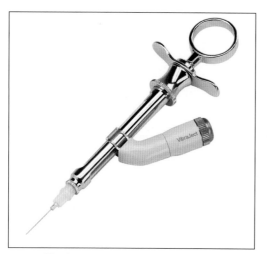

**Fig 1-23** VibraJect is a vibrating unit that is attached to a local anesthetic syringe. (Courtesy of Vibraject.)

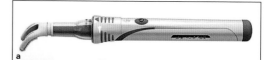
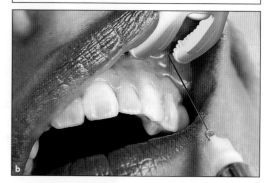

**Fig 1-24** The DentalVibe *(a)* creates vibrations in the tissues around the injection site as well as illumination while anesthesia injections are administered *(b)*. (Courtesy of Bing Innovations.)

The DentalVibe (Bing Innovations) (Fig 1-24) vibrates, illuminates, and retracts the tissue during a dental injection. Ching and coauthors[281] found a significant reduction in self-reported pain in adolescent patients during local anesthesia injection when using the DentalVibe versus a conventional injection. DiFelice and coauthors[282] compared the effectiveness of topical anesthetic to a vibratory device plus topical anesthetic for IANBs. They found that the vibratory device plus topical anesthetic significantly reduced pain (21 mm VAS) compared with topical anesthetic alone (39 mm VAS). Elbay and coauthors[283] compared injection pain of the DentalVibe injection system to a traditional syringe for IANBs in children. They found no statistically significant differences in pain. Patients preferred the traditional procedure to the DentalVibe.

**IN CONCLUSION,** *vibrating devices need further studies to determine if injection pain is decreased.*

## Electronic dental anesthesia and transcutaneous electrical nerve stimulation

Various pediatric studies[284,285] have found that electronic dental anesthesia (EDA) reduced discomfort during local anesthetic administration in young, sedated dental patients and was effective in pain control. Meechan and Winter[286] found that EDA was no more effective than a placebo for pain of palatal injection. However, Meechan and coauthors[287] did find that transcutaneous electrical nerve stimulation (TENS) reduced injection discomfort better than 20% benzocaine for IANBs. Regarding operative procedures, Yap and Ho[288] found that local anesthesia was more effective than EDA. Modaresi and coauthors[289] reported that EDA was no more effective than a placebo treatment and felt that EDA probably worked by distracting the patient. Schäfer and coauthors[290] found that as an alternative to local anesthetics, TENS would not be useful because it offered only minor advantages over a placebo.

**IN CONCLUSION,** *EDA and TENS are not totally effective for pain control.*

# Alternative Instruments

## Lasers

Laser treatment has been advocated as a means of providing analgesia during dental cavity preparation. Hadley and coauthors[291] studied lasers for cavity preparation and found that they decreased the discomfort levels for the patients who declined to receive local anesthesia. Liu and coauthors[292] found that laser cavity preparation was less painful than conventional methods in children. Whitters and coauthors[293] found a small increase in pain thresholds (as measured with the EPT) with laser treatments. Poli and Parker[294] performed single cavity preparation with an erbium, chromium: yttrium-scandium-gallium-garnet (Er,Cr:YSGG) laser. Approximately 80% of the patients felt no pain or only a very slight sensation. Factors that promoted more pain were posterior teeth, greater caries depth, greater use of higher power levels, and longer ablation time. It seems that the laser may help decrease pain but not eliminate it.[295–297]

    **IN CONCLUSION,** *further research is needed to define the pain with laser treatment.*

## Rotary polymer bur

Allen and coauthors[298] found that a number of subjects preferred the rotary polymer bur with no local anesthetic to a carbide bur with local anesthesia. However, the subjects reported more pain and pressure when treated with the polymer instrument.

    **IN CONCLUSION,** *further research may define if a rotary polymer instrument is useful in clinical practice.*

## Air abrasion

The use of air abrasion techniques for restorative dentistry has been advocated over conventional techniques because of a reduced need for anesthesia. One study[299] found that no anesthesia was required when using air abrasion for removing occlusal fissure caries lesions in mandibular premolars.

    **IN CONCLUSION,** *further studies are indicated to objectively evaluate the use of air abrasion to provide pain-free restorative treatment.*

# Final Thoughts

In conclusion, regarding clinical factors related to local anesthesia, we have to look at Evvie Nef's Law: There is a solution to every problem; the only difficulty is finding it!

# References

1. Ågren E, Danielsson K. Conduction block analgesia in the mandible. A comparative investigation of the techniques of Fischer and Gow-Gates. Swed Dent J 1981;5:81–89.

2. Vreeland DL, Reader A, Beck M, Meyers W, Weaver J. An evaluation of volumes and concentrations of lidocaine in human inferior alveolar nerve block. J Endod 1989;15:6–12.

3. Hinkley SA, Reader A, Beck M, Meyers WJ. An evaluation of 4% prilocaine with 1:200,000 epinephrine and 2% mepivacaine with 1:20,000 levonordefrin compared with 2% lidocaine with 1:100,000 epinephrine for inferior alveolar nerve block. Anesth Prog 1991;38:84–89.

4. McLean C, Reader A, Beck M, Meyers WJ. An evaluation of 4% prilocaine and 3% mepivacaine compared with 2% lidocaine (1:100,000 epinephrine) for inferior alveolar nerve block. J Endod 1993;19:146–150.

5. Chaney MA, Kerby R, Reader A, Beck FM, Meyers WJ, Weaver J. An evaluation of lidocaine hydrocarbonate compared with lidocaine hydrochloride for inferior alveolar nerve block. Anesth Prog 1991;38:212–216.

6. Dunbar D, Reader A, Nist R, Beck M, Meyers WJ. Anesthetic efficacy of the intraosseous injection after an inferior alveolar nerve block. J Endod 1996;22:481–486.

7. Nist RA, Reader A, Beck M, Meyers WJ. An evaluation of the incisive nerve block and combination inferior alveolar and incisive nerve blocks in mandibular anesthesia. J Endod 1992;18:455–459.

8. Childers M, Reader A, Nist R, Beck M, Meyers WJ. Anesthetic efficacy of the periodontal ligament injection after an inferior alveolar nerve block. J Endod 1996;22:317–320.

9. Clark S, Reader A, Beck M, Meyers WJ. Anesthetic efficacy of the mylohyoid nerve block and combination inferior alveolar nerve block/mylohyoid nerve block. Oral Surg Oral Med Oral Pathol Oral Radiol Endod 1999;87:557–563.

10. Reitz J, Reader A, Nist R, Beck M, Meyers WJ. Anesthetic efficacy of the intraosseous injection of 0.9 mL of 2% lidocaine (1:100,000 epinephrine) to augment an inferior alveolar nerve block. Oral Surg Oral Med Oral Pathol Oral Radiol Endod 1998;86:516–523.

11. Stabile P, Reader A, Gallatin E, Beck M, Weaver J. Anesthetic efficacy and heart rate effects of the intraosseous injection of 1.5% etidocaine (1:200,000 epinephrine) after an inferior alveolar nerve block. Oral Surg Oral Med Oral Pathol Oral Radiol Endod 2000;89:407–411.

12. Gallatin E, Stabile P, Reader A, Nist R, Beck M. Anesthetic efficacy and heart rate effects of the intraosseous injection of 3% mepivacaine after an inferior alveolar nerve block. Oral Surg Oral Med Oral Pathol Oral Radiol Endod 2000;89:83–87.

13. Guglielmo A, Reader A, Nist R, Beck M, Weaver J. Anesthetic efficacy and heart rate effects of the supplemental intraosseous injection of 2% mepivacaine with 1:20,000 levonordefrin. Oral Surg Oral Med Oral Pathol Oral Radiol Endod 1999;87:284–293.

14. Hannan L, Reader A, Nist R, Beck M, Meyers WJ. The use of ultrasound for guiding needle placement for inferior alveolar nerve blocks. Oral Surg Oral Med Oral Pathol Oral Radiol Endod 1999;87:658–665.

15. Ridenour S, Reader A, Beck M, Weaver J. Anesthetic efficacy of a combination of hyaluronidase and lidocaine with epinephrine in inferior alveolar nerve blocks. Anesth Prog 2001;48:9–15.

16. Mikesell P, Nusstein J, Reader A, Beck M, Weaver J. A comparison of articaine and lidocaine for inferior alveolar nerve blocks. J Endod 2005;31:265–270.

17. Dreven LJ, Reader A, Beck M, Meyers WJ, Weaver J. An evaluation of an electric pulp tester as a measure of analgesia in human vital teeth. J Endod 1987;13:233–238.

18. Certosimo A, Archer R. A clinical evaluation of the electric pulp tester as an indicator of local anesthesia. Oper Dent 1996;21:25–30.

19. Jones V, Rivera E, Walton R. Comparison of carbon dioxide versus refrigerant spray to determine pulpal responsiveness. J Endod 2002;28:531–533.

20. Cohen H, Cha B, Spangberg L. Endodontic anesthesia in mandibular molars: A clinical study. J Endod 1993;19:370–373.

21. Miller SO, Johnson JD, Allemang JD, Strother JM. Cold testing through full-coverage restorations. J Endod 2004;30:695–700.

22. Kitamura T, Takahashi T, Horiuchi H. Electrical characteristics and clinical application of a new automatic pulp tester. Quintessence Int 1983;1:45–53.

23. Black JA, Liu S, Tanaka M, Cummins TR, Waxman SG. Changes in the expression of tetrodotoxin-sensitive sodium channels within dorsal root ganglia neurons in inflammatory pain. Pain 2004;108:237–247.

24. Hargreaves K, Keiser K. Local anesthetic failure in endodontics: Mechanisms and management. Endod Topics 2003;1:26–39.

25. Lai J, Porreca J, Hunter J, Gold M. Voltage-gated sodium channels and hyperalgesia. Ann Rev Pharmacol 2004;44:37–97.

26. Wells JE, Bingham V, Rowland KC, Hatton J. Expression of NaV 1.9 channels in human dental pulp and trigeminal ganglion. J Endod 2007;33:1172–1176.

27. Roy M, Narahashi T. Differential properties of tetrodotoxin-sensitive and tetrodotoxin-resistant sodium channels in rat dorsal root ganglion neurons. J Neurosci 1992;12:2104–2111.

28. Brand HS, Bekker W, Baart JA. Complications of local anaesthesia. An observational study. Int J Dent Hyg 2009;7:270–272.

29. Vika M, Raadal M, Skaret E, Kvale G. Dental and medical injections: Prevalence of self-reported problems among 18-year-old subjects in Norway. Eur J Oral Sci 2006;114:122–127.

30. Kaufman E, Weinstein P, Milgrom P. Difficulties in achieving local anesthesia. J Am Dent Assoc 1984;108:205–208.

31. Simon JF, Peltier B, Chambers D, Dower J. Dentists troubled by the administration of anesthetic injections: Long term stresses and effects. Quintessence Int 1994; 25:641–646.

32. Dower JS Jr, Simon JF, Peltier B, Chambers D. Patients who make a dentist most anxious about giving injections. J Calif Dent Assoc 1995;23(9):35–40.

33. Cohen SP. Compassion fatigue and veterinary health team. Vet Clin North Am Small Anim Pract 2007;37:123–124.

34. Aycock N, Boyle D. Interventions to manage compassion fatigue in oncology nursing. Clin J Oncol Nurs 2009;13:183–191.

35. Malamed S. Handbook of Local Anesthesia, ed 5. St Louis: Mosby, 2004.

36. Zhuang H, Hu D, Singer D, et al. Local anesthetics induce autophagy in young permanent tooth pulp cells [published online 07 September 2015]. Cell Death Discovery doi:10.1038/cddiscovery.2015.24.

37. Robertson D, Nusstein J, Reader A, Beck M, McCartney M. The anesthetic efficacy of articaine in buccal infiltration of mandibular posterior teeth. J Am Dent Assoc 2007;138:1104–1112.

38. Pateromichelakis S, Prokopiou AA. Local anaesthesia efficacy: Discrepancies between in vitro and in vivo studies. Acta Anaesthesiol Scand 1988;32:672–675.

39. Danielsson K, Evers H, Nordenram A. Long-acting local anesthetics in oral surgery: An experimental evaluation of bupivacaine and etidocaine for oral infiltration anesthesia. Anesth Prog 1985;32:65–68.

40. Gross R, McCartney M, Reader A, Beck M. A prospective, randomized, double-blind comparison of bupivacaine and lidocaine for maxillary infiltrations. J Endod 2007;33:1021–1024.

41. Johnson G, Hlava G, Kalkwarf K. A comparison of periodontal intraligamental anesthesia using etidocaine HCl and lidocaine HCl. Anesth Prog 1985;32:202–205.

42. Mason R, Drum M, Reader A, Nusstein J, Beck M. A prospective, randomized, double-blind comparison of 2% lidocaine with 1:100,000 and 1:50,000 epinephrine and 3% mepivacaine for maxillary infiltrations. J Endod 2009;35:1173–1177.

43. Katz S, Drum M, Reader A, Nusstein J, Beck M. A prospective, randomized, double-blind comparison of 2% lidocaine with 1:100,000 epinephrine, 4% prilocaine with 1:200,000 epinephrine and 4% prilocaine for maxillary infiltrations. Anesth Prog 2010;57:45–51.

44. Fishbain DA, Fishbain D, Lewis J, et al. Genetic testing for enzymes of drug metabolism: Does it have clinical utility for pain medicine at the present time? A structured review. Pain Med 2004;5:81–93.

45. Sheets PL, Jackson JO 2nd, Waxman SG, Dib-Haij SD, Cummins TR. A NaV 1.7 channel mutation associated with hereditary erythromelalgia contributes to neuronal hyperexcitability and displays reduced lidocaine sensitivity. J Physiol 2007;581:1019–1031.

46. Kleiber C, Schutte DL, McCartney AM, Floria-Santos M, Murray JC, Hanrahan K. Predictors of topical anesthetic effectiveness in children. J Pain 2006;8:168–174.

47. Diatchenko L, Slade GD, Nackley AG, et al. Genetic basis for individual variations in pain perception and the development of a chronic pain condition. Hum Mol Genet 2005;14:135–143.

48. Liem EB, Joiner TV, Tsueda K, Sessler DI. Increased sensitivity to thermal pain and reduced subcutaneous lidocaine efficacy in redheads. Anesthesiology 2005;102:509–514.

49. Liem EB, Lin CM, Suleman MI, et al. Anesthetic requirement is increased in redheads. Anesthesiology 2004;101:279–283.

50. Binkley CJ, Beacham A, Neace W, Gregg RG, Liem EB, Sessler DI. Genetic variations associated with red hair color and fear of dental pain, anxiety regarding dental care and avoidance of dental care. J Am Dent Assoc 2009;140:896–905.

51. Myles PS, Buchanan FF, Bain CR. The effect of hair colour on anaesthetic requirements and recovery time after surgery. Anaesth Intensive Care 2012;40:683–689.

52. Droll B, Drum M, Nusstein J, Reader A, Beck M. Anesthetic efficacy of the inferior alveolar nerve block in red-haired women. J Endod 2012;38:1564–1569.

53. Dougher MJ, Goldstein D, Leight KA. Induced anxiety and pain. J Anxiety Discord 1987;1:259–264.

54. Fillingim R, Edwards R, Powell T. The relationship of sex and clinical pain to experimental pain responses. Pain 1999;83:419–425.

55. Liddell A, Locker D. Gender and age differences in attitudes to dental pain and dental control. Community Dent Oral Epidemiol 1997;25:314–318.

56. Morin C, Lund JP, Villarroel T, Clokie CM, Feine JS. Differences between the sexes in post-surgical pain. Pain 2000;85:79–85.

57. Tofoli GR, Ramacciato JC, Volpato MC, Meechan JG, Ranali J, Groppo FC. Anesthetic efficacy and pain induced by dental anesthesia: The influence of gender and menstrual cycle. Oral Surg Oral Med Oral Pathol Oral Radiol Endod 2007;103:e34–38.

58. Loyd DR, Sun XX, Locke EE, Salas MM, Hargreaves KM. Sex differences in serotonin enhancement of capsaicin-evoked calcitonin gene-related peptide release from human dental pulp. Pain 2012;153: 2061–2067.

59. Lin CS. Pain catastrophizing in dental patients: Implications for treatment management. J Am Dent Assoc 2013;144:1244–1251.

60. Carter AE, Carter G, Boschen M, AlShwaimi E, George R. Ethnicity and pathways of fear in endodontics. J Endod 2015;41:1437–1440.

61. Haas D, Pynn B, Sands T. Drug use for the pregnant or lactating patient. Gen Dent 2000;48:54–60.

62. Hagai A, Diav-Citrin O, Shechtman S, Ornoy A. Pregnancy outcome after in utero exposure to local anesthetics as part of dental treatment: A prospective comparative cohort study. J Am Dent Assoc 2015;146:572–580 [erratum 2015;146:874].

63. Little J, Falace DA, Miller CS, Rhodus NL. Dental Management of the Medically Compromised Patient, ed 7. St Louis: Mosby Elsevier, 2008.

64. Nordenram A, Danielsson K. Local anesthesia in elderly patients. An experimental study of oral infiltration anaesthesia. Swed Dent J 1990;14:19–24.

65. Harkins SW, Chapman CR. Detection and decision factors in pain perception in young and elderly men. Pain 1976;2:253–264.

66. Harkins SW, Chapman CR. The perception of induced dental pain in young and elderly women. J Gerontol 1977;32:428–435.

67. Stewart SH, Finn PR, Pihl RO. A dose-response study of the effects of alcohol on the perceptions of pain and discomfort due to electric shock in men at high familial-genetic risk for alcoholism. Psychopharmacology (Berl) 1995;119:261–267.

68. Fiset L, Leroux B, Rothen M, Prall C, Zhu C, Ramsay DS. Pain control in recovering alcoholics: Effects of local anesthesia. J Stud Alcohol 1997;58:291–296.

69. Seng G, Kraus K, Cartridge G. Confirmed allergic reactions to amide local anesthetics. Gen Dent 1996;44:52–54.

70. Batinac T, Sotošek Tokmadžić V, Peharda V, Brajac I. Adverse reactions and alleged allergy to local anesthetics: Analysis of 331 patients. J Dermatol 2013;40:522–527.

71. Rood JP. Adverse reaction to dental local anesthetic injection: "Allergy" is not the cause. Br Dent J 2000;189:380–384.

72. Bosco DA, Haas DA, Young ER, Harrop KL. An anaphylactoid reaction following local anesthesia: A case report. Anesth Pain Control Dent 1993;2:87–93.

73. Chiu CY, Lin TY, Hsia SH, Lai SH, Wong KS. Systemic anaphylaxis following local lidocaine administration during a dental procedure. Pediatr Emerg Care 2004;20:178–180.

74. Morais-Almeida M, Gaspar A, Marinho S, Rosado-Pinto J. Allergy to local anesthetics of the amide group with tolerance to procaine. Allergy 2003;58:827–828.

75. Harboe T, Guttormsen AB, Aarebrot S, Dybendal T, Irgens A, Florvaag E. Suspected allergy to local anaesthetics: Follow-up in 135 cases. Acta Anaesthesiol Scand 2010;54:536–542.

76. Shojaei A, Haas D. Local anesthetic cartridges and latex allergy: A literature review. J Can Dent Assoc 2002;68:622–626.

77. Smolinske SC. Review of parenteral sulfite reactions. J Toxicol Clinical Toxicol 1992;30:597–606.

78. Naftalin L, Yagiela J. Vasoconstrictors: Indications and precautions. Dent Clin North Am 2002;46:733–746.

79. Laviola M, McGavin SK, Freer GA, et al. Randomized study of phentolamine mesylate for reversal of local anesthesia. J Dent Res 2008;87:635–639.

80. Hersh EV, Moore PA, Papas AS, et al. Reversal of soft-tissue local anesthesia with phentolamine mesylate in adolescents and adults. J Am Dent Assoc 2008;139:1080–1093.

81. Rutherford B, Zeller JR, Thake D. Local and systemic toxicity of intraoral submucosal injections of phentolamine mesylate (OraVerse). Anesth Prog 2009;56:123–127.

82. Moore PA, Hersh EV, Papas AS, et al. Pharmacokinetics of lidocaine with epinephrine following local anesthesia reversal with phentolamine mesylate. Anesth Prog 2008;55:40–48.

83. Tavares M, Goodson JM, Studen-Pavlovich D, et al; Soft Tissue Anesthesia Reversal Group. Reversal of soft-tissue local anesthesia with phentolamine mesylate in pediatric patients. J Am Dent Assoc 2008;139:1095–1104 [erratum 2008;139:1312].

84. Froum SJ, Froum SH, Malamed SF. The use of phentolamine mesylate to evaluate mandibular nerve damage following implant placement. Compendium 2010;31:520–528.

85. Fowler S, Nusstein J, Drum M, Reader A, Beck M. Reversal of soft-tissue anesthesia in asymptomatic endodontic patients: A preliminary, prospective, randomized, single-blind study. J Endod 2011;37:1353–1358.

86. Saunders TR, Psaltis G, Weston JF, Yanase RR, Rogy SS, Ghalie RG. In-practice evaluation of OraVerse for the reversal of soft-tissue anesthesia after dental procedures. Compend Contin Educ Dent 2011;32:58–62.

87. Prados-Frutos JC, Rojo R, González-Serrano J, et al. Phentolamine mesylate to reverse oral soft-tissue local anesthesia: A systematic review and meta-analysis. J Am Dent Assoc 2015;146:751–759.e3.

88. Elmore S, Nusstein J, Drum M, Reader A, Beck M, Fowler S. Reversal of pulpal and soft tissue anesthesia by using phentolamine: a prospective randomized, single-blind study. J Endod. 2013;39:429–434.

89. Van Wijk AJ, Hoogstraten J. Experience with dental pain and fear of dental pain. J Dent Res 2005;84:947–950.

90. Van Wijk AJ, Hoogstraten J. Anxiety and pain during dental injections. J Dent 2009;37:700–704.

91. Arnzt A, Dreessen L, de Jong. The influence of anxiety on pain: Attentional and attributional mediators. Pain 1994;56:307–314.

92. Vika M, Raadal M, Skaret E, Kvale G. Dental and medical injections: Prevalence of self-reported problems among 18-year-old subjects in Norway. Eur J Oral Sci 2006;114:122–127.

93. Carter LE, McNeil DW, Vowles KE, et al. Effects of emotion on pain reports, tolerance and physiology. Pain Res Manag 2002;7:21–30.

94. Locker D, Liddell AM. Correlates of dental anxiety among older adults. J Dent Res 1991;70:198–203.

95. Kieser J, Herbison P. Clinical anxiety among dental students. N Z Dent J 2000;96:138–139.

96. Corah NL, O'Shea RM, Bissell GD, Thines TJ, Mendola P. The dentist-patient relationship: Perceived dentist behaviors that reduce patient anxiety and increase satisfaction. J Am Dent Assoc 1988;116:73–76.

97. Jackson DL, Johnson BS. Conscious sedation for dentistry: Risk management and patient selection. Dent Clin North Am 2000;46:767–780.

98. Lindemann M, Reader A, Nusstein J, Drum M, Beck M. Effect of sublingual triazolam on the success of inferior alveolar nerve block in patients with irreversible pulpitis. J Endod 2008;34:1167–1170.

99. Khademi AA, Saatchi M, Minaiyan M, Rostamizadeh N, Sharafi F. Effect of preoperative alprazolam on the success of inferior alveolar nerve block for teeth with irreversible pulpitis. J Endod 2012;38:1337–1339.

100. Stanley W, Drum M, Nusstein J, Reader A, Beck M. Effect of nitrous oxide on the efficacy of the inferior alveolar nerve block in patients with symptomatic irreversible pulpitis. J Endod 2012;38:565–569.

101. Schellenberg J, Drum M, Reader A, Nusstein J, Fowler S, Beck M. Effect of buffered 4% lidocaine on the success of the inferior alveolar nerve block in patients with symptomatic irreversible pulpitis: A prospective, randomized, double-blind study. J Endod 2015;41:791–796.

102. Fullmer S, Drum M, Reader A, Nusstein J, Beck M. Effect of preoperative acetaminophen/hydrocodone on the efficacy of the inferior alveolar nerve block in patients with symptomatic irreversible pulpitis: A prospective, randomized, double-blind, placebo-controlled study. J Endod 2014;40:1–5.

103. Click V, Drum M, Reader A, Nusstein J, Beck M. Evaluation of the Gow-Gates and Vazirani-Akinosi techniques in patients with symptomatic irreversible pulpitis: A prospective randomized study. J Endod 2015;41:16–21.

104. Webster S Jr, Drum M, Reader A, Fowler S, Nusstein J, Beck M. How effective is supplemental intraseptal anesthesia in patients with symptomatic irreversible pulpitis? J Endod 2016;42:1453–1457.

105. Gale EN, Carlsson SG, Ericksson A, Jontell M. Effects of dentists' behavior on patients' attitudes. J Am Dent Assoc 1984;109:444–446.

106. Davidhizar R, Shearer R. Improving your bedside manner. J Pract Nurs 1998;48:10–14.

107. Schouten BC, Eijkman MA, Hoogstraten J. Dentists' and patients' communicative behavior and their satisfaction with the dental encounter. Community Dent Health 2003;20:11–15.

108. Fletcher KE, Furney SL, Stern DT. Patients speak: What's really important about bedside interactions with physician teams. Teach Learn Med 2007;19:120–127.

109. Becker DE, Rosenberg M. Nitrous oxide and the inhalation anesthetics. Anesth Prog 2008;55:124–130.

110. Emmanouil DE, Dickens AS, Heckert RW, et al. Nitrous oxide-antinociception is mediated by opioid receptors and nitric oxide in the periaqueductal gray region of the midbrain. Eur Neuropsychopharmacol 2008;18:194–199.

111. Georgiev SK, Baba H, Kohno T. Nitrous oxide and the inhibitory synaptic transmission in rat dorsal horn neurons. Eur J Pain 2010;14:17–22.

112. Duarte R, McNeill A, Drummond G, Tiplady B. Comparison of the sedative, cognitive, and analgesic effects of nitrous oxide, sevoflurane, and ethanol. Br J Anaesth 2008;100:203–210.

113. Furuya A, Ito M, Fukao T, et al. The effective time and concentration of nitrous oxide to reduce venipuncture pain in children. J Clin Anesth 2009;21:190–193.

114. Burnweit C, Diana-Zerpa JA, Nahmad MH, et al. Nitrous oxide analgesia for minor pediatric surgical procedures: An effective alternative to conscious sedation? J Pediatr Surg 2004;39:495–499.

115. Jacobs S, Haas DA, Meechan JG, May S. Injection pain: Comparison of three mandibular block techniques and modulation by nitrous oxide:oxygen. J Am Dent Assoc 2003;134:869–876.

116. Takkar D, Rao A, Shenoy R, Rao A, Saranya BS. Evaluation of nitrous oxide inhalation sedation during inferior alveolar block administration in children aged 7-10 years: A randomized control trial. J Indian Soc Pedod Prev Dent 2015;33:239–244.

117. Kiecolt-Glaser JK, Graham JE, Malarkey WB, Porter K, Lemeshow S, Galser R. Olfactory influences on mood and autonomic, endocrine, and immune function. Psychoneuroendocrinology 2008;33:328–339.

118. Aelig W, Laurence D, O'Neil R, Verrill P. Cardiac effects of adrenaline and felypressin as vasoconstrictors in local anaesthesia for oral surgery under diazepam sedation. Br J Anaesth 1970;42:174–176.

119. Hasse A, Heng M, Garrett N. Blood pressure and electrocardiographic response to dental treatment with use of local anesthesia. J Am Dent Assoc 1986;113:639–642.

120. Knöll-Kohler E, Frie A, Becker J, Ohlendorf D. Changes in plasma epinephrine concentrations after dental infiltration anesthesia with different doses of epinephrine. J Dent Res 1989;68:1098–1101.

121. Salonen M, Forsell H, Sceinin M. Local dental anesthesia with lidocaine and adrenalin: Effects on plasma catecholamines, heart rate, and blood pressure. Int J Oral Maxillofac Surg 1988;17:392–394.

122. Troullos E, Goldstein DS, Hargreaves K, Dionne R. Plasma epinephrine levels and cardiovascular responses to high administered doses of epinephrine contained in local anesthesia. Anesth Prog 1987;34:10–13.

123. Moore PA, Boynes SG, Hersh EV, et al. The anesthetic efficacy of 4% articaine 1:200,000 epinephrine: Two clinical trials. J Am Dent Assoc 2006;137:1572–1581.

124. Hersh EV, Giannakopoulos H, Levin LM, et al. The pharmacokinetics and cardiovascular effects of high-dose articaine with 1:100,000 and 1:200,000 epinephrine. J Am Dent Assoc 2006;137:1562–1571.

125. Wood M, Reader A, Nusstein J, Beck M, Padgett D, Weaver J. Comparison of intraosseous and infiltration injections for venous lidocaine blood concentrations and heart rate changes after injection of 2% lidocaine with 1:100,000 epinephrine. J Endod 2005;31:435–438.

126. Meechan J, Rawlins M. The effects of two different dental local anesthetic solutions on plasma potassium levels during third molar surgery. Oral Surg Oral Med Oral Pathol 1988;66:650–653.

127. Tolas A, Pflug A, Halter J. Arterial plasma epinephrine concentrations and hemodynamic responses after dental injection of local anesthetic with epinephrine. J Am Dent Assoc 1982;104:41–43.

128. Vanderheyden P, Williams R, Sims T. Assessment of ST segment depression in patients with cardiac disease after local anesthesia. J Am Dent Assoc 1989;119:407–412.

129. Replogle K, Reader A, Nist R, Beck M, Weaver J, Meyers WJ. Cardiovascular effects of intraosseous injections of 2 percent lidocaine with 1:100,000 epinephrine and 3 percent mepivacaine. J Am Dent Assoc 1999;130:649–657.

130. Chamberlain T, Davis R, Murchison D, Hansen S, Richardson B. Systemic effects of an intraosseous injection of 2% lidocaine with 1:100,000 epinephrine. Gen Dent 2000;48:299–302.

131. Nusstein J, Berlin J, Reader A, Beck M, Weaver J. Comparison of injection pain, heart rate increase and post-injection pain of articaine and lidocaine in a primary intraligamentary injection administered with a computer-controlled local anesthetic delivery system. Anesth Prog 2004;51:126–133.

132. Niwa H, Sugimura M, Satoh Y, Tanimoto A. Cardiovascular response to epinephrine-containing local anesthesia in patients with cardiovascular disease. Oral Surg Oral Med Oral Pathol Oral Radiol Endod 2001;92:610–616.

133. Elad S, Admon D, Kedmi M, et al. The cardiovascular effect of local anesthesia with articaine plus 1:200,000 adrenalin versus lidocaine plus 1:100,000 adrenalin in medically compromised cardiac patients: A prospective, randomized, double blind study. Oral Surg Oral Med Oral Pathol Oral Radiol Endod 2008;105:725–730.

134. Niwa H, Sato Y, Matsuura H. Safety of dental treatment in patients with previously diagnosed acute myocardial infarction or unstable angina pectoris. Oral Surg Oral Med Oral Pathol Oral Radiol Endod 2000;89:35–41.

135. Isselbacher KJ, Braunwald E, Wilson JD, Martin JB, Fauci AS, Kasper DL (eds). Harrison's Principles of Internal Medicine, ed 13. New York: McGraw-Hill, 1994.

136. Kohase H, Umino M. Allergic reaction to epinephrine preparation in 2% lidocaine: Two case reports. Anesth Prog 2004;51:134–137.

137. Chin KL, Yagiela JA, Quinn CL, Henderson KR, Duperon DF. Serum mepivacaine concentrations after intraoral injection in young children. J Calif Dent Assoc 2003;31:757–764.

138. Becker DE. Preoperative medical evaluation. Part 1: General principles and cardiovascular considerations. Anesth Prog 2009;56:92–103.

139. Yagiela JA, Duffin SR, Hunt LM. Drug interactions and vasoconstrictors used in local anesthetic solutions. Oral Surg Oral Med Oral Pathol 1985;59:565–571.

140. Friedlander AH, Mahler M, Norman KM, Ettinger RL. Parkinson disease. Systemic and orofacial manifestations, medical and dental management. J Am Dent Assoc 2009;140:658–669.

141. Saraghi M, Hersh EV. Potential diversion of local anesthetics from dental offices for use as cocaine adulterants. J Am Dent Assoc 2014;145:256–259.

142. Taddio A, Ilersich AF, Ilersich AN, Wells J. From the mouth of babes: Getting vaccinated doesn't have to hurt. Can J Infect Dis Med Microbiol 2014;25:196–200.

143. Taddio A, Lord A, Hogan ME, et al. A randomized controlled trial of analgesia during vaccination in adults. Vaccine 2010;28:5365–5369.

144. Versloot J, Veerkamp JS, Hoogstraten J. Assessment of pain by the child, dentist, and independent observers. Pediatr Dent 2004;26:445–449.

145. Perry S, Drum M, Reader A, Nusstein J, Beck M. Effect of operator and subject gender on injection pain: A randomized double-blind study. J Endod 2015;41:141–145.

146. Nusstein JM, Beck M. Effectiveness of 20% benzocaine as a topical anesthetic for intraoral injections. Anesth Prog 2003;50:159–163.

147. Nusstein J, Steinkruger G, Reader A, Beck M, Weaver J. The effects of a 2-stage injection technique on inferior alveolar nerve block injection pain. Anesth Prog 2006;53:126–130.

148. Willett J, Reader A, Drum M, Nusstein J, Beck M. The anesthetic efficacy of diphenhydramine and the combination diphenhydramine/lidocaine for the inferior alveolar nerve block. J Endod 2008;34:1446–1450.

149. Kaufman E, Epstein JB, Naveh E, Gorsky M, Cohen G. A survey of pain, pressure, and discomfort induced by commonly used oral local anesthesia injections. Anesth Prog 2005;52:122–127.

150. Aminabadi NA, Farahani RMZ, Oskouei SG. Site-specificity of pain sensitivity to intraoral anesthetic injections in children. J Oral Sci 2009;51:239–243.

151. Wahl MJ, Schmitt MM, Overton DA, Gordon MK. Injection pain of bupivacaine with epinephrine vs. prilocaine plain. J Am Dent Assoc 2002;133:1652–1656.

152. Meechan JG, Howlett PC, Smith BD. Factors influencing the discomfort of intraoral needle penetration. Anesth Prog 2005;52:91–94.

153. Scott J, Drum M, Reader A, Nusstein J, Beck M. The efficacy of a repeated infiltration in prolonging duration of pulpal anesthesia in maxillary lateral incisors. J Am Dent Assoc 2009;140:318–324.

154. Mikesell A, Drum M, Reader A, Beck M. Anesthetic efficacy of 1.8 mL and 3.6 mL of 2% lidocaine with 1:100,000 epinephrine for maxillary infiltrations. J Endod 2008;34:121–125.

155. Fuller NP, Menke RA, Meyers WJ. Perception of pain to three different intraoral penetrations of needles. J Am Dent Assoc 1979;99:822–824.

156. Flanagan T, Wahl MJ, Schmitt MM, Wahl JA. Size doesn't matter: Needle gauge and injection pain. Gen Dent 2007;55:216–217.

157. McPherson JS, Dixon SA, Townsend R, Vandewalle KS. Effect of needle design on pain from dental local anesthetic injections. Anesth Prog 2015;62:2–7.

158. Kramp LF, Eleazer PD, Scheetz JP. Evaluation of prilocaine for the reduction of pain associated with transmucosal anesthetic administration. Anesth Prog 1999;46:52–55.

159. Meechan JG, Day PF. A comparison of intraoral injection discomfort produced by plain and epinephrine-containing lidocaine local anesthetic solutions: A randomized, double-blind, split-mouth, volunteer investigation. Anesth Prog 2002;49:44–48.

160. Wahl MJ, Overton D, Howell J, Siegel E, Schmitt MM, Muldoon M. Pain on injection of prilocaine plain vs. lidocaine with epinephrine. A prospective double-blind study. J Am Dent Assoc 2001;132;1396–1401.

161. Wahl MJ, Schmitt MM, Overton DA. Injection pain of prilocaine plain, mepivacaine plain, articaine with epinephrine, and lidocaine with epinephrine. Gen Dent 2006;54:168–171.

162. Lammers E, Nusstein J, Reader A, Drum M, Beck M, Fowler S. Does the combination of 3% mepivacaine plain plus 2% lidocaine with epinephrine improve anesthesia and reduce the pain of anesthetic injection for the inferior alveolar nerve block? A prospective, randomized, double-blind study. J Endod 2014;40:1287–1292.

163. Evans G, Nusstein J, Drum M, Reader A, Beck M. A prospective, randomized double-blind comparison of articaine and lidocaine for maxillary infiltrations. J Endod 2008;34:389–393.

164. Haase A, Reader A, Nusstein J, Beck M, Drum M. Comparing anesthetic efficacy of articaine versus lidocaine as a supplemental buccal infiltration of the mandibular first molar after an inferior alveolar nerve block. J Am Dent Assoc 2008;139:1228–1235.

165. Sumer M, Misir F, Çelebi N, Mug˘lali M. A comparison of injection pain with articaine with adrenaline, prilocaine with phenylpressin and lidocaine with adrenaline. Med Oral Patol Oral Cir Buccal 2008;13:E427–430.

166. Hochman MN, Friedman MJ, Williams W, Hochman CB. Interstitial tissue pressure associated with dental injections: A clinical study. Quintessence Int 2006;37:469–476.

167. Kudo M. Initial injection pressure for dental local anesthesia: Effects on pain and anxiety. Anesth Prog 2005;52:95–101.

168. Kanaa M, Meechan J, Corbett I, Whitworth J. Speed of injection influences efficacy of inferior alveolar nerve blocks: A double-blind randomized controlled trial in volunteers. J Endod 2006;32:919–923.

169. Hochman M, Chiarello D, Bozzi-Hochman C, Lopatkin R, Pergola S. Computerized local anesthetic delivery vs. traditional syringe technique. N Y State Dent J 1997;63:24–29.

170. Levato C. Giving the Wand a shot. Dent Pract Finance 1998;4:53–57.

171. Gibson RS, Allen K, Hutfless S, Beiraghi S. The Wand vs traditional injection: A comparison of pain related behaviors. Pediatr Dent 2000;22:458–462.

172. Nicholson JW, Berry TG, Summitt JB, Yuan CH, Witten TM. Pain perception and utility: A comparison of the syringe and computerized local injection techniques. Gen Dent 2001;49:167–173.

173. Tan PY, Vukasin P, Chin ID, et al. The Wand local anesthetic delivery system. A more pleasant experience for anal anesthesia. Dis Colon Rectum 2001;44:686–689.

174. Rosenberg ES. A computer-controlled anesthetic delivery system in a periodontal practice: Patient satisfaction and acceptance. J Esthet Restor Dent 2002;14:39–46.

175. Primosch RE, Brooks R. Influence of anesthetic flow rate delivered by the Wand local anesthetic system on pain response to palatal injections. Am J Dent 2002;15:15–20.

176. True RH, Elliott R. Microprocessor-controlled local anesthesia versus the conventional syringe technique in hair transplantation. Dermatol Surg 2002;28:463–468.

177. Allen KD, Kotil D, Larzelere RE, Hutfless S, Beiraghi S. Comparison of a computerized anesthesia device with a traditional syringe in preschool children. Pediatr Dent 2002;24:315–320.

178. Ram D, Peretz B. The assessment of pain sensation during local anesthesia using a computerized local anesthesia (Wand) and a conventional syringe. J Dent Child 2003;70:130–133.

179. Nusstein J, Lee S, Reader A, Beck M, Weaver J. Injection pain and postinjection pain of the anterior middle superior alveolar injection administered with the Wand or conventional syringe. Oral Surg Oral Med Oral Pathol Oral Radiol Endod 2004;98:124–131.

180. Palm AM, Kirkegaard U, Poulsen S. The wand versus traditional injection for mandibular nerve block in children and adolescents: Perceived pain and time of onset. Pediatr Dent 2004;26;481–484.

181. Loomer PM, Perry DA. Computer-controlled delivery versus syringe delivery of local anesthetic injections for therapeutic scaling and root planing. J Am Dent Assoc 2004;135:358–365.

182. Versloot J, Veerkamp JS, Hoogstraten J. Computerized anesthesia delivery system vs. traditional syringe: Comparing pain and pain-related behavior in children. Eur J Oral Sci 2005;113:488–493.

183. Oztas N, Ulusu T, Bodur H, Dougan C. The wand in pulp therapy: An alternative to inferior alveolar nerve block. Quintessence Int 2005;36:559–564.

184. Sumer M, Misir F, Koyuturk AE. Comparison of the Wand with a conventional technique. Oral Surg Oral Med Oral Pathol Oral Radiol Endod 2006;101:106–109.

185. Ashkenazi M, Blumer S, Eli I. Effectiveness of various modes of computerized delivery of local anesthesia in primary maxillary molars. Pediatr Dent 2006;28:29–38.

186. Lee EW, Tucker NA. Pain associated with local anesthetic injection in eyelid procedures: Comparison of microprocessor-controlled versus traditional syringe techniques. Ophthal Plast Reconstr Surg 2007;23:37–38.

187. Yesilyurt C, Bulut G, Taşdemir T. Summary of: Pain perception during inferior alveolar injection administered with the Wand or conventional syringe. Br Dent J 2008;205:258–259.

188. Ram D, Kassirer J. Assessment of a palatal approach-anterior superior alveolar (P-ASA) nerve block with the Wand in paediatric dental patients. Int J Paediatr Dent 2006;16:348–351.

189. Yenisey M. Comparison of the pain levels of computer-controlled and conventional anesthesia techniques in prosthodontics treatment. J Appl Oral Sci 2009;17:414–420.

190. Asarch T, Allen K, Petersen B, Beiraghi S. Efficacy of a computerized local anesthesia device in pediatric dentistry. Pediatr Dent 1999;21:421–424.

191. Saloum FS, Baumgartner JC, Marshall G, Tinkle J. A clinical comparison of pain perception to the Wand and a traditional syringe. Oral Surg Oral Med Oral Pathol Oral Radiol Endod 2000;86:691–695.

192. Tahmassebi JF, Nikolaou M, Duggal MS. A comparison of pain and anxiety associated with the administration of maxillary local analgesia with Wand and conventional technique. Eur Arch Paediatr Dent 2009;10:77–82.

193. Versloot J, Veerkamp JS, Hoogstraten J. Pain behavior and distress in children during two sequential dental visits: Comparing a computerized anaesthesia delivery system and a traditional syringe. Br Dent J 2008;205:30–31.

194. Goodell GG, Gallagher FJ, Nicoll BK. Comparison of a controlled injection pressure system with a conventional technique. Oral Surg Oral Med Oral Pathol Oral Radiol Endod 2000;90:88–94.

195. Sandeep V, Kumar M, Jyostna P, Duggi V. Evaluation of 2-stage injection technique in children. Anesth Prog 2016;63:3–7.

196. Pogrel MA, Thamby S. Permanent nerve involvement resulting from inferior alveolar nerve block. J Am Dent Assoc 2000;131:901–907.

197. Pogrel MA, Thamby S. The etiology of altered sensation in the inferior alveolar, lingual and mental nerves as a result of dental treatment. J Calif Dent Assoc 1999;27:531, 534–538.

198. Krafft TC, Hickel R. Clinical investigation into the incidence of direct damage to the lingual nerve caused by local anaesthesia. J Craniomaxillofac Surg 1994;22:294–296.

199. Rout PG, Saksena A, Fisher SE. An investigation of the effect on 27-gauge needle tips following single local anaesthetic injection. Dent Update 2003;30:370–374.

200. Stacy GC, Hajjar G. Barbed needle and inexplicable paresthesia and trismus after regional anesthesia. Oral Surg Oral Med Oral Pathol 1994;78:680–681.

201. Pogrel MA. Broken local anesthetic needles. A case series of 16 patients, with recommendations. J Am Dent Assoc 2009;140:1517–1522.

202. Milgrom P, Coldwell SE, Getz T, Weinstein P, Ramsey D. Four dimensions of fear of dental injections. J Am Dent Assoc 1997;128:756–762.

203. Kleinknect R, Klepac R, Alexander L. Origins and characteristics of fear of dentistry. J Am Dent Assoc 1993;86:842–848.

204. Milgrom P, Fiset L, Melnick S, Weinstein P. The prevalence and practice management consequences of dental fear in a major US city. J Am Dent Assoc 1988;116:641–647.

205. Rosivack R, Koenigsberg S, Maxwell K. An analysis of the effectiveness of two topical anesthetics. Anesth Prog 1990;37:290–292.

206. Hersh E, Houpt M, Cooper S, Feldman R, Wolff M, Levin L. Analgesic efficacy and safety of an intraoral lidocaine patch. J Am Dent Assoc 1996;127:1626–1634.

207. Hutchins H, Young F, Lackland D, Fishburne C. The effectiveness of topical anesthesia and vibration in alleviating the pain of oral injections. Anesth Prog 1997;44:87–89.

208. Gill C, Orr D. A double-blind crossover comparison of topical anesthetics. J Am Dent Assoc 1979;98:213–214.

209. Keller B. Comparison of the effectiveness of two topical anesthetics and a placebo in reducing injection pain. Hawaii Dent J 1985;16:10–11.

210. Martin M, Ramsay D, Whitney C, Fiset L, Weinstein P. Topical anesthesia: Differentiating the pharmacological and psychological contributions to efficacy. Anesth Prog 1994;41:40–47.

211. Johnson J, Primosch RE. Influence of site preparation methods on the pain reported during palatal infiltration using the Wand Local Anesthetic System. Am J Dent 2003;16:165–169.

212. Vongsavan K, Vongsavan N. Comparison of topical anesthetic gel and TENS in reducing pain [abstract]. J Dent Res 1996;75:248.

213. Meechan JG, Gowans A, Welbury R. The use of patient controlled transcutaneous electronic nerve stimulation (TENS) to decrease the discomfort of regional anesthesia in dentistry: A randomized controlled clinical trial. J Dent 1998;26:417–420.

214. Nakanishi O, Haas D, Ishikawa T, Kameyama S. Nishi M. Efficacy of mandibular topical anesthesia varies with the site of administration. Anesth Prog 1996;43:14–19.

215. Holst A, Evers H. Experimental studies of new topical anesthetics on the oral mucosa. Swed Dent J 1985;9:185–191.

216. Vickers ER, Punnia-Moorthy A. A clinical evaluation of three topical anesthetic agents. Aust Dent J 1992;37:266–270.

217. Carrel R, Friedman L, Binns W. Laboratory and clinical evaluation of a new topical anesthetic. Anesth Prog 1974;21:126–131.

218. Carr MP, Horton J. Clinical evaluation and comparison of 2 topical anesthetics for pain caused by needle sticks and scaling and root planing. J Periodontol 2001;72:479–484.

219. Carr MP, Horton J. Evaluation of a transoral delivery system for topical anesthesia. J Am Dent Assoc 2001;132:1714–1719.

220. Svensson P, Peterson J. Anesthetic effect of EMLA occluded with Orahesive oral bandages on oral mucosa. A placebo-controlled study. Anesth Prog 1992;39:79–82.

221. Meechan JG, Thomason J. A comparison of 2 topical anesthetics on the discomfort of intraligamentary injections. Oral Surg Oral Med Oral Pathol Oral Radiol Endod 1999;87:362–365.

222. de Freiras GC, Pozzobon RT, Blaya DS, Moreira CH. Efficacy of benzocaine 20% topical anesthetic compared to placebo prior to administration of local anesthesia in the oral cavity: A randomized controlled trial. Anesth Prog 2015;62(2):46–50.

223. Ghaderi F, Banakar S, Rostami S. Effect of pre-cooling injection site on pain perception in pediatric dentistry: "A randomized clinical trial." Dent Res (Isfahan) 2013;10:790–794.

224. Franz-Montan M, Silva ALR, Cogo K, et al. Liposome-encapsulated ropivacaine for topical anesthesia of human oral mucosa. Anesth Anal 2007;104:1528–1531.

225. Al-Melh MA, Andersson L. Comparison of topical anesthetics (EMLA/Oraquix vs. benzocaine) on pain experienced during palatal needle insertion. Oral Surg Oral Med Oral Pathol Oral Radiol Endod 2007;103(5):e16–20.

226. Al-Melh MA, Andersson L, Behbehani E. Reduction of pain from needle stick in the oral mucosa by topical anesthetics: A comparative study between lidocaine/prilocaine and benzocaine. J Clin Dent 2005;16:53–56.

227. Al-Melh MA, Andersson L. Reducing pain from palatal needle stick by topical anesthetics: A comparative study between two lidocaine/prilocaine substances. J Clin Dent 2008;19:43–47.

228. Kravitz ND. The use of compound topical anesthetics: A review. J Am Dent Assoc 2007;138:1333–1339.

229. Macdonnel WA. Compounded topical anesthetics more common place in dental offices? Am Dent Soc Anesth Pulse 2008;41(5):4–5.

230. Bhalia J, Meechan JG, Lawrence HP, Grad HA, Haas DA. Effect of time on clinical efficacy of topical anesthesia. Anesth Prog 2009;56:36–41.

231. Jälevik B, Klingberg G. Pain sensation and injection techniques in maxillary dento-alveolar surgery procedures in children—A comparison between conventional and computerized injection techniques (The Wand). Swed Dent J 2014;38:67–75.

232. Sattayut S. Low intensity laser for reducing pain from anesthetic palatal injection. Photomed Laser Surg 2014;32:658–662.

233. Martin S, Jones JS, Wynn BN. Does warming local anesthetic reduce the pain of subcutaneous injection? Am J Emerg Med 1996;14:10–12.

234. Colaric KB, Overton DT, Moore K. Pain reduction in lidocaine administration through buffering and warming. Am J Emerg Med 1998;16:353–356.

235. Sultan J. Towards evidence based emergency medicine: Best BETs from Manchester Royal Infirmary. Effect of warming local anaesthetics on pain of infiltration. Emerg Med J 2007;24:723–725.

236. Fialkov JA, McDougall EP. Warmed local anesthetic reduces pain of infiltration. Ann Plast Surg 1996;36:11–13.

237. Bell RW, Butt ZA, Gardner RF. Warming lignocaine reduces the pain of injection during local anaesthetic eyelid surgery. Eye (London) 1996;10:558–560.

238. Sultan J. Towards evidence based emergency medicine: Best BETs from Manchester Royal Infirmary. The effect of warming local anaesthetics on pain of infiltration. Emerg Med J 2007;24:791–793.

239. Oikarinen VJ, Ylipaavalniemi P, Evers H. Pain and temperature sensations related to local analgesia. Int J Oral Surg 1975;4:151–156.

240. Volk RJ, Gargiulo AV. Local anesthetic cartridge warmer—First in, first out fresh. Ill Dent J 1984;53:92–94.

241. Hijazi R, Taylor D, Richardson J. Effect of topical alkane vapocoolant spray on pain with intravenous cannulation in patients in emergency departments: Randomised double blind placebo controlled trial. BMJ 2009;338:b215.

242. Robinson PA, Carr S, Pearson S, Frampton C. Lignocaine is a better analgesic than either ethyl chloride or nitrous oxide for peripheral intravenous cannulation. Emerg Med Australas 2007;19:427–432.

243. Hartstein BH, Barry JD. Mitigation of pain during intravenous catheter placement using a topical skin coolant in the emergency department. Emerg Med J 2008;25:257–261.

244. Aminabadi NA, Farahani RM. The effect of pre-cooling the injection site on pediatric pain perception during the administration of local anesthesia. J Contemp Dent Pract 2009;10:43–50.

245. Harbert H. Topical ice: A precursor to palatal injections. J Endod 1989;15:27–28.

246. Kosaraju A, Vandewalle KS. A comparison of a refrigerant and a topical anesthetic gel as preinjection anesthetics: A clinical evaluation. J Am Dent Assoc 2009;140:68–72.

247. Wiswall AT, Bowles WR, Lunos S, McClanahan SB, Harris S. Palatal anesthesia: Comparison of four techniques for decreasing injection discomfort. Northwest Dent 2014;93(4):25–29.

248. Davies RJ. Buffering the pain of local anaesthetics: A systematic review. Emerg Med (Fremantle) 2003;15:81–88.

249. Hanna MN, Elhassan A, Veloso PM, et al. Efficacy of bicarbonate in decreasing pain on intradermal injection of local anesthetics: A meta analysis. Reg Anesth Pain Med 2009;34:122–125.

250. Welch MN, Czyz CN, Kalwerisky K, Holck DE, Mihora LD. Double-blind, bilateral pain comparison with simultaneous injection of 2% lidocaine versus buffered 2% lidocaine for periocular anesthesia. Ophthalmology 2012;119:2048–2052.

251. Al-Sultan AF. Effectiveness of pH adjusted lidocaine versus commercial lidocaine for maxillary infiltration anesthesia. Al-Rafidain Dent J 2004;4:34–39.

252. Al-Sultan AF, Fathie WK, Hamid RS. A clinical evaluation on the alkalization of local anesthetic solution in periapical surgery. Al-Rafidain Dent J 2006;6:71–77.

253. Kashyap VM, Desai R, Reddy PB, Menon S. Effect of alkalinisation of lignocaine for intraoral nerve block on pain during injection, and speed of onset of anaesthesia. Br J Oral Maxillofac Surg 2011;49(8):e72–e75.

254. Malamed SF, Tavana S, Falkel M. Faster onset and more comfortable injection with alkalinized 2% lidocaine with epinephrine 1:100,000. Compend Contin Educ Dent 2013;34:10–20.

255. Bowles WH, Frysh H, Emmons R. Clinical evaluation of buffered local anesthetic. Gen Dent 1995;43:182–184.

256. Primosch RE, Robinson L. Pain elicited during intraoral infiltration with buffered lidocaine. Am J Dent 1996;9:5–10.

257. Whitcomb M, Drum M, Reader A, Nusstein J, Beck M. A prospective, randomized double-blind study of the anesthetic efficacy of sodium bicarbonate buffered 2% lidocaine with 1:100,000 epinephrine in inferior alveolar nerve blocks. Anesth Prog 2010;57:59–66.

258. Balasco M, Drum M, Reader A, Nusstein J, Beck M. Buffered lidocaine for incision and drainage: A prospective, randomized double-blind study. J Endod 2013;39:1329–1334.

259. Harreld TK, Fowler S, Drum M, Reader A, Nusstein J, Beck M. Efficacy of a buffered 4% lidocaine formulation for incision and drainage: A prospective, randomized, double-blind study. J Endod 2015;41:1583–1588.

260. Saatchi M, Khademi A, Baghaei B, Noormohammadi H. Effect of sodium bicarbonate-buffered lidocaine on the success of inferior alveolar nerve block for teeth with symptomatic irreversible pulpitis: A prospective, randomized double-blind study. J Endod 2015;41:33–35.

261. Hobeich P, Simon S, Schneiderman E, He J. A prospective, randomized, double-blind comparison of the injection pain and anesthetic onset of 2% lidocaine with 1:100,000 epinephrine buffered with 5% and 10% sodium bicarbonate in maxillary infiltrations. J Endod 2013;39:597–599.

262. Shurtz R, Nusstein J, Reader A, Drum M, Fowler S, Beck M. Buffered 4% articaine as a primary buccal infiltration of the mandibular first molar: A prospective, randomized, double-blind study. J Endod 2015;41:1403–1407.

263. Comerci AW, Maller SC, Townsend RD, Teepe JD, Vandewalle KS. Effect of a new local anesthetic buffering device on pain reduction during nerve block injections. Gen Dent 2015;63(6):74–78.

264. Wennberg E, Haljamäe H, Edwall G, Dhuner KG. Effects of commercial (pH approximately 3.5) and freshly prepared (pH approximately 6.5) lidocaine-adrenaline solutions on tissue pH. Acta Anaesthesiol Scand 1982;26:524–527.

265. Punnia-Moorthy A. Buffering capacity of normal and inflamed tissues following the injection of local anaesthetic solutions. Br J Anaesth 1988;61:154–159.

266. Packer JL, Krall B, Makki A, Torabinejad M. The effect of sonophoresis on topical anesthesia: A pilot project. Anesth Prog 2013;60:37–41.

267. Zsigmond EK, Darby P, Koenig HM, Goll EF. Painless intravenous catheterization by intradermal jet injection of lidocaine: A randomized trial. J Clin Anesth 1999;11:87–94.

268. Cooper JA, Bromley LM, Baranowski AP, Barker SG. Evaluation of a needle-free injection system for local anaesthesia prior to venous cannulation. Anaesthesia 2000;55:247–250.

269. Jimenez N, Bradford H, Seidel KD, Sousa M, Lynn AM. A comparison of a needle-free injection system for local anesthesia versus EMLA for intravenous catheter insertion in the pediatric patient. Anesth Analg 2006;102:411–414.

270. Lysakowski C, Dumont L, Tramèr MR, Tassonyi E. A needle-free jet-injection system with lidocaine for peripheral intravenous cannula insertion: A randomized controlled trial with cost-effectiveness analysis. Anesth Analg 2003;96:215–219.

271. Weiss RS. Re: No-needle jet anesthetic technique for no-scalpel vasectomy. J Urol 2006;176:842–843.

272. Geenen L, Marks LA, Martens LC. Clinical evaluation of the INJEX system, a local anesthesia system without needles: A comfort evaluation study [in French]. Rev Belge Med Dent 2004;59:149–155.

273. Dabarakis NN, Alexander V, Tsirlis AT, Parissis NA, Nikolaos M. Needle-less local anesthesia: Clinical evaluation of the effectiveness of the jet anesthesia Injex in local anesthesia in dentistry. Quintessence Int 2007;38:E572–576.

274. Arapostathis KN, Dabarakis NN, Coolidge T, Tsirlis A, Kotsanos N. Comparison of acceptance, preference, and efficacy between jet injection INJEX and local infiltration anesthesia in 6 to 11 year old dental patients. Anesth Prog 2010;57:3–12.

275. Aminabadi NA, Farahani RMZ, Gajan EB. The efficacy of distraction and counterstimulation in the reduction of pain reaction to intraoral injection by pediatric patients. J Contemp Dent Pract 2008;9(6):33–40.

276. Nanitsos E, Vartuli R, Forte A, Dennison PJ, Peck CC. The effect of vibration on pain during local anaesthesia injections. Aust Dent J 2009;54:94–100.

277. Furman E, Jasinevicius TR, Bissada NF, Victoroff KZ, Skillicorn R, Buchner M. Virtual reality distraction for pain control during periodontal scaling and root planing procedures. J Am Dent Assoc 2009;140:1508–1516.

278. Dahlquist LM, Weiss KE, Law EF, et al. Effects of videogame distraction and a virtual reality type head-mounted display helmet on cold pressor pain in young elementary school-aged children. J Pediatr Psychol 2010;35:617–625.

279. Saijo M, Ito E, Ichinohe T, Kaneko Y. Lack of pain reduction by a vibrating local anesthetic attachment: A pilot study. Anesth Prog 2005;52:62–64.

280. Roeber B, Wallace DP, Rothe V, Salama F, Allen KD. Evaluation of the effects of the VibraJect attachment on pain in children receiving local anesthesia. Pediatr Dent 2011;33:46–50.

281. Ching D, Finkelman M, Loo CY. Effect of the DentalVibe injection system on pain during local anesthesia injections in adolescent patients. Pediatr Dent 2014;36:51–55.

282. DiFelice MG, Vandewalle KS, Maller SC, Hancock RH. Effects of a vibratory device on pain from anesthetic injections. Compend Contin Educ Dent 2014;35:246–251.

283. Elbay M, Şermet Elbay Ü, Yıldırım S, Uğurluel C, Kaya C, Baydemir C. Comparison of injection pain caused by the DentalVibe Injection System versus a traditional syringe for inferior alveolar nerve block anaesthesia in paediatric patients. Eur J Paediatr Dent 2015;16:123–128.

284. Wilson S, Molina Lde L, Preisch J, Weaver J. The effect of electronic dental anesthesia on behavior during local anesthetic injection in the young, sedated dental patient. Pediatr Dent 1999;21:12–17.

285. Munshi AK, Hegde AM, Girdhar D. Clinical evaluation of electronic dental anesthesia for various procedures in pediatric dentistry. J Clin Pediatr Dent 2000;24:199–204.

286. Meechan JG, Winter RA. A comparison of topical anaesthesia and electronic nerve stimulation for reducing the pain of intra-oral injections. Br Dent J 1996;181:333–335.

287. Meechan JG, Gowans AJ, Welbury RR. The use of patient-controlled transcutaneous nerve stimulation (TENS) to decrease the discomfort of regional anaesthesia in dentistry: A randomized controlled clinical trial. J Dent 1998;26:417–420.

288. Yap AU, Ho HC. Electronic and local anesthesia: A clinical comparison for operative procedures. Quintessence Int 1996;27:549–553.

289. Modaresi A, Lindsay SJ, Gould A, Smith P. A partial double-blind, placebo-controlled study of electronic dental anaesthesia in children. Int J Paediatr Dent 1996;6:245–251.

290. Schäfer E, Finkensiep H, Kaup M. Effect of transcutaneous electrical nerve stimulation on pain perception threshold of human teeth: A double-blind, placebo-controlled study. Clin Oral Investig 2000;4:81–86.

291. Hadley J, Young DA, Eversole LR, Gornbein JA. A laser-powered hydrokinetic system for caries removal and cavity preparation. J Am Dent Assoc 2000;131:777–785.

292. Liu JF, Lai YL, Shu WY, Lee SY. Acceptance and efficiency of Er:YAG laser for cavity preparation in children. Photomed Laser Surg 2006;24:489–493.

293. Whitters CJ, Hall A, Creanor SL, et al. A clinical study of pulsed Nd:YAG laser-induced pulpal analgesia. J Dent 1995;23:145–150.

294. Poli R, Parker S. Achieving dental analgesia with the erbium chromium yttrium scandium gallium garnet laser (2780 nm): A protocol for painless conservative treatment. Photomed Laser Surg 2015;33:364–371.

295. Giza S. Comparative studies of carious defects filling using the classical method and dental drill, and using the Carisolv chemomechanical method and YAG:Er CTL-1601 laser [in Polish]. Ann Acad Med Stetin 2007;53(3):88–99.

296. Matsumoto K, Hossain M, Hossain MM, Kawano H, Kimura Y. Clinical assessment of Er,Cr:YSGG laser application for cavity preparation. J Clin Laser Med Surg 2002;20:17–21.

297. Matsumoto K, Nakamura Y, Mazeki K, Kimura Y. Clinical dental application of Er:YAG laser for class V cavity preparation. J Clin Laser Med Surg 1996;14:123–127.

298. Allen KL, Salgado TL, Janal MN, Thompson VP. Removing carious dentin using a polymer instrument without anesthesia versus a carbide bur with anesthesia. J Am Dent Assoc 2005;136:643–651.

299. Malmström HS, Chaves Y, Moss ME. Patient preference: Conventional rotary handpieces or air abrasion for cavity preparation. Oper Dent 2003;28:667–671.

# Mandibular Anesthesia

**2**

### After reading this chapter, the practitioner should be able to:

- Describe success, failure, onset, and duration of pulpal anesthesia using 2% lidocaine with 1:100,000 epinephrine for the inferior alveolar nerve block (IANB).
- Discuss alternate anesthetic solutions for the IANB.
- Evaluate alternate mandibular injection locations.
- Describe attempts to increase success of the IANB.
- Explain mechanisms of failure with the IANB.
- Discuss why asymptomatic patients do not achieve pulpal anesthesia with the IANB.
- Describe methods that have increased success of mandibular anesthesia.

Because failure occurs most often with the inferior alveolar nerve block (IANB), we will first concentrate on mandibular anesthesia.[1] Additionally, while anesthesia requirements vary among dental procedures, the following discussion will concentrate on pulpal anesthesia. The technique for administering an IANB can be reviewed in available textbooks.

## Conventional IANB

As a frame of reference, we will review the expected outcomes following administration of a conventional IANB to pain-free patients using 1.8 mL of 2% lidocaine with 1:100,000 epinephrine.

### Anesthetic success

One way to define *anesthetic success* for a nerve block is by the percentage of patients who have no response to an electric pulp tester (EPT) (two consecutive 80 readings) within 15 minutes of injection and continuously sustain the 80 reading for 60 minutes.[2–19] In other words, the objective is to achieve anesthesia within 15 minutes and have anesthesia that lasts 1 hour, which is within range for the length of an appointment (most likely between

| Table 2-1 | | Anesthetic success and failure rates using 1.8 mL of 2% lidocaine with 1:100,000 epinephrine for the IANB | | | |
|---|---|---|---|---|---|
| Tooth | Success rate[a] (%) | References | Failure rate[b] (%) | References |
| Second molar | 65 | 6–8,11–13,15,16 | 17 | 6–9,11,21,22,24,28 |
| First molar | 51 | 2–8,10–18,23 | 23 | 4–9,11,21,22,24–26,28 |
| Second premolar | 58 | 6–8,11–13,15,16 | 19 | 6–9,11,21,22 |
| First premolar | 60 | 2–8,10–18 | 21 | 3,7,9,11,21,24,28 |
| Canine | 52 | 2,23 | 32 | 2,23 |
| Lateral incisor | 34 | 2–5,7,10–14,16–18,23 | 44 | 3–5,7,9,11,21–23,27 |
| Central incisor | 10 | 7,11,12,16,23 | 58 | 7,9,11,21–23,27 |

[a]Percentage of patients who have no response to two consecutive 80 readings with the EPT within 15 minutes and sustain the reading for 60 minutes.
[b]Percentage of patients who never achieve two consecutive 80 readings with the EPT within 60 minutes.

46 and 60 minutes[20]) among general practitioners, and unless otherwise indicated, this will be the standard definition of *success* throughout this chapter.

The objective of profound pulpal anesthesia is important to restorative dentistry but also has relevance for endodontic treatment. Table 2-1 shows the percentage of success rates in various mandibular teeth. It is important to realize that 100% of the subjects in these studies had profound lip numbness.[2–19,21–23] Success occurs most often in the molars and premolars and less often in the incisors.

**IN CONCLUSION,** *anesthetic success varies from 51% in the first molar to 10% in the central incisor even though patients have profound lip numbness.*

## Anesthetic failure

Anesthetic failure is a factor in the total definition of anesthetic success. *Anesthetic failure* has been defined as the percentage of patients who never achieve two consecutive 80 EPT readings at any time during a 60-minute period. These patients have the highest potential for pain during a dental procedure. Table 2-1 also shows the percentage of failure rates in various mandibular teeth.[2–19,21–28] Again, all of these subjects had profound lip numbness. While these patients did not achieve complete pulpal anesthesia, their results are as expected from the population at large.

**IN CONCLUSION,** *anesthetic failure varies from 23% in the first molar to 58% in the central incisor even though patients have profound lip numbness.*

### How do we react to failure?
Failure to obtain pulpal anesthesia will occur in clinical practice (see Table 2-1). It happens to every dentist. If we think every injection must result in 100% pulpal anesthesia, then we carry a significant burden into clinical practice. Instead, when failure occurs, we need to be able to add the supplemental techniques necessary to overcome initial failure.

**IN CONCLUSION,** *failure of pulpal anesthesia occurs for every dentist.*

## Onset of pulpal anesthesia

In most cases, following the conventional IANB, the onset of pulpal anesthesia occurs within 5 to 19 minutes.[2–5,12–14] The onset of pulpal anesthesia is generally slower than the onset of lip numbness, which usually occurs within 4.5 to 6 minutes.[2–5,18] Table 2-2 shows the various onset times for the

| Table 2-2 | Approximate onset of pulpal anesthesia for the IANB | | | |
|---|---|---|---|---|
| Tooth | Time of onset[a] (min) | Reference(s) | Occurrence of slow onset[b] (%) | Reference(s) |
| Second molar | 5.2 | 12,13 | 12 | 6,11 |
| First molar | 9.2 | 2–5,12–14 | 14 | 2–6,11 |
| Second premolar | 9.5 | 12,13 | 19 | 6,11 |
| First premolar | 9.9 | 3–5,12,13 | 20 | 3–5,11 |
| Canine | 13.6 | 2 | 20 | 2 |
| Lateral incisor | 13.8 | 2–5,12–14 | 20 | 2–5,11 |
| Central incisor | 19.2 | 12 | 16 | 11 |

[a]Time of first of two consecutive 80 readings with the EPT.
[b]Percentage of patients who achieve an 80 reading with the EPT after 15 minutes.

teeth after an IANB using 1.8 mL of 2% lidocaine with 1:100,000 epinephrine. Notice that the anterior teeth have a slower onset than the posterior teeth. This is what happens in the majority of patients.

IN CONCLUSION, *onset of pulpal anesthesia varies from approximately 9 minutes in the first molar to 19 minutes in the central incisor.*

## Slow onset

In some patients, onset will be delayed. Slow onset is a factor in the total definition of success. *Slow onset* is defined as the percentage of patients who achieve an 80 EPT reading after 15 minutes. Table 2-2 also shows the percentage of slow onset of anesthesia, which occurs about 12% to 20% of the time in mandibular teeth; approximately 8% of patients have onset after 30 minutes.[2–6,10,29] We have all had patients who are not anesthetized during the restorative appointment but state, "I think my teeth are starting to get numb," as they walk out the door at the completion of the appointment. To determine if pulpal anesthesia has been obtained, simply test the tooth for pulpal anesthesia with a cold refrigerant.

IN CONCLUSION, *about 12% to 20% of patients have slow onset of pulpal anesthesia.*

## Noncontinuous anesthesia

In addition to success and failure, there are other considerations in mandibular anesthesia such as noncontinuous anesthesia, which is a factor in the total definition of anesthetic success. *Noncontinuous anesthesia* means that the patient does not have a continuous duration of anesthesia during the appointment and reports episodes of anesthesia followed by a lack of pulpal anesthesia. This may possibly relate to the action of the anesthetic solution on the nerve membrane (blocking and unblocking of the sodium channels) and occurs about 12% to 20% of the time in mandibular teeth.[2–6,10]

IN CONCLUSION, *patients may go in and out of pulpal anesthesia during an appointment.*

## Duration of pulpal anesthesia

Duration of pulpal anesthesia in the mandible is very good.[2–19,21–29] Therefore, if patients are anesthetized initially, anesthesia with a cartridge of 2% lidocaine with 1:100,000 epinephrine usually persists for approximately 2.5 hours.[13] Table 2-3 shows the duration of pulpal anesthesia for various anesthetic formulations.

| Table 2-3 | Approximate duration of pulpal and soft tissue anesthesia for the IANB | |
|---|---|---|
| Local anesthetic agent (1.8 mL) | Pulpal anesthesia | Soft tissue anesthesia |
| 2% lidocaine with 1:100,000 epinephrine | 2 h 24 min[13] | Over 3 h[13] |
| 2% lidocaine with 1:50,000 epinephrine | At least 60 min[18] | Not studied |
| 2% mepivacaine with 1:20,000 levonordefrin | At least 60 min[3] | Not studied[a] |
| 3% mepivacaine plain | At least 50 min[4] | Over 3 h[b] |
| 4% prilocaine with 1:200,000 epinephrine | At least 60 min[3] | Not studied[a] |
| 4% prilocaine plain | At least 50 min[4] | Over 3 h[b] |
| 0.5% bupivacaine with 1:200,000 epinephrine | 3 to 4 h[13] | Over 8 h[13] |
| 4% articaine with 1:100,000 epinephrine | At least 60 min[11] | Not studied[a] |
| 4% articaine with 1:200,000 epinephrine | Not studied | Not studied |

[a]Time should be similar to 2% lidocaine with 1:100,000 epinephrine.
[b]Data extrapolated from Hersh et al[30] and Fernandez et al[13] data.

## Time course of pulpal anesthesia

The information discussed thus far should be complemented by looking at specific graphs.

As stated by Fiedler's Rule: Always state your results using complex, detailed graphs—this proves you have a sense of humor.

In the following graphs of time course of pulpal anesthesia, the incidence of pulpal anesthesia was defined by the percentage of patients who did not respond to an 80 stimulus (maximum output) with the EPT over time for 60 minutes.

### First and second molars
Figures 2-1 and 2-2 depict the time course for complete pulpal anesthesia of asymptomatic first and second molars. As one can see, the majority of patients achieved pulpal anesthesia within 15 minutes. However, some patients (12% to 20%) had slow onset as indicated by the sloping plateau of anesthesia after 15 minutes. The duration of anesthesia was very good for at least 1 hour, but the success rate was not 100% because of anesthetic failure. The second molar, while similar to the first molar, had a slightly higher incidence of pulpal anesthesia.

### First and second premolars
Figures 2-3 and 2-4 depict the time course for complete pulpal anesthesia of asymptomatic first and second premolars. The time course of pulpal anesthesia is similar to that for the first molar with a slightly higher incidence of pulpal anesthesia.

### Canines and central and lateral incisors
Figures 2-5 to 2-7 depict the time course for complete pulpal anesthesia of asymptomatic canines and central and lateral incisors. The success rate is lower for the canines than the premolars and is the lowest for the lateral and central incisors.

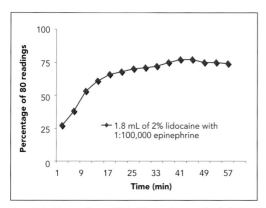

**Fig 2-1** Incidence of mandibular first molar anesthesia following an IANB. Results determined by lack of response to an EPT at maximum reading (80 reading) across 60 minutes.

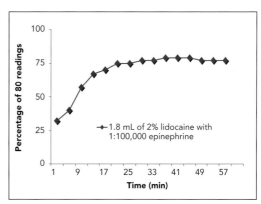

**Fig 2-2** Incidence of mandibular second molar anesthesia following an IANB. Results determined by lack of response to an EPT at maximum reading (80 reading) across 60 minutes.

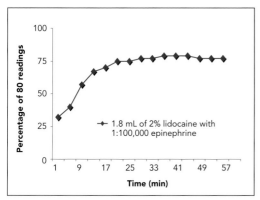

**Fig 2-3** Incidence of mandibular first premolar anesthesia following an IANB. Results determined by lack of response to an EPT at maximum reading (80 reading) across 60 minutes.

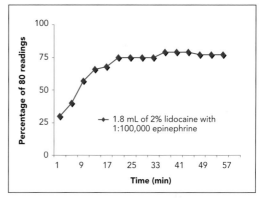

**Fig 2-4** Incidence of mandibular second premolar anesthesia following an IANB. Results determined by lack of response to an EPT at maximum reading (80 reading) across 60 minutes.

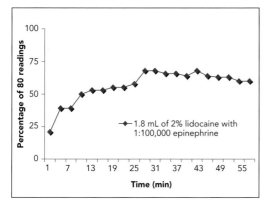

**Fig 2-5** Incidence of mandibular canine anesthesia following an IANB. Results determined by lack of response to an EPT at maximum reading (80 reading) across 60 minutes.

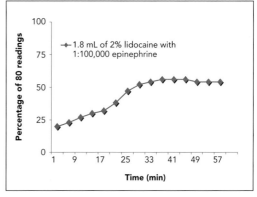

**Fig 2-6** Incidence of mandibular lateral incisor anesthesia following an IANB. Results determined by lack of response to an EPT at maximum reading (80 reading) across 60 minutes.

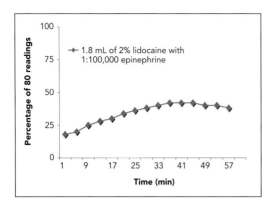

## Soft tissue anesthesia

The presence of soft tissue anesthesia (usually measured by lip numbness or lack of mucosal responsiveness to a sharp explorer) does not adequately indicate pulpal anesthesia.[2–19,21–29] However, the lack of soft tissue anesthesia is a useful indicator that the block injection was not administered accurately for that patient. Missed blocks occur less than 10% of the time with experienced clinicians and should prompt readministration of the nerve block before continuing with treatment.[17] If successful lip numbness is achieved after administering an IANB, do not change technique. That is, be careful in trying to improve the IANB, because there is an old saying: If it isn't broke, fix it until it is and really be in trouble. You, along with the majority of practitioners, are accurately locating the inferior alveolar nerve. However, not all patients achieve pulpal anesthesia. This is completely normal.

**IN CONCLUSION,** *lip numbness or soft tissue sticks do not indicate pulpal anesthesia, and not all patients achieve pulpal anesthesia after achieving lip numbness.*

### Missed blocks

A *missed block* is defined as not obtaining profound lip numbness within 15 to 20 minutes after an IANB.[31] No pulpal anesthesia will be present with a missed block. A missed IANB is mostly likely due to placing the anesthetic solution outside the pterygomandibular space. The missed block differs from a failed IANB, where lip numbness is achieved but not pulpal anesthesia. Malamed[32] discusses the factors for failure as technical errors (needle insertion below the mandibular foramen, needle insertion too far anteriorly, needle insertion too far posteriorly) and anatomical variation. The occurrence of missed IANBs occurs often with inexperienced operators (for example, dental students). However, Krediet and coauthors[33] found that even experts missed intraneural injections for regional anesthesia.

We have all been in the position where we have missed three blocks in a row and have other patients waiting to be treated. We have no rationale for this but have observed it clinically. Add another cartridge of 2% lidocaine with 1:100,000 epinephrine to decrease the incidence of missed block.

In a study of 2,450 asymptomatic subjects, Fowler and coauthors[31] found that missed blocks occurred 6% of the time with a one-cartridge volume of lidocaine with epinephrine and 4% of the time with a two-cartridge volume. Using a two-cartridge volume significantly decreases the incidence of missed IANBs. A missed IANB should prompt readministration of the nerve block because pulpal anesthesia will not be obtained without lip numbness.

**IN CONCLUSION**, *missed blocks occur in asymptomatic patients from 4% (two-cartridge volume) to 6% (one-cartridge volume) of the time. Using a two-cartridge volume significantly decreases the incidence of missed IANBs.*

## Onset of lip anesthesia

Onset of lip anesthesia using 1.8 mL of 2% lidocaine with 1:100,000 epinephrine for the IANB will range from 4.5 to 6 minutes.[2–5,18] However, the onset of lip numbness may not indicate the onset of pulpal anesthesia.

**IN CONCLUSION**, *onset of lip numbness is usually within 4.5 to 6 minutes.*

## Duration of lip numbness

Table 2-3 shows the approximate duration of lip numbness for various local anesthetic formulations. Dentists commonly believe that plain 3% mepivacaine and 4% prilocaine formulations provide a shorter duration of lip numbness than 2% lidocaine with 1:100,000 epinephrine for IANBs.[30] However, Hersh and coauthors[30] found no reduction in the length of lip numbness for the three anesthetic formulations. Therefore, there is no advantage to using a plain solution to decrease lip numbness duration for an IANB.

**IN CONCLUSION**, *duration of lip numbness does not seem to be different for plain solutions versus 2% lidocaine with 1:100,000 epinephrine.*

## Buccal nerve anesthesia with an IANB

The contribution of buccal anesthesia from the IANB would not normally be expected without a separate long buccal injection.[2] However, Vreeland and colleagues[2] showed that buccal soft tissue anesthesia could be obtained 30% to 63% of the time with only an IANB using 1.8 to 3.6 mL of lidocaine with epinephrine. Goldberg and coauthors[14] found an 81% incidence of buccal nerve anesthesia when using 3.6 mL of 2% lidocaine with 1:100,000 epinephrine for an IANB. Regardless of the incidence reported in these studies, buccal nerve anesthesia was not 100%.

**IN CONCLUSION**, *a separate long buccal injection should be given when soft tissue anesthesia is required in the molars.*

# Positive aspirations

Aspiration before administration of local anesthetics reduces the incidence of adverse reactions. Various authors[34–39] have found that positive aspirations occur from 4% to 16% of the time. Delgado-Molina[38] found a positive aspiration rate ranging from 3.6% to 22% in 14 previous publications from 1957 to 1995.

**IN CONCLUSION**, *positive aspirations occur from 4% to 22% of the time with an IANB.*

# Trismus

Studies of postoperative trismus following an IANB using 2% lidocaine with 1:100,000 epinephrine have shown an incidence of 2% to 9%.[11,22,40] Add another cartridge of 2% lidocaine with 1:100,000 epinephrine to decrease the incidence of missed block. Improvement usually occurs over a few days.

Generally, trismus is treated by the application of heat, muscle stretches, analgesic medications, possibly muscle relaxants, and a physical therapy referral.[41] The severity and duration of the trismus will dictate the scope of therapy.

**IN CONCLUSION**, *trismus may occur after an IANB but generally improves over a few days.*

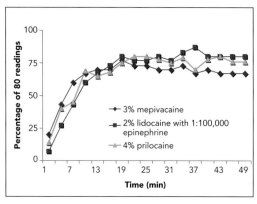

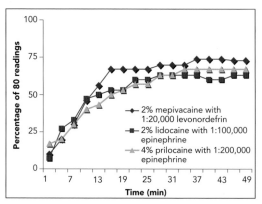

**Fig 2-8** Incidence of mandibular first molar anesthesia: comparison of 3% mepivacaine, 4% prilocaine, and 2% lidocaine with 1:100,000 epinephrine in an IANB. Results determined by lack of response to an EPT at maximum reading (80 reading) across 60 minutes. No significant difference among the three solutions was noted. (Reprinted from McLean et al[4] with permission.)

**Fig 2-9** Incidence of mandibular first molar anesthesia: comparison of 2% mepivacaine with 1:20,000 levonordefrin, 4% prilocaine with 1:200,000 epinephrine, and 2% lidocaine with 1:100,000 epinephrine in an IANB. Results determined by lack of response to an EPT at maximum reading (80 reading) across 60 minutes. No significant difference among the three solutions was noted. (Reprinted from Hinkley et al[3] with permission.)

# Alternate Anesthetic Solutions for the IANB

## Plain solutions: Mepivacaine and prilocaine

McLean and coauthors[4] have shown that 3% mepivacaine plain (Polocaine, Dentsply) and 4% prilocaine plain (Citanest Plain, Dentsply) are as effective as 2% lidocaine with 1:100,000 epinephrine in an IANB for 50 minutes (Fig 2-8). In a clinical study of patients with irreversible pulpitis, Cohen and coauthors[42] also found that 3% mepivacaine and 2% lidocaine with 1:100,000 epinephrine were equivalent for IANBs.

**IN CONCLUSION,** *3% mepivacaine plain and 4% prilocaine plain are equivalent to 2% lidocaine with 1:100,000 epinephrine for pulpal anesthesia of approximately 50-minute duration.*

### Importance of using 3% mepivacaine (Carbocaine)
Plain anesthetic solutions are indicated when medical conditions or drug therapies suggest caution in administering epinephrine-containing solutions, and 3% mepivacaine can be used as an alternative for the IANB.

**IN CONCLUSION,** *3% mepivacaine is an excellent alternative for the IANB when medical conditions or drug therapies suggest caution in administering epinephrine-containing solutions.*

## Prilocaine with epinephrine and mepivacaine with levonordefrin

In an experimental study, Hinkley and coauthors[3] have shown that 4% prilocaine with 1:200,000 epinephrine (Citanest Forte, Dentsply) and 2% mepivacaine with 1:20,000 levonordefrin (Carbocaine with Neo-Cobefrin, Cook-Waite) are equivalent to 2% lidocaine with 1:100,000 epinephrine in achieving pulpal anesthesia for an IANB (Fig 2-9).

**IN CONCLUSION,** *4% prilocaine with 1:200,000 epinephrine and 2% mepivacaine with 1:20,000 levonordefrin are equivalent to 2% lidocaine with 1:100,000 epinephrine for pulpal anesthesia in an IANB.*

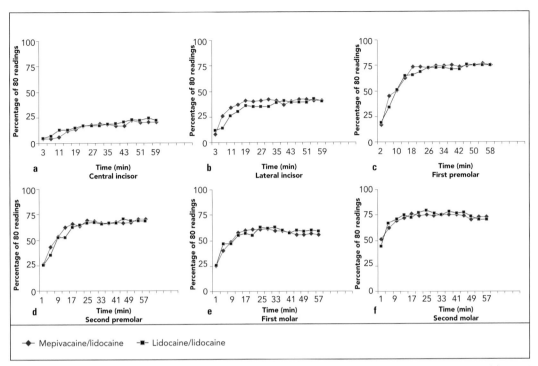

**Fig 2-10** Incidence of pulpal anesthesia following an IANB for the central incisor *(a)*, lateral incisor *(b)*, first premolar *(c)*, second premolar *(d)*, first molar *(e)*, and second molar *(f)* as determined by lack of response to an EPT at maximum reading (percentage of 80 readings), at each postinjection time interval, for the mepivacaine/lidocaine and lidocaine/lidocaine combinations. There were no significant differences between the two combinations for any of the teeth. (Reprinted from Lammers et al[43] with permission.)

## Combinations of plain solutions and lidocaine with epinephrine

Some clinicians initially administer 3% mepivacaine plain and then add 2% lidocaine with 1:100,000 epinephrine for IANBs. The rationale is that 3% mepivacaine has a higher pH because it does not contain epinephrine and has more anesthetic molecules than 2% lidocaine because of its higher concentration.[43] In theory, using 3% mepivacaine initially would provide a quicker onset of anesthesia, increase anesthetic success, and possibly potentiate the effect of giving a second cartridge of 2% lidocaine with epinephrine for IANBs. Two studies found that 3% mepivacaine was equivalent to 2% lidocaine with 1:100,000 epinephrine for an IANB.[4,42] Rood and coauthors[44] found that there was no potentiation of lidocaine with epinephrine by adding 4% prilocaine plain for dental extractions.

Lammers and coauthors[43] found that onset times and anesthetic success with the initial administration of 3% mepivacaine plain (Carbocaine) followed by 2% lidocaine with 1:100,000 epinephrine were not significantly different than those from initially administering 2% lidocaine with 1:100,000 epinephrine followed by 2% lidocaine with 1:100,000 epinephrine for an IANB (Fig 2-10). The mean pH of the mepivacaine formulation averaged 6.7, and the mean pH of the lidocaine formulation averaged 4.3.

**IN CONCLUSION,** *there is no clinical advantage in initially administering 3% mepivacaine plain followed by 2% lidocaine with epinephrine for IANBs.*

## Levonordefrin as a vasoconstrictor

The manufacturer of 2% mepivacaine with 1:20,000 levonordefrin (Neo-Cobefrin, Cook-Waite) states that it is a vasoconstrictor that causes less cardiac and central nervous system stimulation than epinephrine. This is true for the basic pharmacology of the drug. Levonordefrin has 75% α activity and only 25% β activity while epinephrine has 50% α activity and 50% β activity.[45] However, levonordefrin is marketed as a 1:20,000 concentration in dental cartridges, which is five times the concentration of 1:100,000.[45] Clinically, the higher concentration of levonordefrin makes it equipotent to epinephrine in clinical and systemic effects.[3,28] Guglielmo and coauthors[28] measured the heart rate (pulse rate) after the intraosseous injection of 1.8 mL of 2% mepivacaine with 1:20,000 levonordefrin and 1.8 mL of 2% lidocaine with 1:100,000 epinephrine. They demonstrated that both anesthetic formulations increased heart rate (mean increase of approximately 23 to 24 beats per minute from baseline) in 80% of the subjects, with no significant difference between the two anesthetic formulations. Because Guglielmo and coauthors[28] found no difference in heart rate and Hinkley and coauthors[3] found no difference in anesthetic success between 1.8 mL of 2% mepivacaine with 1:20,000 levonordefrin and 1.8 mL of 2% lidocaine with 1:100,000 epinephrine, it would appear that 1:20,000 levonordefrin offers no clinical advantage over 1:100,000 epinephrine.

**IN CONCLUSION,** *1:20,000 levonordefrin offers no clinical advantage over 1:100,000 epinephrine.*

## Articaine

Articaine was cleared for use in the United States in April 2000.[46] The formulation is known as Septocaine (Septodont), Articadent (Dentsply), and Zorcaine (Cook-Waite) and is available as a 4% solution with 1:100,000 and 1:200,000 epinephrine. Articaine is classified as an amide and contains a thiophene ring instead of a benzene ring like other amide local anesthetics.[46] Being an amide and not an ester of para-aminobenzoic acid (PABA), there is no concern for cross-allergy to PABA derivatives. A second molecular difference between articaine and other amide local anesthetics is the extra ester linkage incorporated into the articaine molecule, which results in hydrolysis of articaine by plasma esterases.[46] Because of this, articaine has a shorter half-life than lidocaine (lidocaine requires hepatic clearance).

### Safety
A number of studies have evaluated articaine and concluded that it is safe when used in appropriate doses.[46–56] Both lidocaine and articaine have the same maximum dose of 500 mg (recommended dose of 6.6 to 7.0 mg/kg) for an adult patient.[45] Because articaine is marketed as a 4% solution, the maximum manufacturer recommended dose for a healthy 70-kg adult would be 7 cartridges of a 4% articaine solution compared with 13 cartridges of a 2% lidocaine solution[45] (see Table 1-1). (See chapter 1 for a discussion of cartridge volumes [1.8 mL versus 1.7 mL].)

**IN CONCLUSION,** *articaine is a safe local anesthetic agent.*

### Paresthesia and methemoglobinemia
Articaine, like prilocaine, has the potential to cause methemoglobinemia and neuropathies.[46] While the incidence of methemoglobinemia is rare, dentists should be aware of this complication in patients who are at an increased risk of developing this condition, for example patients with breathing problems (asthma, emphysema).[57]

Haas and Lennon[58] and Miller and Lennon[59] investigated the incidence of local anesthetic–induced neuropathies. The incidence of neuropathies (ones that involved the lip and/or tongue) associated with articaine and prilocaine was approximately five times that found with either lidocaine or mepivacaine.[58,59] In the Haas and Lennon retrospective study,[58] the incidence of paresthesia was only 14 cases out of 11 million injections or approximately one in 785,000 injections.

Gaffen and Haas[60] and Garisto and coauthors[61] found that articaine and prilocaine had a higher incidence of paresthesias: one in 2,070,678 injections for prilocaine, one in 4,159,848 injections for articaine, and one in 181,076,673 injections for lidocaine. Therefore, according to these retrospective studies, the paresthesia incidence is higher for articaine and prilocaine but is still a clinically rare event.

Pogrel[62] evaluated patients referred with a diagnosis of damage to the inferior alveolar and/or lingual nerve that could only have resulted from an IANB. He found that 35% were caused by a lidocaine formulation and 30% were caused by an articaine formulation. He concluded that there was not a disproportionate nerve involvement from articaine. In an update, Pogrel[63] found that permanent nerve involvement of the IANB occurred in 25% of cases with lidocaine, in 33% with articaine, and in 34% with prilocaine.

Therefore, fear of paresthesia should not limit the clinical use of articaine. However, with any paresthesia, documentation of the patient's reported area of altered sensation, the type of altered sensation (eg, anesthesia, paresthesia, or dysesthesia), and regular follow-up are important.

Note that because some attorneys are aware of the proposed association between articaine and paresthesia with nerve block, and because there is no difference in anesthetic success between lidocaine and articaine formulations for nerve blocks,[11] it seems reasonable to use articaine for infiltrations and other solutions for nerve blocks.

**IN CONCLUSION,** *paresthesias with articaine are rare.*

## Irritation

Hoffmeister,[64] Leuschner and Leblanc,[54] and Ribeiro and coauthors[65] found that articaine was not cytotoxic to nerves and was similar to other anesthetic agents (mepivacaine, bupivacaine, and lidocaine) in tissue tolerance. Baroni and coauthors[66] evaluated the toxicity of articaine (using histology) in rat mental nerve injections. The authors found that articaine was not toxic to the nervous structures.

**IN CONCLUSION,** *articaine is similar to other local anesthetic agents regarding tissue tolerance and toxicity.*

## Mechanism of action of articaine

A number of studies have shown the superiority of 4% articaine with 1:100,000 epinephrine over 2% lidocaine with 1:100,000 epinephrine when used as a primary buccal infiltration of the mandibular first molar[67–69] and as a supplemental buccal infiltration of the first molar following an IANB.[70,71] The exact mechanism of articaine's increased efficacy is not known. Borchard and Drouin[72] found that a lower concentration of articaine was sufficient to block an action potential when compared with other amide anesthetics. Potocnik and coauthors,[73] in a study of sensory nerve conduction in rats, found that both 2% and 4% articaine were superior to 2% lidocaine in blocking nerve conduction. It may be that factors other than the concentration are responsible for articaine's clinical efficacy. For instance, the unique chemical structure of articaine (the thiophene ring), which is not possessed by other local anesthetic agents, may facilitate better diffusion of the anesthetic solution.[74] One study suggested that it is the intramolecular hydrogen bond that gives articaine its favorable properties.[74]

Nydegger and coauthors[75] determined if the 4% concentration was responsible for articaine effectiveness by comparing the degree of pulpal anesthesia obtained with 1.8 mL of 4% articaine with 1:100,000 epinephrine, 4% lidocaine with 1:100,000 epinephrine, and 4% prilocaine with 1:200,000 epinephrine as a primary buccal infiltration in the mandibular first molar. The success rates were 55%, 33%, and 32%, respectively (Fig 2-11). They found that the 4% articaine with epinephrine formulation (pH of 3.3) was statistically better than both 4% lidocaine with epinephrine (pH of 6.1) and 4% prilocaine with epinephrine (pH of 4.0) formulations. Rather than a 4% concentration or pH, it is likely the chemical structure of articaine that results in better anesthesia for mandibular buccal infiltrations.

**IN CONCLUSION,** *factors other than concentration are responsible for articaine's clinical efficacy.*

## Insurance carrier warning

A letter was sent to thousands of US dentists by the insurance company Emery and Webb/ACE USA stating:

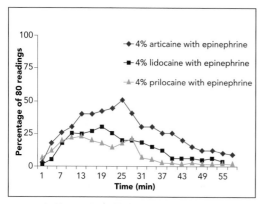

**Fig 2-11** Incidence of mandibular first molar pulpal anesthesia as determined by lack of response to an EPT at maximum reading (percentage of 80 readings), at each postinjection time interval, for the articaine, lidocaine, and prilocaine formulations. A 4% articaine formulation was statistically better than both 4% lidocaine and 4% prilocaine formulations. However, the success rate of 55% is not high enough to support its use as a primary buccal infiltration technique in the mandibular first molar. (Reprinted from Nydegger et al[75] with permission.)

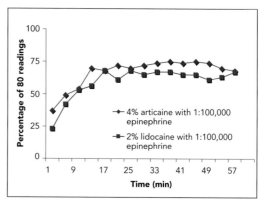

**Fig 2-12** Incidence of mandibular first molar anesthesia: comparison of 4% articaine with 1:100,000 epinephrine to 2% lidocaine with 1:100,000 epinephrine in an IANB. Results determined by lack of response to an EPT at maximum reading (80 reading) across 60 minutes. No significant difference between the two formulations was noted. (Reprinted from Mikesell et al[11] with permission.)

We at Emery and Webb have had a recent increase in anesthetic related malpractice incidents.… We have noticed an increase in reversible and, in some cases, nonreversible paresthesias (with articaine).… We are writing you to alert you to these events in hopes that you will not fall victim to one of these incidents.[76]

Knowledgeable dentists and educators communicated their concerns, and a notice of retraction was issued:

Unfortunately, we at Emery and Webb discovered upon further review, and subsequent to the mailings, that both documents contained inaccuracies and an alarmist tone, which was not warranted. . . . Emery and Webb has not noted an increase in malpractice claims or lawsuits in connection with articaine. . . . It should be made clear that Emery and Webb has not conducted any scientific investigation, sampling, testing, or other investigation of the articaine anesthetic, and has no independent knowledge or data which would restrict the use of the product.[76]

**IN CONCLUSION,** *dentists should consult authoritative sources for correct information regarding articaine.*

## Clinical effectiveness for IANBs

Articaine has a reputation of providing an improved local anesthetic effect.[77] The available literature indicates that articaine is equally effective for an IANB when statistically compared with other local anesthetics.[11,55,78–85] When comparing the anesthetic efficacy of 4% articaine with 1:100,000 epinephrine and 2% lidocaine with 1:100,000 epinephrine for IANBs, Mikesell and coauthors[11] found that the two formulations were not significantly different (Fig 2-12).

Tofoli and coauthors[86] found that 4% articaine with 1:100,000 epinephrine was equivalent to 4% articaine with 1:200,000 epinephrine in IANBs. Moore and coauthors[87] also found no difference in clinical efficacy between 4% articaine with 1:100,000 and 1:200,000 epinephrine in clinical studies. Brandt and coauthors[88] and Kung and coauthors[89] performed a meta-analysis of articaine versus lidocaine in dentistry. The authors found that articaine was not better than lidocaine for IANBs.

**IN CONCLUSION,** *articaine and lidocaine are equivalent for IANBs.*

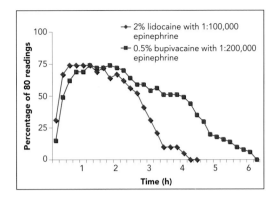

**Fig 2-13** Incidence of mandibular first molar anesthesia: comparison of 0.5% bupivacaine with 1:200,000 epinephrine to 2% lidocaine with 1:100,000 epinephrine in an IANB. Results determined by lack of response to an EPT at maximum reading (80 reading) across 60 minutes. The bupivacaine solution showed a longer duration of anesthesia than the lidocaine solution. (Reprinted from Fernandez et al[13] with permission.)

## Long-acting anesthetic agents

### Bupivacaine and etidocaine

Clinical trials with bupivacaine (Marcaine, Cook-Waite; Vivacaine, Septodont) and etidocaine (Duranest, AstraZeneca) have been performed in oral surgery,[90,91] endodontics,[92,93] and periodontics.[94,95] Etidocaine has been withdrawn from the market by Dentsply.

Fernandez and coauthors[13] compared 0.5% bupivacaine with 1:100,000 epinephrine to 2% lidocaine with 1:100,000 epinephrine in an IANB and found a similar success rate for the first molar between the two formulations. However, a lower success rate was found for the second molars, premolars, and lateral incisors with bupivacaine. A portion of the lower success rate with bupivacaine was related to a slower onset of pulpal anesthesia.[13] The bupivacaine formulation had an average duration of pulpal anesthesia of 4 hours while the lidocaine formulation averaged 2 hours and 24 minutes[13] (Fig 2-13).

Duration of mandibular lip anesthesia will be significantly prolonged with bupivacaine when compared with lidocaine.[13] Other studies have reported similar results.[92,93,96–106] While lip numbness lasts longer than pulpal anesthesia, there is little advantage to having lip numbness for extended periods of time. Difficulty in eating and speaking and the possibility of soft tissue trauma are viewed as nuisances by the patient. Rosenquist and Nystrom[103] found that 34% of patients commented that the long-acting anesthesia produced by a bupivacaine solution was unpleasant. In a follow-up study, Rosenquist and coauthors[104] found that some patients were willing to sustain some pain after oral surgery if lip sensation was regained sooner. Therefore, patients should be questioned regarding their preference for extended lip anesthesia and not be given a long-acting anesthetic routinely.

It is well known that bupivacaine prolongs the analgesic period following an IANB.[95,102,105–107] While bupivacaine reduces initial postoperative pain and the need for analgesics, it does not completely eliminate pain or the need for any analgesic medication.[92,93,103–105,108] Therefore, the longevity of the postoperative pain should also be considered when extending the analgesic period with bupivacaine. Neal and coauthors[107] found that a significant decrease in pain occurred on the first postoperative day when bupivacaine was used compared with lidocaine. However, on subsequent days, lidocaine and bupivacaine pain scores were comparable. Rosenquist and Nystrom[103] found that pain scores were lower for a bupivacaine solution when compared with a lidocaine/diflunisal regimen at 2 and 3 hours postoperatively, whereas at 6 hours the bupivacaine solution had higher pain scores. This means that the analgesic period does not usually extend long enough to cover the whole time of postoperative discomfort and that prescribing analgesic medication for the entire postoperative period would be warranted when using a bupivacaine solution.

In maxillary endodontic surgery, Meechan and Blair[109] found that a long-acting anesthetic used for infiltration anesthesia did not decrease postoperative pain or analgesic intake when compared with a lidocaine solution. The authors also found that the lidocaine solution provided better anesthesia and

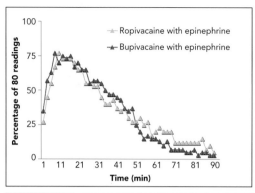

**Fig 2-14** Incidence of maxillary lateral incisor anesthesia: comparison of 0.5% bupivacaine with 1:200,000 epinephrine to 0.5% ropivacaine with 1:200,000 epinephrine in an infiltration injection. Results determined by lack of response to an EPT at maximum reading (80 reading) across 60 minutes. No significant difference between the two solutions was noted. (Reprinted from Kennedy et al[110] with permission.)

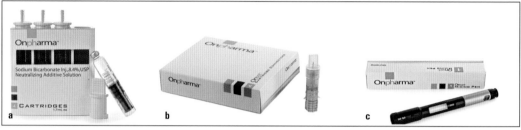

**Fig 2-15** The Onpharma Onset system consists of a neutralizing additive (8.4% sodium bicarbonate) *(a)*, an Onset cartridge connector *(b)*, and an Onset mixing pen *(c)*. (Courtesy of Onpharma.)

less hemorrhaging than the bupivacaine solution. Therefore, bupivacaine is less effective for maxillary endodontic surgery using infiltration.

**IN CONCLUSION,** *bupivacaine has a slower onset of pulpal anesthesia and prolongs the duration of pulpal anesthesia when compared with lidocaine. Soft tissue anesthesia is prolonged with bupivacaine when compared with lidocaine.*

### Other long-acting agents

A long-acting local anesthetic is ropivacaine. It is a structural homologue of bupivacaine.[110] A number of studies have demonstrated that ropivacaine has a lower potential for central nervous system and cardiovascular toxic effects than bupivacaine.[110] Kennedy and coauthors[110] concluded that 0.5% ropivacaine with 1:200,000 epinephrine was equivalent to 0.5% bupivacaine with 1:200,000 epinephrine in pharmacologic action (Fig 2-14). El-Sharrawy and Yagiela[111] found that 0.5% and 0.75% concentrations of ropivacaine without epinephrine were effective for IANBs. Another study evaluated levobupivacaine (a long-acting local anesthetic) for IANBs and found that it was equivalent to bupivacaine.[112] Therefore, ropivacaine and levobupivacaine have the potential to replace bupivacaine in clinical dental practice due to the decreased potential for cardiac and central nervous system toxicity.

**IN CONCLUSION,** *other long-acting anesthetics may sometime in the future replace bupivacaine in dental practice.*

## Buffering of anesthetic solutions

Two systems are commercially available to buffer local anesthetics: the Onset system (Onpharma) and the Anutra system (Anutra Medical). The Onset system buffers a local anesthetic solution using a unique dispensing system (Fig 2-15) and includes an Onset mixing pen, an Onset cartridge connector, and an Onset sodium bicarbonate neutralizing additive solution. The Anutra system (Fig 2-16), consists of a dispenser, a 5-mL multiple-dose syringe, and a cassette.

**Fig 2-16** Anutra buffering system. The dispenser *(a)* and syringe *(b)* are shown. (Courtesy of Anutra Medical.)

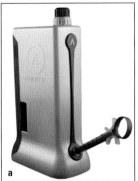

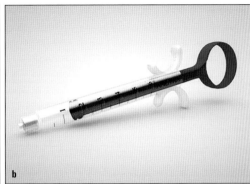

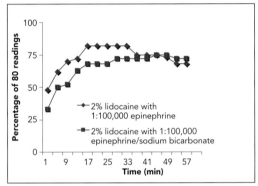

**Fig 2-17** Incidence of mandibular first molar anesthesia: comparison of buffered 2% lidocaine with 1:100,000 epinephrine to 2% lidocaine with 1:100,000 epinephrine in an IANB. Results determined by lack of response to an EPT at maximum reading (80 reading) across 60 minutes. No significant difference between the two solutions was noted. (Reprinted from Whitcomb et al[116] with permission.)

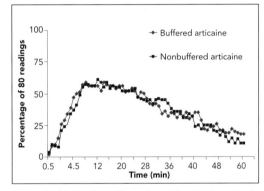

**Fig 2-18** Incidence of mandibular first molar pulpal anesthesia as determined by lack of response to an EPT at maximum reading (80 reading), at each postinjection time interval, for the buffered and nonbuffered formulations. Anesthetic success for buffered articaine and nonbuffered articaine were 71% and 65%, respectively. There was no significant difference between the formulations. (Reprinted from Shurtz et al[119] with permission.)

Buffering an anesthetic should in theory increase anesthetic success by providing a greater number of deionized, uncharged base anesthetic molecules. With a greater number of base molecules, more anesthetic should be able to penetrate the nerve sheath and block the sodium channels. Galindo[113] used pH-adjusted local anesthetic solutions (pH of 7.4) in epidurals, peripheral nerve blocks, and regional anesthesia. He found that higher pH solutions established anesthesia of better quality.

In dentistry, while buffering lidocaine has been shown by Al-Sultan and coauthors[114,115] to improve efficacy for extractions and periapical surgery, Whitcomb and coauthors[116] did not find an increased efficacy with buffered lidocaine for asymptomatic subjects with the IANB (Fig 2-17), nor did Saatchi and coauthors[117] or Schellenberg and coauthors[118] find a significant difference for IANBs in patients presenting with symptomatic irreversible pulpitis. Shurtz and coauthors[119] did not find a buffered articaine solution superior to a nonbuffered articaine solution for buccal infiltration of the mandibular first molar (Fig 2-18). Additionally, Balasco and coauthors[120] and Harreld and coauthors[121] did not find decreased pain for an incision and drainage procedure with a buffered lidocaine formulation.

Regarding onset of anesthesia, some authors[114,115,122,123] have found a faster onset with buffered lidocaine formulations, while others have not.[116,119,124] Malamed and coauthors[123] proposed that the clinician could administer an IANB and go to work immediately. This belief was based on a study of the IANB in 18 subjects. The authors found an onset of pulpal anesthesia of around 2 minutes for a buffered lidocaine formulation and around 6½ minutes for the nonbuffered lidocaine. Wow! However, these times did not include onset of lip numbness. That is, pulpal anesthesia was measured after lip numbness occurred. Lip numbness times were not included in the study by Malamed and coauthors.[123] Therefore, we would still have to wait for lip numbness, which could range from 4½ to 6 minutes, adding additional waiting time. Besides lip numbness, failure of pulpal anesthesia for an IANB (estimated to be around 23% for the first molar) and slow onset of anesthesia (which occurs around 14% of the time) will also occur. Because of the small number of subjects sampled, neither of these events occurred.

Theoretically, the higher pH should have resulted in faster onset of anesthesia and a higher success rate. However, the body intrinsically has an efficient buffering system that maintains tissues at physiologic pH. The pH conversion buffering process, as reported by Wennberg and coauthors,[125] could occur within several minutes. Punnia-Moorthy[126] reported a freshly prepared 2% lignocaine with adrenaline formulation (pH 5.25) being converted to a pH of 7.17 within 3 minutes following an intradermal injection. This physiologic conversion may help explain why buffering an anesthetic did not demonstrate any benefit in increasing anesthetic success.

Some clinicians think buffering is better for IANBs. I think that if they were to compare a buffered solution with a nonbuffered solution and objectively evaluate success of the block (blind the solutions), the results would be surprising.

**IN CONCLUSION,** *buffering anesthetic solutions does not seem to increase success or speed the onset of pulpal anesthesia.*

# Alternate Injection Locations

## Gow-Gates and Vazirani-Akinosi techniques

The Gow-Gates technique[127] (Fig 2-19) has been reported to have a higher success rate than the conventional IANB.[45,128] However, experimental studies have failed to show that the Gow-Gates technique is superior[14,29,129–132] (Fig 2-20).

Akinosi introduced his technique for mandibular anesthesia in 1977,[133] while Vazirani had also described a similar technique in 1960,[134] so the name was changed to reflect both contributions.[45] The Vazirani-Akinosi[45,133] technique (Fig 2-21) has also not been found to be superior to the standard IANB.[14,129,135–137] Goldberg and coauthors[14] compared the degree of pulpal anesthesia obtained with the conventional, the Gow-Gates, and the Vazirani-Akinosi techniques in vital, asymptomatic teeth using 3.6 mL of 2% lidocaine with 1:100,000 epinephrine. They found that for the subjects who achieved lip numbness, the conventional IANB was similar to the Gow-Gates and Vazirani-Akinosi techniques regarding anesthetic success (Fig 2-22). However, the Gow-Gates and Vazirani-Akinosi techniques had a slower onset of pulpal anesthesia when compared with the conventional technique. These techniques do not replace the conventional IANB.

When a patient presents with trismus or limited mandibular opening, the Vazirani-Akinosi technique can be used because the mouth is closed during the injection. Neither technique is better than the conventional IANB in reducing the pain of injection.[14,129,130,138]

**IN CONCLUSION,** *neither the Gow-Gates technique nor Vazirani-Akinosi technique is better than the conventional IANB.*

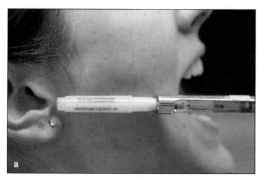

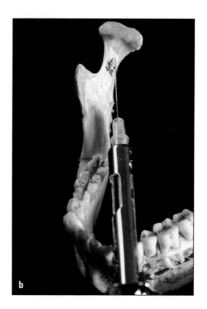

**Fig 2-19** *(a)* Extraoral landmark for the Gow-Gates technique: the lower border of the tragus of the ear and the corner of the mouth. *(b)* Intraoral target site for the Gow-Gates technique: the neck of the mandibular condyle.

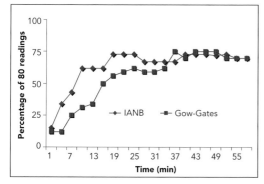

**Fig 2-20** Incidence of mandibular first molar anesthesia: comparison of the IANB and Gow-Gates techniques. Results determined by lack of response to an EPT at maximum reading (80 reading) across 60 minutes. No significant difference between the two techniques was noted. (Reprinted from Goldberg et al[14] with permission.)

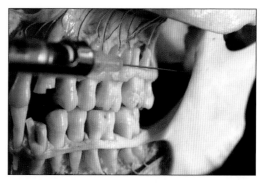

**Fig 2-21** Vazirani-Akinosi technique. This closed-mouth technique has the landmark for needle insertion on line with the mucogingival junction of the maxillary second molar.

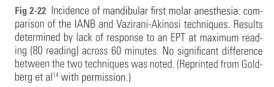

**Fig 2-22** Incidence of mandibular first molar anesthesia: comparison of the IANB and Vazirani-Akinosi techniques. Results determined by lack of response to an EPT at maximum reading (80 reading) across 60 minutes. No significant difference between the two techniques was noted. (Reprinted from Goldberg et al[14] with permission.)

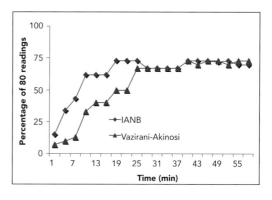

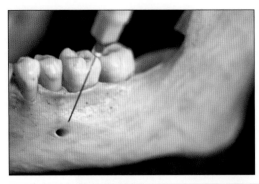

**Fig 2-23** Incisive nerve block. The needle is directed distal to the long axis of the second premolar in an anterior-inferior orientation.

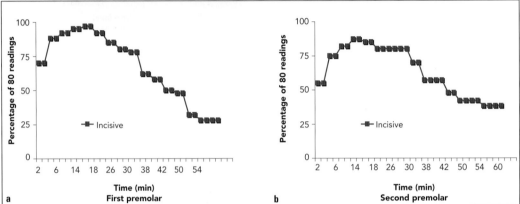

**Fig 2-24** Incidence of mandibular first premolar *(a)* and second premolar *(b)* anesthesia for the incisive nerve block. Results determined by lack of response to an EPT at maximum reading (80 reading) across 60 minutes. (Reprinted from Nist et al[7] with permission.)

## Incidence of buccal nerve anesthesia

Gow-Gates[127] and Akinosi[133] state that a separate buccal injection is not required for soft tissue anesthesia with their techniques. Goldberg and coauthors[14] reported the incidence of buccal nerve anesthesia at 84% with the Gow-Gates technique and 80% with the Vazirani-Akinosi technique using 3.6 mL of 2% lidocaine with 1:100,000 epinephrine. Previous studies have found an incidence of 62%,[139] 68%,[132] 77%,[128] 78%,[140] 20%,[130] and 89%[131] for buccal nerve anesthesia with the Gow-Gates technique. For the Vazirani-Akinosi technique, previous studies have found that buccal nerve anesthesia occurred 80%[135] and 71%[141] of the time. Generally, some buccal nerve anesthesia can be obtained with these techniques because the long buccal nerve can be anesthetized as it crosses the anterior border of the mandibular ramus[142] if anesthetic solution is deposited as the needle is inserted or withdrawn or if enough volume is injected to diffuse to the nerve. Regardless of the incidence reported for these techniques, buccal nerve anesthesia was not 100%. Therefore, a separate long buccal injection should be given when soft tissue anesthesia is required in the molar teeth.

**IN CONCLUSION,** *buccal nerve anesthesia is not complete with the Gow-Gates or Vazirani-Akinosi technique.*

## Incisive nerve block at the mental foramen

Nist and coauthors,[7] Joyce and Donnelly,[143] and Whitworth and coauthors[144] demonstrated that the incisive nerve block (Fig 2-23) alone is reasonably successful in anesthetizing premolars whether the mental foramen is entered or not. The duration of pulpal anesthesia was 20 to 30 minutes[7,143] (Fig 2-24). Batista da Silva and coauthors[145] demonstrated that a 4% articaine formulation was better than

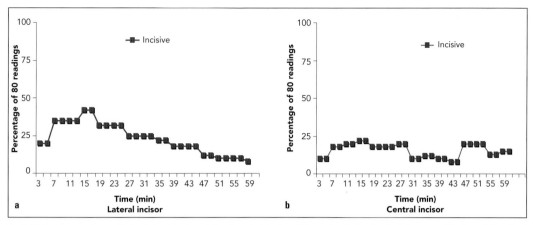

**Fig 2-25** Incidence of mandibular lateral incisor *(a)* and central incisor *(b)* anesthesia for the incisive nerve block as determined by lack of response to an EPT at maximum reading (80 reading) across 60 minutes. (Reprinted from Nist et al[7] with permission.)

a lidocaine formulation for the incisive nerve block but only used a volume of 0.6 mL, which resulted in a duration of anesthesia of approximately 10 minutes.

Nist and coauthors[7] and Whitworth and coauthors[144] showed that this technique did not effectively anesthetize the mandibular lateral and central incisors (Fig 2-25). Additionally, Nist and coauthors[7] found no difficulty entering the foramen, while Joyce and Donnelly[143] found that the foramen could be located only 57% of the time. Jaber and coauthors[146] studied the effects of soft tissue massage (60 seconds) on the efficacy of the mental and incisive nerve block. The authors concluded that soft tissue massage did not influence success or onset of an incisive/mental nerve block.

Phillips[147] stated that the incisive nerve block is more painful than the traditional technique; however, Pampush[148] found that it is less painful than the traditional IANB. Nist and coauthors[7] found that needle insertion into the foramen is mildly discomforting (5% to 8% moderate pain) whether given alone or following an IANB. They showed that solution deposition for the incisive nerve block alone resulted in an incidence of moderate-to-severe pain 18% of the time. The IANB had a 25% incidence of moderate-to-severe pain. Therefore, according to this study, the incisive nerve block is less painful than the IANB.

Joyce and Donnelly[143] recorded low pain ratings and no difference in pain perception whether the injection is given inside or outside the mental foramen. Whitworth and coauthors[144] found that a slow incisive nerve injection (60 seconds) is less painful than a fast injection (15 seconds).

Northrop[149] felt there is more postoperative discomfort with the incisive nerve block than the IANB. Nist and coauthors[7] found that the incisive nerve block had less potential for postoperative pain (2% moderate pain) than the IANB (17% moderate pain) and also recorded no paresthesias, whereas Joyce and Donnelly[143] had two patients with altered mental nerve sensations.

**IN CONCLUSION,** *the incisive nerve block is somewhat successful in the premolars, but the duration is around 20 to 30 minutes.*

## Incisive nerve block plus a repeat articaine infiltration

Dressman and coauthors[150] determined the degree of pulpal anesthesia obtained with a primary infiltration of one cartridge of articaine in the incisive/mental nerve region of the mandibular second premolar as well as the anesthetic efficacy of a repeat articaine infiltration 20 minutes following the primary infiltration. In a randomized, single-blind study, 100 asymptomatic adults received two sets

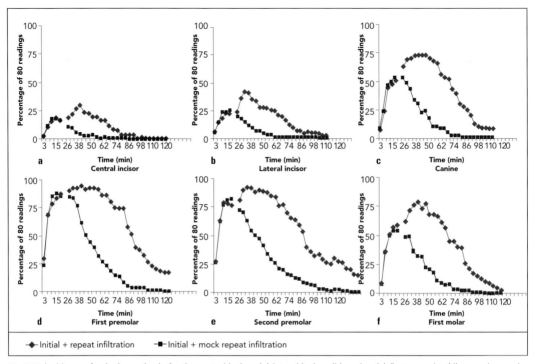

**Fig 2-26** Incidence of pulpal anesthesia for the central incisor *(a)*, lateral incisor *(b)*, canine *(c)*, first premolar *(d)*, second premolar *(e)*, and first molar *(f)* as determined by lack of response to an EPT at maximum reading (80 reading), at each postinjection time interval, for initial infiltration of one cartridge of 4% articaine with 1:100,000 epinephrine plus a repeat infiltration at 20 minutes of one cartridge of 4% articaine with 1:100,000 epinephrine or a mock infiltration. The initial infiltration in the incisive/mental nerve area was not effective in anesthetizing the first molar, canine, or incisors and was only moderately successful in the premolars. While the repeat infiltration significantly increased success and duration of pulpal anesthesia in the premolars, the initial infiltration success rates were too low to make this regimen useful as an alternate anesthetic technique. (Reprinted from Dressman et al[150] with permission.)

of injections: *(1)* a primary mandibular second premolar infiltration of one cartridge of 4% articaine with 1:100,000 epinephrine, and then *(2)* either a repeat infiltration 20 minutes later (using the same volume of articaine) or a mock repeat infiltration. These injections were given in two separate appointments scheduled at least 1 week apart. An EPT was used to test the first molar, premolars, canine, and incisors for anesthesia in 4-minute cycles for 120 minutes.

For the first molar, canine, and incisors, success rates for the initial infiltrations ranged from 19% to 59% (Fig 2-26). Success rates for the premolars were higher (80% to 87%), but anesthesia declined after 20 to 25 minutes. The repeat infiltration given at 20 minutes significantly increased success (92% to 94%) and duration of pulpal anesthesia for the premolars. Despite these moderate success rates with repeat infiltration, the initial infiltration success rates were too low to make this regimen useful as an alternate anesthetic technique.

**IN CONCLUSION,** *the initial infiltration of articaine was not effective in anesthetizing the first molar, canine, or incisors and was only moderately successful in the premolars. While the repeat infiltration increased success and duration of pulpal anesthesia in the premolars, the initial infiltration success rates were too low to make this regimen useful as an alternate anesthetic technique.*

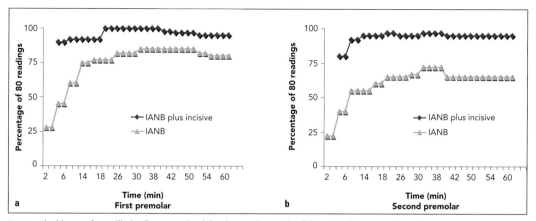

**Fig 2-27** Incidence of mandibular first premolar *(a)* and second premolar *(b)* anesthesia: comparison of the combination IANB and incisive nerve block to the IANB alone. Results determined by lack of response to an EPT at maximum reading (80 reading) across 60 minutes. The combination technique improved anesthesia. (Reprinted from Nist et al[7] with permission.)

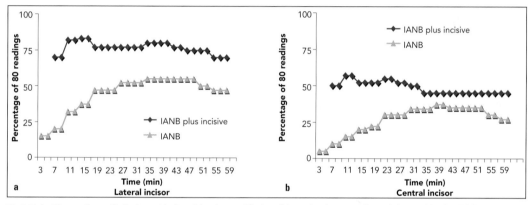

**Fig 2-28** Incidence of mandibular lateral incisor *(a)* and central incisor *(b)* anesthesia: comparison of the combination IANB and incisive nerve block to the IANB alone. Results determined by lack of response to an EPT at maximum reading (80 reading) across 60 minutes. The combination technique improved anesthesia, but anesthesia was not 100%. (Reprinted from Nist et al[7] with permission.)

## IANB plus the incisive nerve block

Nist and coauthors[7] found that the combination of the IANB plus the incisive nerve block resulted in good success rates in the premolars (Fig 2-27) but not in the central and lateral incisors (Fig 2-28). Although Nist and coauthors[7] demonstrated an increased success rate in the first molar when the incisive nerve block was combined with the IANB, an infiltration of a cartridge of 4% articaine with 1:100,000 epinephrine or an intraosseous injection would be a better choice for supplemental anesthesia of the first molar if the IANB fails.

**IN CONCLUSION,** *combining the incisive nerve block with an IANB is effective for pulpal anesthesia in the premolars.*

## Mandibular infiltrations

### Lidocaine infiltrations

Labial or lingual infiltration injections of a lidocaine solution alone are not very effective for pulpal anesthesia in mandibular teeth[80,81,151,152] (Fig 2-29). Meechan and coauthors[153] found that using 1.8 mL

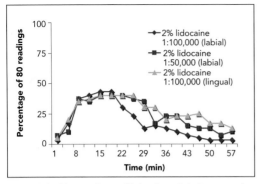

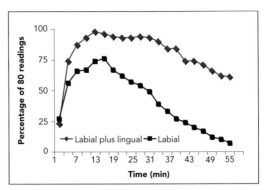

**Fig 2-29** Incidence of mandibular lateral incisor anesthesia: comparison of labial infiltrations of 2% lidocaine with 1:100,000 and 1:50,000 epinephrine and a lingual infiltration of 2% lidocaine with 1:100,000 epinephrine. Results determined by lack of response to an EPT at maximum reading (80 reading) across 60 minutes. All anesthetic solutions had pulpal anesthesia below 50% and showed a declining duration of anesthesia over the hour. (Reprinted from Yonchak et al[151] with permission.)

**Fig 2-30** Incidence of mandibular lateral incisor anesthesia: comparison of a labial plus lingual infiltration to a labial infiltration using 4% articaine with 1:100,000 epinephrine. Results determined by lack of response to an EPT at maximum reading (80 reading) across 60 minutes. Significant differences were shown from 4 to 58 minutes for the combination infiltrations. (Reprinted from Nuzum et al[154] with permission.)

of 2% lidocaine with 1:100,000 epinephrine for either a buccal or buccal plus lingual infiltration of the mandibular first molar resulted in low success rates (no patient response to the EPT) of 32% to 39%.

**IN CONCLUSION,** *lidocaine infiltrations alone are not very effective for mandibular anesthesia.*

### Labial and lingual infiltrations of articaine for anterior teeth

Nuzum and coauthors[154] found that the labial infiltration of a cartridge of 4% articaine with 1:100,000 epinephrine plus a lingual infiltration of a cartridge of 4% articaine with 1:100,000 epinephrine significantly improves the success rate (no patient response to two consecutive 80 readings with the EPT) to 98% compared with a labial infiltration of a cartridge of the same articaine formulation (76% success).[154] The combination of labial and lingual infiltrations did not provide pulpal anesthesia for 60 minutes (Fig 2-30).

Jaber and coauthors[155] found that 4% articaine was more effective than 2% lidocaine (both with 1:100,000 epinephrine) in anesthetizing mandibular incisors after labial or labial plus lingual infiltrations. However, neither solution sustained anesthesia for 45 minutes.

**IN CONCLUSION,** *buccal and lingual infiltrations of an articaine formulation in anterior teeth provide predictable pulpal anesthesia, but anesthesia declines over 60 minutes.*

### Lidocaine infiltration of anterior teeth following an IANB

Adding a labial infiltration (1.8 mL of 2% lidocaine with 1:100,000 epinephrine) to a conventional IANB increases the success of anterior pulpal anesthesia, but success is not 100%[23] (Fig 2-31). However, adding a labial and a lingual infiltration of articaine to an IANB or using a supplemental intraosseous injection should result in a higher success rate.[6,154]

**IN CONCLUSION,** *adding a labial infiltration of lidocaine to an IANB increases success in anterior teeth over an infiltration alone, but adding a labial and a lingual infiltration of articaine or using a supplemental intraosseous injection should result in a higher success rate.*

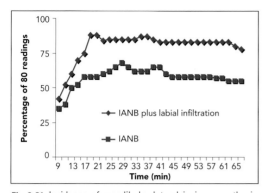

**Fig 2-31** Incidence of mandibular lateral incisor anesthesia: comparison of a combination IANB plus labial infiltration of 1.8 mL of 2% lidocaine with 1:100,000 epinephrine to an IANB alone. Results determined by lack of response to an EPT at maximum reading (80 reading) across 60 minutes. The labial infiltration improved pulpal anesthesia, but success was not 100%. (Reprinted from Clark et al[23] with permission.)

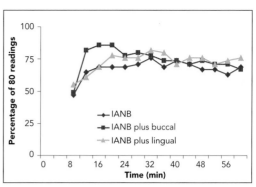

**Fig 2-32** Incidence of mandibular first molar anesthesia: comparison of the IANB alone, the IANB plus buccal infiltration, and the IANB plus lingual infiltration using a cartridge of 2% lidocaine with 1:100,000 epinephrine. Results determined by lack of response to an EPT at maximum reading (80 reading) across 60 minutes. No significant difference among the three techniques was noted. (Reprinted from Foster et al[15] with permission.)

## Lidocaine infiltration of the first molar following an IANB

Foster and coauthors[15] found that adding a buccal or lingual infiltration injection, using 1.8 mL of 2% lidocaine with 1:100,000 epinephrine, following an IANB did not significantly result in more profound pulpal anesthesia in the first molar (Fig 2-32). If the mylohyoid nerve contributed to failure of first molar anesthesia, a lingual infiltration of 1.8 mL of a lidocaine solution would be expected to significantly increase the success of IANB. Because this did not occur, it is unlikely that the mylohyoid nerve contributes significantly to posterior teeth innervation. Clark and coauthors[9] also studied the contribution of the mylohyoid nerve to mandibular pulpal anesthesia and found no significant support for an active role of the mylohyoid nerve in pulpal anesthesia.

**IN CONCLUSION,** *adding a buccal or lingual infiltration of the first molar using a lidocaine formulation following an IANB will not predictably increase pulpal anesthesia over the IANB alone.*

## Articaine infiltration of the first molar

Kanaa and coauthors[69] showed that a cartridge of 4% articaine with 1:100,000 epinephrine was significantly better than a cartridge of 2% lidocaine with 1:100,000 epinephrine for a primary buccal infiltration of the mandibular first molar. However, articaine only had a 64% success rate (no patient response to two consecutive 80 readings with the EPT). Jung and coauthors[156] and Corbett and coauthors[157] also used a primary first molar buccal infiltration of an articaine formulation and found success rates of 54% and 64% to 70% (no patient response to two consecutive 80 readings with the EPT), respectively. Robertson and coauthors[68] found an 87% success rate (no patient response to two consecutive 80 readings with the EPT) for a primary articaine buccal infiltration of the mandibular first molar versus a 57% success rate (no patient response to two consecutive 80 readings with the EPT) for a lidocaine solution. The superiority of articaine over lidocaine may be related to the intramolecular hydrogen bonding allowing better bone penetration.[74] Pabst and coauthors[158] found a 64% to 69% success rate (no patient response to two consecutive 80 readings with the EPT) for a primary buccal

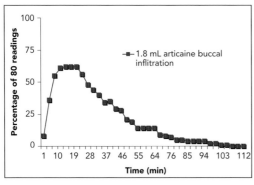

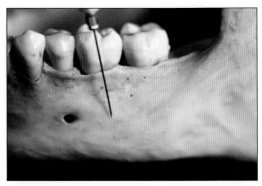

**Fig 2-33** Incidence of mandibular first molar anesthesia using a buccal infiltration of a cartridge of 4% articaine with 1:100,000 epinephrine. Results determined by lack of response to an EPT at maximum reading (80 reading) across 60 minutes. Pulpal anesthesia did not reach 70%. (Reprinted from Pabst et al[158] with permission.)

**Fig 2-34** Proximity of the incisive canal to the first molar buccal infiltration site.

infiltration of an articaine formulation in the first molar (Fig 2-33). The duration of pulpal anesthesia declined over 60 minutes. Meechan and coauthors[159] found that a buccal first molar infiltration of 1.8 mL of 4% articaine with 1:100,000 epinephrine was more successful (65% success rate) than a lingual infiltration (10% success rate) of the same amount of anesthesia.

Robertson and coauthors[68] found that onset of pulpal anesthesia was faster with the articaine formulation compared with the lidocaine formulation. They also found that adjacent teeth were anesthetized by the buccal infiltration of the first molar. The anesthetic solution appeared to move anteriorly from the first molar site; ie, a higher success rate was recorded in the premolars and first molar than in the second molar for both anesthetic formulations. Additionally, the authors speculated that the anesthetic solution may have entered the mental foramen, which led to the higher success rates in the premolars and first molar. They also found a high incidence (98% to 100%) and duration (60 minutes) of unilateral lip numbness with both formulations, which indicates that a buccal infiltration of a cartridge over the first molar can result in subjective lip numbness. However, because pulpal anesthesia was not always obtained, lip numbness should not be considered an indicator of pulpal anesthesia for a buccal infiltration of the first molar. The most likely reason for subjective lip numbness is the close proximity of the mental nerve to the first molar injection site (Fig 2-34).

Robertson and coauthors[68] also found that the pain of the three phases of the buccal infiltration injection were not different between the articaine and lidocaine formulations. Likewise, Kanaa and coauthors[69] found no significant difference in injection discomfort between articaine and lidocaine formulations for mandibular buccal infiltrations of the first molar. The pain ratings of the three phases of injection were generally reported as faint to weak. Kanaa and coauthors,[69] Pabst and coauthors,[158] and McEntire and coauthors[160] also found the pain of buccal infiltrations of the first molar to be in the mild range when using articaine or lidocaine formulations.

Robertson and coauthors[68] found that postoperative pain was reported as faint pain, and there was no difference in pain ratings between articaine and lidocaine formulations. Pabst and coauthors[158] and McEntire and coauthors[160] reported postoperative pain as faint to mild, with no significant differences between articaine formulations with 1:100,000 and 1:200,000 epinephrine. There were no reports of paresthesias in any of the patients in these three studies.

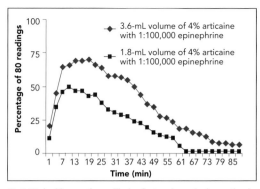

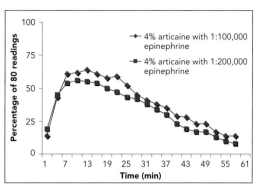

**Fig 2-35** Incidence of mandibular first molar pulpal anesthesia as determined by lack of response to an EPT at maximum reading (80 reading), at each postinjection time interval, for 1.8 mL and 3.6 mL of 4% articaine with 1:100,000 epinephrine. Significant differences between the anesthetic volumes occurred between 7 and 49 minutes. The anesthetic efficacy of the 3.6-mL volume was better than that of the 1.8-mL volume, but the success rate of 70% is not high enough to support its use as a primary injection technique in the mandibular first molar. (Reprinted from Martin et al[161] with permission.)

**Fig 2-36** Incidence of mandibular first molar anesthesia: comparison of a buccal infiltration using 4% articaine with 1:100,000 and 1:200,000 epinephrine. Results determined by lack of response to an EPT at maximum reading (80 reading) across 60 minutes. No significant difference between the two solutions was noted. Pulpal anesthesia did not reach 70%. (Reprinted from McEntire et al[160] with permission.)

Brandt and coauthors[88] and Kung and coauthors[89] performed a meta-analysis of articaine versus lidocaine in dentistry. The authors found that articaine was better than lidocaine for buccal infiltrations in the mandible.

**IN CONCLUSION,** *mandibular buccal infiltration of articaine is better than lidocaine. However, when used alone, an articaine infiltration will not predictably provide pulpal anesthesia in the first molar.*

## 1.8 mL versus 3.6 mL of 4% articaine with 1:100,000 epinephrine as a primary buccal infiltration of the mandibular first molar

Martin and coauthors[161] compared the degree of pulpal anesthesia obtained with 1.8 mL and 3.6 mL of 4% articaine with 1:100,000 epinephrine as a primary infiltration in the mandibular first molar. They found that the 3.6-mL volume showed a statistically higher success rate (70%) than the 1.8-mL volume (50% success rate) (Fig 2-35). However, a success rate of 70% is not high enough to support use of 3.6 mL of 4% articaine with 1:100,000 epinephrine as a primary injection technique in the mandibular first molar.

**IN CONCLUSION,** *the success rate (70%) is better using 3.6 mL of articaine but is still not high enough to support its use as a primary buccal infiltration technique.*

## Epinephrine concentration for buccal infiltration of the mandibular first molar
McEntire and coauthors[160] reported no difference between a cartridge of 4% articaine with 1:100,000 or 1:200,000 epinephrine for a primary buccal infiltration of the mandibular first molar (Fig 2-36). However, for maxillary periodontal surgery, Moore and coauthors[162] found that the 1:100,000 epinephrine concentration of 4% articaine provided better visualization of the surgical field and less bleeding. de Morais and coauthors[163] did not find perceptible clinical changes in hemodynamic parameters between 4% articaine with 1:100,000 or 1:200,000 epinephrine.

**IN CONCLUSION,** *there is no difference in clinical efficacy for buccal infiltration of the mandibular first molar between 4% articaine with 1:100,000 or 1:200,000 epinephrine.*

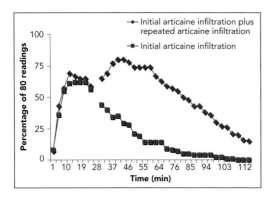

**Fig 2-37** Incidence of mandibular first molar anesthesia: comparison of a buccal infiltration of a cartridge of 4% articaine with 1:100,000 epinephrine and a combination initial buccal articaine infiltration plus a repeated articaine buccal infiltration at 25 minutes. Results were determined by lack of response to an EPT at maximum reading (80 reading) across 112 minutes. The repeated infiltration of articaine significantly increased the duration of pulpal anesthesia, but the overall success was not 100%. (Reprinted from Pabst et al[158] with permission.)

## A 0.9-mL volume of anesthetic for mandibular first molar infiltrations

The previous studies discussed used 1.8 mL of 2% lidocaine with 1:100,000 epinephrine or 1.8 mL of 4% articaine with 1:100,000 epinephrine. Abdulwahab and coauthors[67] evaluated a volume of 0.9 mL using six local anesthetic formulations for mandibular first molar infiltrations. They found that the articaine formulations (4% articaine with either 1:100,000 or 1:200,000 epinephrine) had the highest success rates (no patient response to two consecutive 80 readings with the EPT) compared with other formulations (lidocaine, prilocaine, mepivacaine, and bupivacaine). However, the success rates were less than 40% for the articaine formulations and would not provide an adequate level of pulpal anesthesia for most dental procedures. The success rates were lower than the previously discussed studies using 1.8 mL of an articaine formulation.

**IN CONCLUSION,** *a buccal infiltration of the first molar using a volume of 0.9 mL of an articaine formulation will not provide predictable pulpal anesthesia.*

## Repeated articaine infiltration in the mandibular first molar

Previous studies have shown declining rates of pulpal anesthesia over 60 minutes when using a cartridge of 4% articaine with 1:100,000 epinephrine for buccal infiltration in the mandibular first molar. Pabst and coauthors[158] found that a repeated infiltration of a cartridge of 4% articaine with 1:100,000 epinephrine given 25 minutes after an initial infiltration of the same type and dose of anesthetic significantly improved the duration of pulpal anesthesia (from 28 through 109 minutes) when compared with only an initial buccal infiltration in the mandibular first molar (Fig 2-37). However, the initial injection of articaine was only 64% to 69% successful. If the success of the initial injection could be increased, the addition of a repeated infiltration could provide a duration of pulpal anesthesia that would be clinically predictable.

**IN CONCLUSION,** *a repeated infiltration of a cartridge of articaine significantly improved the duration of pulpal anesthesia in the mandibular first molar.*

## Articaine infiltration of the first molar following an IANB

In a prospective, randomized, double-blind crossover study, Haase and coauthors[70] compared the degree of pulpal anesthesia achieved by mandibular first molar buccal infiltrations of two anesthetic solutions—4% articaine with 1:100,000 epinephrine and 2% lidocaine with 1:100,000 epinephrine—following an IANB (using 4% articaine with 1:100,000 epinephrine). They found that 4% articaine with 1:100,000 epinephrine resulted in a higher success rate (88%) than 2% lidocaine with 1:100,000 epinephrine (71%). Success was defined as achieving two consecutive 80 readings within 10 minutes following the IANB plus infiltration injections and continuously sustaining the 80 readings through

Fig 2-38 Incidence of mandibular first molar anesthesia for a combination IANB plus a buccal infiltration of 4% articaine with 1:100,000 epinephrine. Results determined by lack of response to an EPT at maximum reading (80 reading) across 60 minutes. The articaine infiltration resulted in a fairly high incidence of pulpal anesthesia through 50 minutes. (Reprinted from Haase et al[70] with permission.)

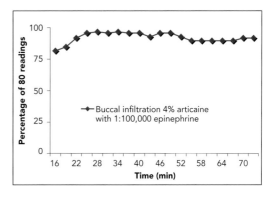

60 minutes. For the 4% articaine formulation, pulpal anesthesia reached a plateau following the initial injection and maintained a fairly high percentage of 80 readings through 50 minutes (Fig 2-38). Therefore, for dental procedures requiring profound pulpal anesthesia, fairly high success rates will be obtained at least through 50 minutes. This is a very important clinical finding. Kanaa and coauthors[71] also found that the IANB supplemented with a buccal articaine infiltration was more successful (no patient response to two consecutive 80 readings with the EPT) (92% success rate) than an IANB (56% success rate).

It may be prudent for the clinician to wait for signs of lip numbness following the IANB before giving the buccal infiltration because without an effective IANB, buccal infiltration alone would not be totally effective and would have a short duration of pulpal anesthesia.[75,158,160] An additional consideration would be that buccal infiltration of a full cartridge of anesthetic in the vicinity of the mandibular first molar could produce mental nerve anesthesia in some patients as a result of anterior diffusion of anesthetic[68] and thus produce a numb lip even if the block was missed.

The relatively thick mandibular bone in the second molar region may hinder anesthetic diffusion. Performing a buccal infiltration over the second molar following an IANB needs further investigation to determine the success of this injection.

Haase and coauthors[70] also found that the pain of three phases of the buccal infiltration injection were not different between the articaine and lidocaine formulations. The pain ratings of the three phases of injection were generally reported as faint to weak. Postoperative pain was reported as faint pain, and there was no difference in pain between articaine and lidocaine formulations. There were no reports of paresthesias in any of the patients.

**IN CONCLUSION,** *an articaine infiltration of the first molar following an IANB should provide pulpal anesthesia for approximately 1 hour.*

# Intraseptal Anesthesia

Intraseptal anesthesia is the deposition of the anesthetic solution directly into the interdental septum, allowing the solution to flow through the porous crestal alveolar bone and hence into the medullary bone surrounding the tooth. The injection is further described by Saadoun and Malamed[164] as being given in buccal keratinized tissue at a point "located at the center of the papillary triangle...equal distance from the adjacent teeth." In a 2005 review of the injection technique by Woodmansey,[165] the author suggests advancing the needle "until it contacts the underlying bone," impaling the osseous crest, and then firmly advancing into the interdental septum where the anesthetic should be delivered. Woodmansey also recommended repeating the intraseptal injection at the mesial and distal

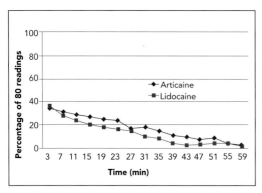

**Fig 2-39** Incidence of mandibular first molar pulpal anesthesia as determined by lack of response to an EPT at maximum reading (80 reading), at each postinjection time interval, for the articaine and lidocaine formulations. Success of the intraseptal injection was 28% for lidocaine and 35% for articaine. There were no significant differences between the two formulations. (Reprinted from Bonar et al[171] with permission.)

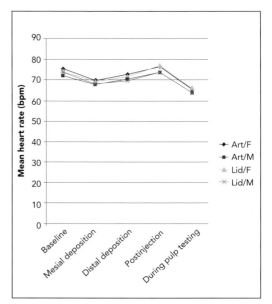

**Fig 2-40** Mean heart rate of males and females at baseline, during mesial and distal solution deposition, and at postinjection periods for each anesthetic solution. There were no significant differences between articaine (Art) and lidocaine (Lid) or between males (M) and females (F) during any of the testing periods. Intraseptal anesthesia does not appear to have a significant effect on heart rate. (Reprinted from Bonar et al[171] with permission.)

aspects of the tooth to gain complete pulpal anesthesia.[165] Success rates of intraseptal anesthesia have ranged from 76% to 90% depending on how success was measured (extractions, restorative procedures, and experimental monitoring with an EPT).[164,166–170]

Bonar and coauthors[171] compared the anesthetic efficacy of a primary intraseptal injection of articaine and lidocaine, administered with a computer-controlled local anesthetic delivery (CCLAD) system, in asymptomatic mandibular first molars. Using a crossover design, 100 subjects randomly received intraseptal injections of 1.4 mL of 4% articaine and 2% lidocaine, both with 1:100,000 epinephrine, at two separate appointments. Injections were given in the interdental papillae, mesial (0.7 mL) and distal (0.7 mL) to the first molar. An EPT was used to test for pulpal anesthesia. Pain of injection, postoperative pain, and heart rate were also evaluated.

The anesthetic success rate (no patient response to two consecutive 80 readings with the EPT) for the mandibular first molar was 35% for the articaine solution and 28% for the lidocaine solution (Fig 2-39), with no statistically significant difference between the two. No significant differences were found between articaine and lidocaine for pain of injection. Moderate pain was reported by 22% to 28% of the patients for needle insertion and 7% to 18% for solution deposition, which would indicate that some pain might be experienced during primary intraseptal anesthesia. The intraseptal injection did not increase the heart rate (Fig 2-40). Postoperative pain decreased each day, with no significant differences between the two solutions. The most common complications were injection site soreness/redness, bruising, and gingival discoloration.

**IN CONCLUSION,** *the anesthetic efficacy of articaine was not significantly better than that of lidocaine for primary intraseptal anesthesia of the mandibular first molar. The primary intraseptal injection does not achieve high success rates (28% to 35%) of pulpal anesthesia.*

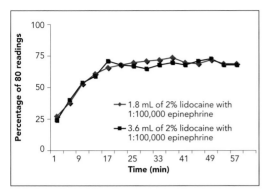

**Fig 2-41** Incidence of mandibular first molar anesthesia: comparison of 3.6 mL and 1.8 mL of 2% lidocaine with 1:100,000 epinephrine. Results determined by lack of response to an EPT at maximum reading (80 reading) across 60 minutes. No significant difference between the two volumes was noted. (Reprinted from Nusstein et al[10] with permission.)

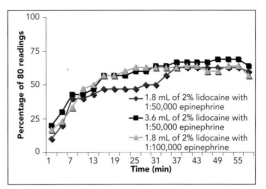

**Fig 2-42** Incidence of mandibular first molar anesthesia: comparison of 3.6 mL of 2% lidocaine with 1:50,000 epinephrine, 1.8 mL of 2% lidocaine with 1:50,000 epinephrine, and 1.8 mL of 2% lidocaine with 1:100,000 epinephrine. Results determined by lack of response to an EPT at maximum reading (80 reading) across 60 minutes. No significant difference among the three volumes was noted. (Reprinted from Wali et al[18] with permission.)

# Attempts to Increase the Success of the IANB in Asymptomatic Patients

The following discussion reviews several methods that have been tried to increase the success of the IANB.

## Increasing the anesthetic volume

One potential method to increase anesthetic success is to double the injection volume of local anesthetic solution. However, increasing the volume of 2% lidocaine with epinephrine to 3.6 mL (two cartridges) does not increase the incidence of pulpal anesthesia with the IANB[2,9,10,14,27,172] (Fig 2-41). Camarda and coauthors[173] reported an increase in success rate with a two-cartridge volume delivered with the CCLAD CompuDent unit (Milestone Scientific), formerly called the *Wand*. However, pulpal anesthesia was not measured—only soft tissue anesthesia. As pointed out earlier, soft tissue anesthesia does not indicate pulpal anesthesia.

**IN CONCLUSION,** *increasing the volume to two cartridges of a lidocaine formulation does not increase pulpal anesthesia in an IANB.*

## Increasing the epinephrine concentration

A second approach for increasing the success of IANBs is to increase the concentration of epinephrine. However, when evaluated in clinically normal teeth, there was no advantage to using a higher concentration (1:50,000) of epinephrine in an IANB.[18,174]

Wali and coauthors[18] concluded that increasing the epinephrine concentration to 1:50,000 in a 2% lidocaine solution or increasing the volume to 3.6 mL of 2% lidocaine with 1:50,000 epinephrine did not result in more successful pulpal anesthesia when compared with 1.8 mL of 2% lidocaine with 1:100,000 epinephrine utilizing the IANB (Fig 2-42).

**IN CONCLUSION,** *increasing the epinephrine concentration in a lidocaine formulation does not increase pulpal anesthesia in an IANB.*

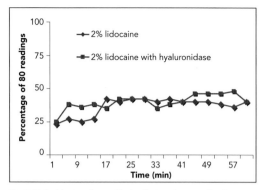

**Fig 2-43** Incidence of mandibular first molar anesthesia: comparison of 2% lidocaine with 1:100,000 epinephrine and a combination of hyaluronidase and 2% lidocaine with 1:100,000 epinephrine in an IANB. Results determined by lack of response to an EPT at maximum reading (80 reading) across 60 minutes. No significant difference between the two solutions was noted. (Reprinted from Ridenour et al[22] with permission.)

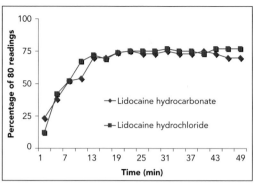

**Fig 2-44** Incidence of mandibular first molar anesthesia: comparison of 2% lidocaine hydrochloride with 1:100,000 epinephrine and 2% lidocaine hydrocarbonate with 1:100,000 epinephrine in an IANB. Results determined by lack of response to an EPT at maximum reading (80 reading) across 60 minutes. No significant difference between the two solutions was noted. (Reprinted from Chaney et al[5] with permission.)

## Hyaluronidase

Hyaluronidase decreases the viscosity of the injected tissue and permits a wider spread of injected fluids.[175] Early studies in dentistry[175,176] found that an IANB was more easily attained and was more complete when hyaluronidase was added to an anesthetic solution. However, Ridenour and coauthors[22] found that adding hyaluronidase to a lidocaine solution with epinephrine did not statistically increase the incidence of pulpal anesthesia in IANBs (Fig 2-43). Additionally, the combined lidocaine/hyaluronidase solution resulted in a significant increase in postoperative pain and trismus.

IN CONCLUSION, *adding hyaluronidase to a lidocaine formulation does not increase pulpal anesthesia in an IANB.*

## Carbonated anesthetic solutions

Experimentally, carbonated anesthetic solutions are more effective due to the trapping of the anesthetic within the nerve.[5] Additionally, carbon dioxide has a synergistic relationship with local anesthetics and a direct depressant action on nerves.[5] However, Chaney and coauthors[5] were not able to demonstrate a superior effect of a carbonated lidocaine formulation in IANBs (Fig 2-44).

According to the Onpharma literature on buffering a local anesthetic, when a sodium bicarbonate solution is mixed with a local anesthetic like lidocaine with epinephrine, carbon dioxide is formed. However, creating carbon dioxide with buffering is very different than a truly carbonated anesthetic solution where the carbon dioxide content is very high.

IN CONCLUSION, *a truly carbonated lidocaine solution does not increase pulpal anesthesia in an IANB.*

## Frequency-dependent conduction blockade of the IANB

Local anesthetic action has been shown to be potentiated by the application of repetitive high-frequency electrical stimulation.[177–180] This action is known as *frequency-dependent, use-dependent,* or *phasic blockade.*[177–179] Despite this evidence, only a few in vivo studies of frequency-dependent blockade have been reported.[181] Stevens and coauthors[181] found that non-noxious electrical stimulation with high frequencies accelerated onset of anesthesia and extended the spread of sensory block

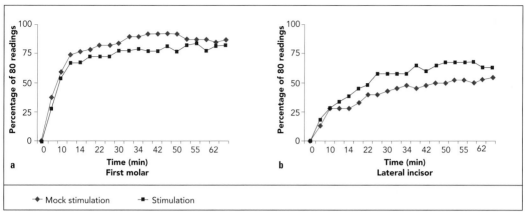

**Fig 2-45** Incidence of first molar (a) and lateral incisor (b) anesthesia as determined by lack of response to an EPT at maximum reading (80 reading), at each postinjection testing interval, for the stimulated and mock-stimulated IANBs. There were no significant differences between the two nerve blocks. Therefore, stimulation of nerves in the presence of local anesthesia (frequency-dependent nerve block) was not statistically superior to an IANB without stimulation. (Reprinted from Hutchison et al[183] with permission.)

for the ulnar nerve. Watson and coauthors[182] demonstrated frequency-dependent conduction block of the median nerve in patients with carpal tunnel syndrome. However, it is unknown how other nerves are affected by frequency-dependent blockade. Differences in the nerve anatomy, physiology, and conductivity as well as in the application of the stimulation may affect the clinical efficacy of frequency-dependent blockade.

Hutchison and coauthors[183] evaluated the degree of pulpal anesthesia obtained with frequency-dependent conduction blockade of the inferior alveolar nerve. In a randomized, single-blind study, 80 adult volunteers received two IANBs: (1) an IANB followed by six 3-minute cycles of continuous electrical stimulation of the first molar or lateral incisor over a period of 64 minutes, and then (2) an IANB followed by mock electrical stimulation using the same cycles. An EPT was used to test for anesthesia (two consecutive 80 readings within 15 minutes and maintained through the 60th minute) of the first molar and lateral incisor.

For the stimulated IANB, the authors found success rates of 35% and 48% for the lateral incisor and first molar, respectively (Fig 2-45). For the mock-stimulated IANB, success was 18% for the lateral incisor and 62% for the first molar. There was no significant difference between the two IANB techniques.

**IN CONCLUSION,** *stimulation of nerves in the presence of local anesthesia (frequency-dependent nerve block) did not statistically increase the success rate of pulpal anesthesia for an IANB.*

## Diphenhydramine as a substitute local anesthetic agent

Diphenhydramine (Benadryl, Johnson & Johnson) has been advocated for patients who are allergic to commonly used local anesthetics. Two older studies found that diphenhydramine was less effective than lidocaine for extractions.[184,185] Willett and coauthors[186] found that diphenhydramine with epinephrine was significantly less effective for pulpal anesthesia than lidocaine with epinephrine for IANBs (Fig 2-46). They also found that the diphenhydramine solution was more painful upon injection and had a high incidence of moderate postoperative pain.

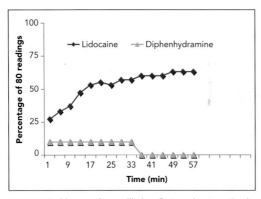

Fig 2-46 Incidence of mandibular first molar anesthesia: comparison of 2% lidocaine with 1:100,000 epinephrine and diphenhydramine with 1:100,000 epinephrine in an IANB. Results determined by lack of response to an EPT at maximum reading (80 reading) across 60 minutes. The solution of diphenhydramine with epinephrine resulted in a very low success rate of pulpal anesthesia. (Reprinted from Willett et al[186] with permission.)

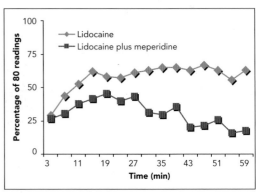

Fig 2-47 Incidence of mandibular first molar anesthesia: comparison of a combination of 2% lidocaine with 1:100,000 epinephrine plus 36 mg meperidine and 2% lidocaine with 1:100,000 epinephrine in an IANB. Results determined by lack of response to an EPT at maximum reading (80 reading) across 60 minutes. The lidocaine with meperidine formulation did not improve pulpal anesthesia and resulted in a declining rate of anesthesia when compared with 2% lidocaine with 1:100,000 epinephrine. (Reprinted from Goodman et al[16] with permission.)

Clause and Zach[187] reported an adverse postoperative reaction to the maxillary anterior injection of 1.8 mL of 1% diphenhydramine with 1:100,000 epinephrine in a dental patient allergic to local anesthetics. Facial edema, extensive nasal swelling with complete occlusion of the nasal passageway, and infraorbital ecchymosis occurred, all of which resolved by 2 weeks.

**IN CONCLUSION,** *diphenhydramine is a poor choice for local anesthesia in patients allergic to common local anesthetic agents.*

## Combination anesthetic solution of meperidine and lidocaine

Investigational and clinical studies in medicine have shown that meperidine (Demerol, Sanofi-Aventis) has local anesthetic effects and may not compete for the same binding site as lidocaine.[16] Therefore, there is a potential for enhancement of a local anesthetic effect if lidocaine is combined with meperidine. However, Goodman and coauthors[16] found that a meperidine and lidocaine combination was less effective than the use of a lidocaine solution in IANBs (Fig 2-47). Bigby and coauthors[188] found that meperidine and lidocaine did not provide better pulpal anesthesia in patients presenting with irreversible pulpitis.

**IN CONCLUSION,** *adding meperidine to lidocaine does not increase pulpal anesthesia in an IANB.*

### Anterior approach for the IANB

Takasugi and coauthors[189] used an anterior approach to the mandibular foramen within the pterygomandibular space. The success rates with this anterior technique were similar to those achieved with the conventional technique.

**IN CONCLUSION,** *the anterior approach to the IANB yielded similar success rates as the conventional approach.*

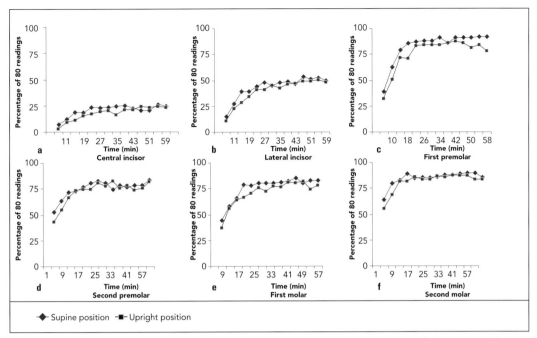

**Fig 2-48** Incidence of pulpal anesthesia following an IANB for the central incisor *(a)*, lateral incisor *(b)*, first premolar *(c)*, second premolar *(d)*, first molar *(e)*, and second molar *(f)* as determined by lack of response to an EPT at maximum reading (80 reading), at each postinjection time interval, for patients in a supine or upright position. There was no significant difference between the two positions. (Reprinted from Crowley[190] with permission.)

## Upright position for administering the IANB

Some clinicians may think that placing the patient in an upright or semiupright position following an IANB allows more of the anesthetic to diffuse in an inferior direction, resulting in better pulpal anesthesia. Crowley[190] compared the degree of pulpal anesthesia obtained with placing the patient in an upright or supine position for an IANB. They found that there was no significant difference between the two positions (Fig 2-48). Takasugi and coauthors[189] also found that a supine position yielded similar success rates as a sitting position for an anterior technique.

    **IN CONCLUSION,** *there is no difference in success of the IANB between a sitting and a supine position.*

## 5% anesthetic formulation for the IANB

Previous studies[191–194] have advocated use of 5% lidocaine with epinephrine to increase the success rate of the IANB. A 5% solution would contain 50 mg per mL or 90 mg per 1.8-mL cartridge. Smith and coauthors[195] studied success of the IANB using 127 mg of lidocaine with epinephrine and found that complete pulpal anesthesia was not obtained (Fig 2-49).

    **IN CONCLUSION,** *a 5% lidocaine solution would still not provide complete pulpal anesthesia.*

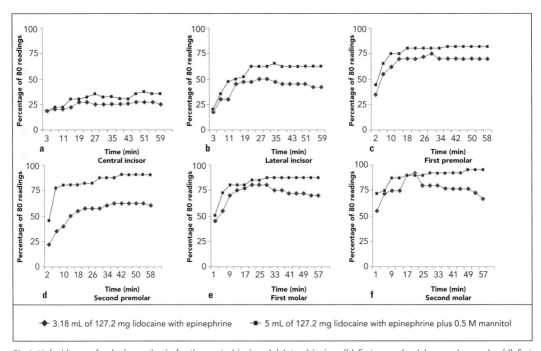

**Fig 2-49** Incidence of pulpal anesthesia for the central incisor *(a)*, lateral incisor *(b)*, first premolar *(c)*, second premolar *(d)*, first molar *(e)*, and second molar *(f)* as determined by lack of response to an EPT at maximum reading (80 reading), at each postinjection time interval, for the two anesthetic formulations. Adding 0.5 M mannitol to 127.2 mg of lidocaine with 50 µg epinephrine was significantly more effective in achieving a greater percentage of total pulpal anesthesia than the same anesthetic formulation without mannitol. (Reprinted from Smith et al[195] with permission.)

# Evaluating Mechanisms of Failure with the IANB

## Accessory innervation—Mylohyoid nerve

Judging from clinical and anatomical studies,[196,197] the mylohyoid nerve is the accessory nerve most often cited as a cause for failure with mandibular anesthesia. Clark and coauthors[9] compared the IANB alone with a combination injection of the IANB plus the mylohyoid nerve block (Fig 2-50), which was aided by the use of a peripheral nerve stimulator (Fig 2-51). The peripheral nerve stimulator was attached to the needle, and the subjects had movement in the floor of the mouth (the mylohyoid muscle) from stimulation of the nerve. The investigators found that the mylohyoid injection did not significantly enhance pulpal anesthesia of the IANB (Figs 2-52 and 2-53). Therefore, the results of the study demonstrate that the mylohyoid nerve is not a major factor in failure with the IANB.

Stein and coauthors[198] felt that bony bridging over the mylohyoid groove may have prevented complete neural blockade in the study by Clark and coauthors.[9] Unfortunately, the authors failed to point out that the injection by Clark and coauthors[9] was aided by a peripheral nerve stimulator, which would not have resulted in mylohyoid muscle activation if there was a bony covering at the target site.

Additionally, a study by Foster and coauthors[15] showed that using a lingual injection of a cartridge of 2% lidocaine with 1:100,000 epinephrine of the first molar following an IANB did not statistically increase pulpal anesthesia. Therefore, the mylohyoid nerve is not a major factor in failure with the IANB.

This follows Fetridge's Law: Important things that are supposed to happen do not happen, especially when people are looking.

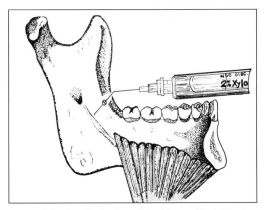

**Fig 2-50** Injection site for the mylohyoid nerve block. (Reprinted from Clark et al[9] with permission.)

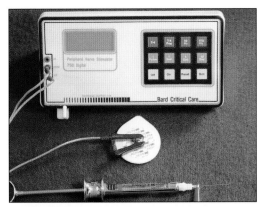

**Fig 2-51** Peripheral nerve stimulator *(top)*, electrocardiograph pad *(middle)*, and syringe with attached needle *(bottom)*. (Reprinted from Simon et al[17] with permission.)

**Fig 2-52** Incidence of mandibular first molar anesthesia: comparison of the IANB plus a mylohyoid injection, a mylohyoid injection alone, and a conventional IANB. Results determined by lack of response to an EPT at maximum reading (80 reading) across 60 minutes. No significant difference between the two IANB techniques was noted. The mylohyoid injection alone resulted in a very poor rate of pulpal anesthesia. (Reprinted from Clark et al[9] with permission.)

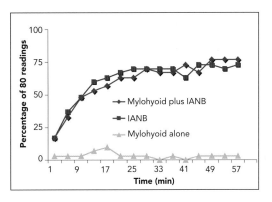

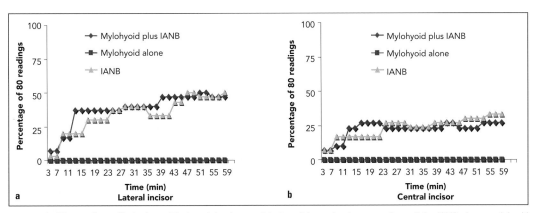

**Fig 2-53** Incidence of mandibular lateral incisor *(a)* and central incisor *(b)* anesthesia: comparison of the IANB plus a mylohyoid injection, a mylohyoid injection alone, and a conventional IANB. Results determined by lack of response to an EPT at maximum reading (80 reading) across 60 minutes. No significant difference between the two IANB techniques was noted. The mylohyoid injection alone resulted in no incidences of pulpal anesthesia. (Reprinted from Clark et al[9] with permission.)

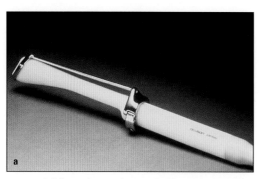
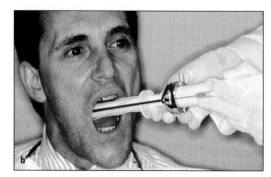

**Fig 2-54** *(a)* Ultrasonic transducer probe. The probe is used rectally to locate the prostate gland. The accompanying needle guide is used to accurately biopsy the prostate tissue. In the study, the needle guide was used to place the needle and anesthetic solution next to the inferior alveolar neurovascular bundle. *(b)* Ultrasonic transducer probe with attached needle guide in the mouth.

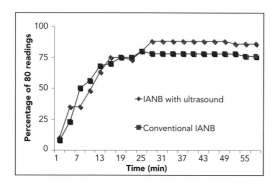

**Fig 2-55** Incidence of mandibular first molar anesthesia: comparison of the IANB using ultrasound location to a conventional IANB. Results determined by lack of response to an EPT at maximum reading (80 reading) across 60 minutes. No significant difference between the two techniques was noted. (Reprinted from Hannan et al[21] with permission.)

Other nerves (buccal, lingual, cervical plexus, and facial) have been cited for failure. Based on the premise that supplementary innervation is supplied by the cervical plexus, Bitner and coauthors[199] described and evaluated an intraoral cervical plexus anesthetic technique. The supplemental injection, using 2% lidocaine with epinephrine, was given on the buccal surface below the roots of the mandibular molars at a 45-degree anterior-posterior inclination. The authors found that the technique resulted in more successful anesthesia than a saline injection. However, the authors did not prove that the cervical nerves were blocked, because a similar supplemental buccal infiltration of the molars will also result in pulpal anesthesia. Further research would be needed to confirm the contribution of the cervical plexus in anesthetic failure in the mandible. The magnitude of failure with the IANB is very difficult to explain by accessory innervation as a major contributor.

**IN CONCLUSION,** *the mylohyoid nerve is not a major factor in failure with the IANB.*

## Accuracy of the injection

It has been theorized that an inaccurate injection contributes to inadequate mandibular anesthesia. While accurate knowledge of anatomy is required for a nerve block, anatomical variation and the fact that the nerves are deeply placed may not allow objective location of the neurovascular bundle. Hannan and coauthors[21] used a medical ultrasound unit to guide needle placement for IANBs. The transducer probe with attached needle guide (Fig 2-54a) was used to place the needle next to the neurovascular bundle using the doppler feature of the unit for direct visualization. Figure 2-54b shows the probe within the mouth. Notice the attached needle guide. While the authors found that the nerve block administered with ultrasound was accurate, it did not result in more successful pulpal anesthesia than a conventionally administered IANB (Fig 2-55). Chanpong and coauthors[200] were able to

**Fig 2-56** Incidence of mandibular first molar anesthesia: comparison of the IANB using a peripheral nerve stimulator to a conventional IANB. Results determined by lack of response to an EPT at maximum reading (80 reading) across 60 minutes. No significant difference between the two techniques was noted. (Reprinted from Simon et al[17] with permission.)

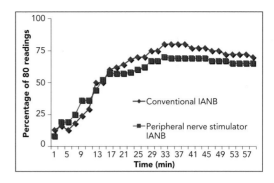

visualize the inferior alveolar nerve with ultrasound. However, they did not perform a clinical study to confirm that the technique resulted in more successful anesthesia.

In medicine, peripheral nerve stimulators are used for regional nerve blocks and to assess the degree of neuromuscular blockade achieved.[201] Peripheral nerve stimulators produce an electrical current through the needle tip to stimulate the nerve. Simon and coauthors[17] compared the degree of pulpal anesthesia obtained with the IANB administered using a peripheral nerve stimulator (see Fig 2-51) compared with a conventional IANB using a cartridge of 2% lidocaine with 1:100,000 epinephrine. They found that the IANB administered using a peripheral nerve stimulator did not increase the success rate of pulpal anesthesia when compared with a conventional IANB (Fig 2-56). Therefore, inaccurate needle placement is not the primary reason for anesthetic failure with this block.

Two studies performed over 30 years ago reached similar conclusions. Berns and Sadove[202] and Galbreath[203] used radiopaque dyes and radiographs to locate the mandibular foramen and found that accurate needle location did not guarantee successful anesthesia. Twenty-five percent of accurate blocks resulted in anesthetic failure. The authors speculated that migration of the anesthetic solution followed the path of least resistance. This was determined by fascial planes and structures encountered in the pterygomandibular space. Using magnetic resonance imaging (MRI) to evaluate the distribution and absorption of local anesthetic solutions after an IANB, Ay and coauthors[204] concluded that "one cannot show a correlation between area of distribution and rate of absorption as detected on MRI with onset and duration." These studies provide an important clinical point: The lack of pulpal anesthesia is not necessarily due to an inaccurate injection.

And yet many clinicians blame failure on an inaccurate injection. But you want to remember Mencken's Meta-law: For every human problem, there is a neat, plain solution—and it is usually wrong.

**IN CONCLUSION,** *once lip numbness is achieved, lack of pulpal anesthesia is not due to an inaccurate IANB.*

## It is not your fault!

One important fact to remember is that even though profound lip anesthesia is achieved, patients do not always achieve pulpal anesthesia. However, it is not your fault of giving an inaccurate injection.

## Average needle depth for an IANB

Malamed[45] recommends a depth of needle penetration of 20 to 25 mm for an IANB. Bremer[205] found the mean needle depth to be 24 mm. Menke and Gowgiel[206] found a mean depth of 16 mm. Therefore, there is some variation in the recommendations for needle depth. Hannan and coauthors[21] compared depth of needle penetration for an IANB using ultrasound location and a conventional technique.

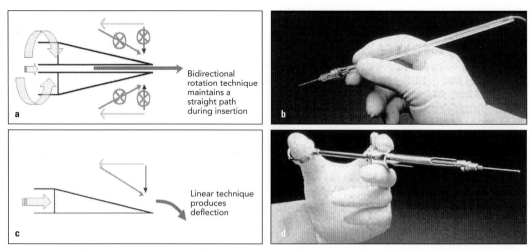

a    Bidirectional rotation technique maintains a straight path during insertion

b

c    Linear technique produces deflection

d

**Fig 2-57** *(a and b)* The clockwise-counterclockwise movement of the bidirectional rotation technique is only possible using the handpiece assembly of the CompuDent CCLAD system. *(c and d)* The thumb grasp on a traditional syringe does not allow rotation. (Reprinted from Kennedy et al[214] with permission.)

They found that the average depth of needle penetration was 19 mm for the conventional IANB and 17 mm for the IANB using ultrasound. Hutchison and coauthors[183] found an average depth of 18 mm. Simon and coauthors[17] reported that the mean depth of needle penetration was 19 mm for both the IANB administered with the peripheral nerve stimulator and the conventional IANB. The results obtained with the peripheral nerve stimulator are closer to the findings of Hannan and coauthors[21] using ultrasound location. Thangavelu and coauthors[207] found that the foramen was 19 ± 2.34 mm from the coronoid notch of the anterior border of the mandible. Chanpong and coauthors[200] were able to visualize the inferior alveolar nerve with ultrasound and found that the average depth to the inferior alveolar nerve measured around 20 mm.

    **IN CONCLUSION,** *the exact needle depth for an IANB varies between studies. The best estimate is approximately 19 mm.*

## Needle deflection and the bidirectional technique

Needle deflection has been theorized as a cause for failure with the IANB.[208–210] Various authors using in vitro methods have reported that beveled needles, when passed through substances of varying densities, will deflect toward the nonbeveled side; ie, the needle will deflect away from the bevel.[208–213] Recently, Hochman and Friedman[210] developed a bidirectional needle rotation technique using the CompuDent CCLAD system. A conventional syringe cannot be rotated because of the ring assembly (Fig 2-57). The bidirectional technique rotates the CCLAD system handpiece assembly and needle in a manner similar to rotation of an endodontic hand file. The technique was found to reduce needle deflection during needle insertion. Kennedy and coauthors[214] compared the anesthetic efficacy of the conventional IANB, administered with the needle bevel oriented away from the mandibular ramus (so the needle would deflect toward the mandibular foramen), and the bidirectional needle rotation technique, administered using the CCLAD anesthesia system, in patients diagnosed with irreversible pulpitis. There were no significant differences between the success rates (50% for the conventional and 56% for the bidirectional) of the two techniques. Neither technique resulted in an acceptable rate of anesthetic success in patients with irreversible pulpitis.

    **IN CONCLUSION,** *the bidirectional technique with the CCLAD system does not increase the success of the IANB.*

**Fig 2-58** Incidence of mandibular first molar anesthesia: comparison of the IANB using a needle bevel oriented away from the mandibular foramen and toward the mandibular foramen. Results determined by lack of response to an EPT at maximum reading (80 reading) across 60 minutes. No significant difference between the two needle bevels was noted. (Reprinted from Steinkruger et al[12] with permission.)

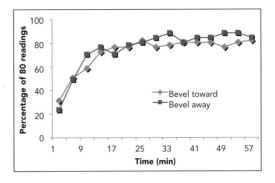

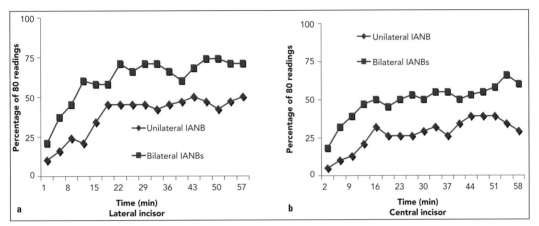

**Fig 2-59** Incidence of mandibular lateral incisor (a) and central incisor (b) anesthesia: comparison of bilateral IANBs versus a unilateral IANB. Results determined by lack of response to an EPT at maximum reading (80 reading) across 60 minutes. While the bilateral IANBs showed a higher incidence of success, pulpal anesthesia was less than 75%. (Reprinted from Yonchak et al[27] with permission.)

## Needle bevel

In pain-free subjects, Steinkruger and coauthors[12] found that the orientation of the needle bevel (away or toward the mandibular ramus) for an IANB did not affect anesthetic success or failure (Fig 2-58). Therefore, the use of commercial needles with markers to indicate needle bevel is not necessary.

**IN CONCLUSION,** *the orientation of the needle bevel does not affect the success of the IANB.*

## Cross innervation

Cross innervation from the contralateral inferior alveolar nerve has been implicated in failure to achieve anesthesia in anterior teeth after an IANB. Experimentally, cross innervation does occur in mandibular central and lateral incisors[27,215] but plays a very small role in failure with the IANB. Cross innervation is not the major reason for failure in incisor teeth—it is the failure of the IANB to adequately anesthetize these teeth. Administering bilateral IANBs does not anesthetize the central and lateral incisors[27] (Fig 2-59).

**IN CONCLUSION,** *cross innervation is not the major reason for failure in incisor teeth with the IANB.*

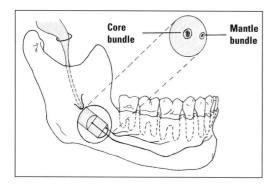

**Fig 2-60** Central core theory. The axons in the mantle bundle supply the molars, and those in the core bundle supply the anterior teeth. The extraneural local anesthetic solution diffuses from the mantle to the core. (Concept borrowed from de Jong.[220])

### Bifid mandibular canals

Langlais and coauthors[216] reported an incidence of 0.95% bifid canals in panoramic radiographs. More recent studies[217,218] using cone beam computed tomography have reported an incidence ranging from 16% to 65%.

Although case reports of inadequate mandibular anesthesia due to bifid canals have been reported,[219] the exact relationship of bifid canals to anesthetic failure needs further study.

**IN CONCLUSION,** *while bifid canals have been reported in the mandible, the exact relationship to failure needs further research.*

# Why Do Asymptomatic Patients Not Achieve Pulpal Anesthesia with the IANB?

The central core theory may be the best explanation for why asymptomatic patients do not achieve pulpal anesthesia with the IANB.[220,221] The theory states that nerves on the outside of the nerve bundle supply molars, while nerves on the inside of the bundle supply anterior teeth (Fig 2-60). The anesthetic solution may not diffuse into the nerve trunk to reach all nerves to produce an adequate block, even if deposited at the correct site. The theory may explain the higher experimental failure rates in anterior teeth with the IANB.[2–5,9,23]

Remember Stephen's Soliloquy: Nothing is perfect. There are usually lumps in it.

Additionally, even if deposited at the correct site, the anesthetic solution may move away from the nerve and follow the path of least resistance within the pterygomandibular space, which makes accurate needle placement moot.[202,203]

**IN CONCLUSION,** *the best explanation for failure with the IANB relates to the central core theory and the movement of anesthetic solution to follow the path of least resistance.*

# Methods to Increase the Success of Mandibular Anesthesia in Asymptomatic Patients

### Buccal infiltration of articaine to the first molar following an IANB

As discussed previously, Haase and coauthors[70] found that an infiltration of 1.8 mL of 4% articaine with 1:100,000 epinephrine resulted in a higher success rate (two consecutive 80 readings were achieved

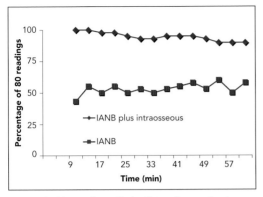

Fig 2-61 Incidence of mandibular first molar anesthesia: comparison of the combination intraosseous injection of 2% lidocaine with 1:100,000 epinephrine plus the IANB and the IANB alone. Results determined by lack of response to an EPT at maximum reading (80 reading) across 60 minutes. The combination technique was significantly better at all postinjection times. (Reprinted from Dunbar et al[6] with permission.)

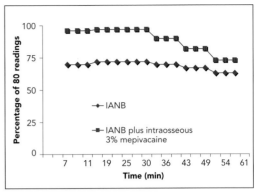

Fig 2-62 Incidence of mandibular first molar anesthesia: comparison of the combination intraosseous injection with 3% mepivacaine plus the IANB and the IANB alone. Results determined by lack of response to an EPT at maximum reading (80 reading) across 60 minutes. The combination technique proved significantly better for approximately 30 minutes. (Reprinted from Gallatin et al[26] with permission.)

within 10 minutes following the IANB plus infiltration injections, and the 80 reading was continuously sustained through 60 minutes) of 88% when compared with an infiltration of 1.8 mL of 2% lidocaine with 1:100,000 epinephrine (71% success rate) in the first molar following an IANB (see Fig 2-38).

IN CONCLUSION, *an articaine infiltration of the first molar following an IANB should provide pulpal anesthesia for approximately 1 hour.*

## Supplemental intraosseous injections

### *Local anesthetic agents with vasoconstrictors*

Dunbar and coauthors[6] and Guglielmo and coauthors[28] studied the contribution of the supplemental intraosseous injection after an IANB. Using common local anesthetic agents with vasoconstrictors and the Stabident intraosseous system (Fairfax Dental), anesthetic success was significantly increased for 60 minutes in the first molar (Fig 2-61). Additionally, the intraosseous injection significantly decreased the incidence of slow onset of pulpal anesthesia to 0% when compared with the IANB alone (18% incidence).[6] Therefore, when pulpal anesthesia is required in asymptomatic teeth, the addition of the intraosseous injection to the IANB in the first molar will provide a quick onset and a high incidence of pulpal anesthesia for 60 minutes.

IN CONCLUSION, *when used as supplemental intraosseous injections, lidocaine and mepivacaine formulations with vasoconstrictors allow quick onset and increase the success of the IANB for approximately 60 minutes.*

### *3% mepivacaine plain*

Gallatin and coauthors[26] found that the use of 3% mepivacaine as a supplemental intraosseous injection following an IANB resulted in statistically increased pulpal anesthesia for 30 minutes (Fig 2-62). The shorter duration of the 3% mepivacaine when compared with 2% lidocaine with 1:100,000 epinephrine[6] was related to the lack of a vasoconstrictor.

IN CONCLUSION, *when used as a supplemental intraosseous injection, 3% mepivacaine increases the success of the IANB, but the duration is approximately 30 minutes.*

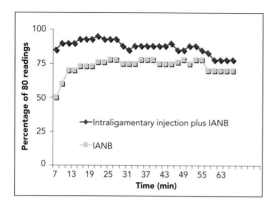

Fig 2-63 Incidence of mandibular first molar anesthesia: comparison of the combination intraligamentary injection plus the IANB and the IANB alone. Results determined by lack of response to an EPT at maximum reading (80 reading) across 60 minutes. The combination technique proved significantly better for approximately 23 minutes. (Reprinted from Childers et al[8] with permission.)

## Supplemental intraligamentary injection

Childers and coauthors[8] studied the contribution of the supplemental intraligamantary injection after an IANB. Using 2% lidocaine with 1:100,000 epinephrine and a high-pressure syringe, anesthetic success was significantly increased for 23 minutes in the first molar (Fig 2-63). The short incidence of anesthesia was related to the small amount of anesthetic solution administered.

IN CONCLUSION, *a supplemental intraligamentary injection of 2% lidocaine with 1:100,000 epinephrine increases the success of the IANB, but the duration is approximately 23 minutes.*

### Injection speed

Kanaa and coauthors[222] found that a slow IANB injection (60 seconds) resulted in higher success rates than a rapid injection (15 seconds) in asymptomatic subjects, and it was less painful. de Souza and coauthors[223] found no difference in pain between a slow injection over 60 seconds and even slower injection over 100 seconds for IANB.

IN CONCLUSION, *a slow IANB (60 seconds) increases success of the IANB in asymptomatic subjects and is less painful.*

### Effect of administration of anesthetic solution during needle placement

McCartney and coauthors[224] found that deposition of 0.2 to 0.4 mL of anesthetic solution during needle placement, using a standard syringe, for the IANB did not result in significant anesthesia of the soft tissue ahead of the needle path in patients with irreversible pulpitis. Further research needs to address ways to reduce pain during needle placement.

IN CONCLUSION, *depositing anesthetic solution during needle placement using a standard syringe does not reduce pain of the IANB.*

### Mannitol

In an experimental study of an isolated nerve, Popitz-Bergez and coauthors[225] found that the concentration of lidocaine within the nerve was only 2% of the injected dose during full block. Therefore, only a small amount of injected local anesthesia penetrates into the nerve. It is possible that trying to increase this amount would lead to better anesthesia.

**Fig 2-64** Incidence of mandibular first molar anesthesia: comparison of 2% lidocaine with epinephrine plus 0.5 M mannitol and 2% lidocaine with 1:100,000 epinephrine in an IANB. Results determined by lack of response to an EPT at maximum reading (80 reading) across 60 minutes. The combination technique improved anesthetic success.

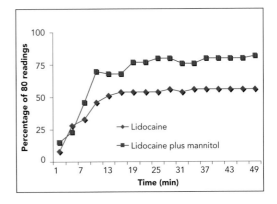

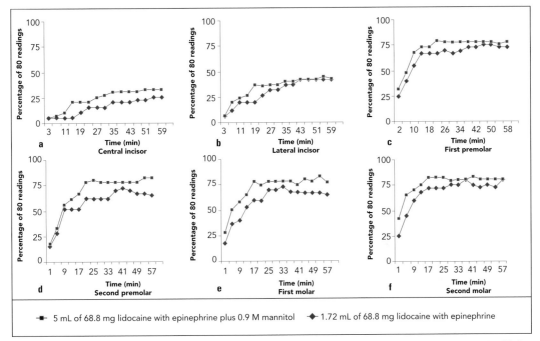

**Fig 2-65** Incidence of pulpal anesthesia for the central incisor (a), lateral incisor (b), first premolar (c), second premolar (d), first molar (e), and second molar (f) as determined by lack of response to an EPT at maximum reading (80 reading), at each postinjection time interval, for the two anesthetic formulations. Adding 0.9 M mannitol to 68.8 mg of lidocaine with 50 µg epinephrine was significantly more effective in achieving a greater percentage of total pulpal anesthesia than the same anesthetic formulation without mannitol. However, the 0.9 M mannitol/lidocaine formulation would not provide complete pulpal anesthesia for the mandibular teeth. (Reprinted from Cohen et al[227] with permission.)

The Ohio State University group studied the use of mannitol to increase the efficacy of nerve blocks. Mannitol (a hyperosmotic sugar solution) temporarily disrupts the protective covering (perineurium) of sensory nerves, allowing the local anesthetic agent to gain entry to the innermost part of the nerve.[226] Without the mannitol, the perineurium is a barrier to the diffusion of the local anesthetic into the nerve. They found that mannitol in combination with lidocaine increased anesthetic success approximately 15% to 20% (Figs 2-64 to 2-66; see also Fig 2-49).[40,195,227] Therefore, there is an effect, but mannitol does not provide complete pulpal anesthesia and is not available clinically.

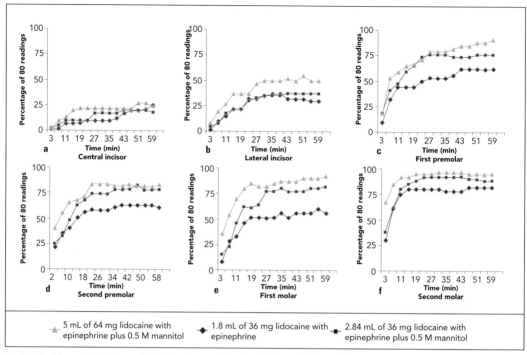

5 mL of 64 mg lidocaine with epinephrine plus 0.5 M mannitol

1.8 mL of 36 mg lidocaine with epinephrine

2.84 mL of 36 mg lidocaine with epinephrine plus 0.5 M mannitol

**Fig 2-66** Incidence of pulpal anesthesia for the central incisor *(a)*, lateral incisor *(b)*, first premolar *(c)*, second premolar *(d)*, first molar *(e)*, and second molar *(f)* as determined by lack of response to an EPT at maximum reading (80 reading), at each postinjection time interval, for the three anesthetic formulations. Adding 0.5 M mannitol to lidocaine with epinephrine formulations was significantly more effective in achieving a greater percentage of total pulpal anesthesia than a lidocaine formulation without mannitol. (Reprinted from Wolf et al[40] with permission.)

For a maxillary infiltration, Younkin and coauthors[228] found that the addition of 0.5 M mannitol to a lidocaine formulation did not increase pulpal anesthesia. Mannitol only has an effect for nerve blocks, not infiltration anesthesia.

**IN CONCLUSION,** *mannitol increases the success of the IANB by 15% to 20%, but it is not available clinically.*

# Final Thoughts

One additional solution to achieving mandibular anesthesia was offered by Dr Guido Fischer[229] in 1914—the stasis bandage. He described the technique as follows:

> The band is fitted around the patient's neck and adjusted by means of a number of eyelets [Fig 2-67]. The bandage should be tight enough to cause the face to be reddened but not bluish in coloration. The bandage produces blood stasis thus retaining the anesthetic solution in the desired field and improving anesthesia.[229]

There is no proof that the bandage works, and we should be glad we can administer supplemental injections instead.

Further research is still indicated to increase the success of the IANB. We think we can summarize the need to continue to study mandibular anesthesia by stating Soderquist's Conclusion: A bird doesn't stop looking even if the worms are scarce. And one day we will succeed if we put our ingenuity and minds to the task, which leads to Offenberger's Corollary: The early bird may get the worm, but the second mouse gets the cheese.

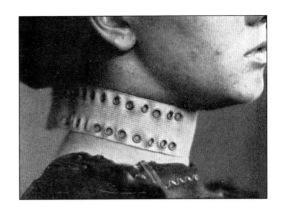

**Fig 2-67** Stasis bandage applied around the patient's neck. (Reprinted from Fischer and Riethmuller.[229])

# References

1. Kaufman E, Weinstein P, Milgrom P. Difficulties in achieving local anesthesia. J Am Dent Assoc 1984;108:205–208.
2. Vreeland DL, Reader A, Beck M, Meyers W, Weaver J. An evaluation of volumes and concentrations of lidocaine in human inferior alveolar nerve block. J Endod 1989;15:6–12.
3. Hinkley SA, Reader A, Beck M, Meyers WJ. An evaluation of 4% prilocaine with 1:200,000 epinephrine and 2% mepivacaine with 1:20,000 levonordefrin compared with 2% lidocaine with 1:100,000 epinephrine for inferior alveolar nerve block. Anesth Prog 1991;38:84–89.
4. McLean C, Reader A, Beck M, Meyers WJ. An evaluation of 4% prilocaine and 3% mepivacaine compared with 2% lidocaine (1:100,000 epinephrine) for inferior alveolar nerve block. J Endod 1993;19:146–150.
5. Chaney MA, Kerby R, Reader A, Beck FM, Meyers WJ, Weaver J. An evaluation of lidocaine hydrocarbonate compared with lidocaine hydrochloride for inferior alveolar nerve block. Anesth Prog 1991;38:212–216.
6. Dunbar D, Reader A, Nist R, Beck M, Meyers WJ. Anesthetic efficacy of the intraosseous injection after an inferior alveolar nerve block. J Endod 1996;22:481–486.
7. Nist RA, Reader A, Beck M, Meyers WJ. An evaluation of the incisive nerve block and combination inferior alveolar and incisive nerve blocks in mandibular anesthesia. J Endod 1992;18:455–459.
8. Childers M, Reader A, Nist R, Beck M, Meyers WJ. Anesthetic efficacy of the periodontal ligament injection after an inferior alveolar nerve block. J Endod 1996;22:317–320.
9. Clark S, Reader A, Beck M, Meyers WJ. Anesthetic efficacy of the mylohyoid nerve block and combination inferior alveolar nerve block/mylohyoid nerve block. Oral Surg Oral Med Oral Pathol Oral Radiol Endod 1999;87:557–563.
10. Nusstein J, Reader A, Beck FM. Anesthetic efficacy of different volumes of lidocaine with epinephrine for inferior alveolar nerve blocks. Gen Dent 2002;50:372–377.
11. Mikesell P, Nusstein J, Reader A, Beck M, Weaver J. A comparison of articaine and lidocaine for inferior alveolar nerve blocks. J Endod 2005;31:265–270.
12. Steinkruger G, Nusstein J, Reader A, Beck M, Weaver J. The significance of needle bevel orientation in success of the inferior alveolar nerve block. J Am Dent Assoc 2006;137:1685–1691.
13. Fernandez C, Reader A, Beck M, Nusstein J. A prospective, randomized, double-blind comparison of bupivacaine and lidocaine for inferior alveolar nerve blocks. J Endod 2005;31:499–503.
14. Goldberg S, Reader A, Drum M, Nusstein J, Beck M. Comparison of the anesthetic efficacy of the conventional inferior alveolar, Gow-Gates, and Vazirani-Akinosi techniques. J Endod 2008;34:1306–1311.
15. Foster W, McCartney M, Reader A, Beck M. Anesthetic efficacy of buccal and lingual infiltrations of lidocaine following an inferior alveolar nerve block in mandibular posterior teeth. Anesth Prog 2007;54:163–169.
16. Goodman A, Reader A, Nusstein J, Beck M. Anesthetic efficacy of lidocaine/meperidine for inferior alveolar nerve blocks. Anesth Prog 2006;53:131–139.
17. Simon F, Reader A, Drum M, Nusstein J, Beck M. A prospective, randomized single-blind study of the anesthetic efficacy of the inferior alveolar nerve block administered with a peripheral nerve stimulator. J Endod 2010;36:429–433.
18. Wali M, Drum M, Reader A, Nusstein J. Prospective, randomized, single-blind study of the anesthetic efficacy of 1.8 and 3.6 milliliters of 2% lidocaine with 1:50,000 epinephrine for the inferior alveolar nerve block. J Endod 2010;36:1459–1462.
19. Lai TN, Lin CP, Kok SH, et al. Evaluation of mandibular block using a standardized method. Oral Surg Oral Med Oral Pathol Oral Radiol Endod 2006;102:462–468.
20. American Dental Association Survey Center. Snapshots of American dentistry: Appointment length. ADA News 2009;40(16):4.
21. Hannan L, Reader A, Nist R, Beck M, Meyers WJ. The use of ultrasound for guiding needle placement for inferior alveolar nerve blocks. Oral Surg Oral Med Oral Pathol Oral Radiol Endod 1999;87:658–665.

22. Ridenour S, Reader A, Beck M, Weaver J. Anesthetic efficacy of a combination of hyaluronidase and lidocaine with epinephrine in inferior alveolar nerve blocks. Anesth Prog 2001;48:9–15.

23. Clark K, Reader A, Beck M, Meyers WJ. Anesthetic efficacy of an infiltration in mandibular anterior teeth following an inferior alveolar nerve block. Anesth Prog 2002;49:49–55.

24. Reitz J, Reader A, Nist R, Beck M, Meyers WJ. Anesthetic efficacy of the intraosseous injection of 0.9 mL of 2% lidocaine (1:100,000 epinephrine) to augment an inferior alveolar nerve block. Oral Surg Oral Med Oral Pathol Oral Radiol Endod 1998;86:516–523.

25. Stabile P, Reader A, Gallatin E, Beck M, Weaver J. Anesthetic efficacy and heart rate effects of the intraosseous injection of 1.5% etidocaine (1:200,000 epinephrine) after an inferior alveolar nerve block. Oral Surg Oral Med Oral Pathol Oral Radiol Endod 2000;89:407–411.

26. Gallatin E, Stabile P, Reader A, Nist R, Beck M. Anesthetic efficacy and heart rate effects of the intraosseous injection of 3% mepivacaine after an inferior alveolar nerve block. Oral Surg Oral Med Oral Pathol Oral Radiol Endod 2000;89:83–87.

27. Yonchak T, Reader A, Beck M, Meyers WJ. Anesthetic efficacy of unilateral and bilateral inferior alveolar nerve blocks to determine cross innervation in anterior teeth. Oral Surg Oral Med Oral Pathol Oral Radiol Endod 2001;92:132–135.

28. Guglielmo A, Reader A, Nist R, Beck M, Weaver J. Anesthetic efficacy and heart rate effects of the supplemental intraosseous injection of 2% mepivacaine with 1:20,000 levonordefrin. Oral Surg Oral Med Oral Pathol Oral Radiol Endod 1999;87:284–293.

29. Ågren E, Danielsson K. Conduction block analgesia in the mandible: A comparative investigation of the techniques of Fischer and Gow-Gates. Swed Dent J 1981;5:81–89.

30. Hersh EV, Hermann DG, Lamp CJ, Johnson PD, MacAfee KA. Assessing the duration of mandibular soft tissue anesthesia. J Am Dent Assoc 1995;126:1531–1536.

31. Fowler S, Reader A, Beck M. Incidence of missed inferior alveolar nerve blocks in vital asymptomatic subjects and in patients with symptomatic irreversible pulpitis. J Endod 2015;41:637–639.

32. Malamed S. Handbook of Local Anesthesia, ed 6. St Louis: Mosby, 2012:387.

33. Krediet AC, Moayeri N, Bleys RL, Groen GJ. Intraneural or extraneural: Diagnostic accuracy of ultrasound assessment for localizing low-volume injection. Reg Anesth Pain Med 2014;39:409–413.

34. Brownbill JW, Walker PO, Bourcy BD, Keenan KM. Comparison of inferior dental nerve block injections in child patients using 30-gauge and 25-gauge short needles. Anesth Prog 1987;34:215–219.

35. Vasconcellos RJ, Vasconcelos BC, Genú PR. Influence of local anesthethics with adrenalina 1:100.000 in basic vital constants during third molar surgery. Med Oral Patol Oral Cir Bucal 2008;13:E431–E437.

36. Danielsson K, Evers H, Nordenram A. Aspiration in oral local anaesthesia. Frequency of blood in cartridges in an undergraduate student material. Swed Dent J 1984;8:265–269.

37. Kuster CG, Udin RD. Frequency of accidental intravascular injection of local anesthetics in children. ASDC J Dent Child 1985;52:183–187.

38. Delgado-Molina E, Bueno-Lafuente S, Berini-Aytés L, Gay-Escoda C. Comparative study of different syringes in positive aspiration during inferior alveolar nerve block. Oral Surg Oral Med Oral Pathol Oral Radiol Endod 1999;88:557–560.

39. Delgado-Molina E, Tamarit-Borrás M, Berini-Aytés L, Gay-Escoda C. Evaluation and comparison of 2 needle models in terms of blood aspiration during truncal block of the inferior alveolar nerve. J Oral Maxillofac Surg 2003;61:1011–1015.

40. Wolf R, Reader A, Drum M, Nusstein J, Beck M. Anesthetic efficacy of combinations of 0.5 m mannitol and lidocaine with epinephrine in inferior alveolar nerve blocks: A prospective randomized, single-blind study. Anesth Prog 2011;58:157–165.

41. Wright EF. Medial pterygoid trismus (myospasm) following inferior alveolar nerve block: Case report and literature review. Gen Dent 2011;59:64–67.

42. Cohen H, Cha B, Spangberg L. Endodontic anesthesia in mandibular molars: A clinical study. J Endod 1993;19:370–373.

43. Lammers E, Nusstein J, Reader A, Drum M, Beck M, Fowler S. Does the combination of 3% mepivacaine plain plus 2% lidocaine with epinephrine improve anesthesia and reduce the pain of anesthetic injection for the inferior alveolar nerve block? A prospective, randomized, double-blind study. J Endod 2014;40:1287–1292.

44. Rood JP, Caruana PE, Danford M, Pateromichelakis S. Prilocaine—An investigation into its use in the presence of inflammation and in combination with lignocaine. J Dent 1981;9:240–247.

45. Malamed S. Handbook of Local Anesthesia, ed 5. St Louis: Mosby, 2004.

46. Malamed SF, Gagnon F, Leblanc D. Articaine hydrochloride: A study of the safety of a new amide local anesthetic. J Am Dent Assoc 2001;132:177–185.

47. Wright G, Weinberger S, Friedman C, Plotzke O. The use of articaine local anesthesia in children under 4 years of age—A retrospective report. Anesth Prog 1989;36:268–271.

48. Hidding J, Khoury F. General complications in dental local anesthesia [in German]. Dtsch Zahnarztl Z 1991;46:834–836.

49. Moller R, Covino B. Cardiac electrophysiologic effects of articaine compared with bupivacaine and lidocaine. Anesth Analg 1993;76:1266–1273.

50. Jakobs W, Ladwig B, Cichon P, Ortel R, Kirch W. Serum levels of articaine 2% and 4% in children. Anesth Prog 1995;42:113–115.

51. Daublander M, Muller R, Lipp M. The incidence of complications associated with local anesthesia in dentistry. Anesth Prog 1997;44:132–144.

52. Simon M, Gielen M, Alberink N, Vree T, van Egmond J. Intravenous regional anesthesia with 0.5% articaine, 0.5% lidocaine, or 0.5% prilocaine. A double-blind randomized clinical study. Reg Anesth 1997;22:29–34.

53. Oertel R, Ebert U, Rahn R, Kirch WT. The effect of age on pharmacokinetics of the local anesthetic drug articaine. Reg Anesth Pain Med 1999;24:524–528.

54. Leuschner J, Leblanc D. Studies on the toxicological profile of the local anesthetic articaine. Arzneimittelforschung 1999;49:126–132.

55. Malamed S, Gagnon S, Leblanc D. A comparison between articaine HCl and lidocaine HCl in pediatric dental patients. Pediatr Dent 2000;22:307–311.

56. Dogan N, Uçok C, Korkmaz C, Uçok O, Karasu HA. The effects of articaine hydrochloride on wound healing: An experimental study. J Oral Maxillofac Surg 2003;61:1467–1470.

57. Wilburn-Goo D, Lloyd L. When patients become cyanotic: Acquired methemoglobinemia. J Am Dent Assoc 1999;130:826–831.

58. Haas DA, Lennon D. A 21-year retrospective study of reports of paresthesia following local anesthetic administration. J Can Dent Assoc 1995;61:319–320,323–326,329–330.

59. Miller P, Lennon D. Incidence of local anesthetic-induced neuropathies in Ontario from 1994–1998 [abstract]. J Dent Res 2000;79:627.

60. Gaffen AS, Haas DA. Retrospective review of voluntary reports of nonsurgical paresthesia in dentistry. J Canadian Dent Assoc 2009;75:579.

61. Garisto GA, Gaffen AS, Lawrence HP, Tenenbaum HC, Haas DA. Occurence of paresthesia after dental local anesthetic administration in the United States. J Am Dent Assoc 2010;141:836–844.

62. Pogrel M. Permanent nerve damage from inferior alveolar nerve blocks—An update to include articaine. J Calif Dent Assoc 2007;35:271–273.

63. Pogrel MA. Permanent nerve damage from inferior alveolar nerve blocks: A current update. J Calif Dent Assoc 2012;40:795–797.

64. Hoffmeister B. Morphological changes of peripheral nerves following intraneural injection of local anesthetic [in German]. Dtsch Zahnarztl Z 1991;46:828–830.

65. Ribeiro PD Jr, Sanches MG, Okamoto T. Comparative analysis of tissue reactions to anesthetic solutions: Histological analysis in subcutaneous tissue of rats. Anesth Prog 2003;50:169–180.

66. Baroni DB, Franz-Montan M, Cogo K, et al. Effect of articaine on mental nerve anterior portion: Histological analysis in rats. Acta Odontol Scand 2013;71:82–87.

67. Abdulwahab M, Boynes S, Moore P, et al. The efficacy of six local anesthetic formulations used for posterior mandibular buccal infiltration anesthesia. J Am Dent Assoc 2009;140:1018–1024.

68. Robertson D, Nusstein J, Reader A, Beck M, McCartney M. The anesthetic efficacy of articaine in buccal infiltration of mandibular posterior teeth. J Am Dent Assoc 2007;138:1104–1112.

69. Kanaa MD, Whitworth JM, Corbett IP, Meechan JG. Articaine and lidocaine mandibular buccal infiltration anesthesia: A prospective randomized double-blind cross-over study. J Endod 2006;32:296–298.

70. Haase A, Reader A, Nusstein J, Beck M, Drum M. Comparing anesthetic efficacy of articaine versus lidocaine as a supplemental buccal infiltration of the mandibular first molar after an inferior alveolar nerve block. J Am Dent Assoc 2008;139:1228–1235.

71. Kanaa MD, Whitworth JM, Corbett IP, Meechan JG. Articaine buccal infiltration enhances the effectiveness of lidocaine inferior alveolar nerve block. Int Endod J 2009;42:238–246.

72. Borchard U, Drouin H. Carticaine: Action of the local anesthetic on myelinated nerve fibres. Eur J Pharmacol 1980;62:73–79.

73. Potocnik I, Tomsic M, Sketelj J, Bajrovic FF. Articaine is more effective than lidocaine or mepivacaine in rat sensory nerve conduction block in vitro. J Dent Res 2006;85:162–166.

74. Skjevik AA, Haug BE, Lygre H, Teigen K. Intramolecular hydrogen bonding in articaine can be related to superior bone tissue penetration: A molecular dynamics study. Biophys Chem 2011;154:18–25.

75. Nydegger B, Nusstein J, Reader A, Drum M, Beck M. Anesthetic comparisons of 4% concentrations of articaine, lidocaine, and prilocaine as primary buccal infiltrations of the mandibular first molar: A prospective randomized, double-blind study. J Endod 2014;40:1912–1916.

76. Malamed S. Articaine versus lidocaine: The author responds. J Calif Dent Assoc 2007;35:383–385.

77. Schertzer E, Malamed S. Articaine vs lidocaine. J Am Dent Assoc 2000;131:1248,1250.

78. Malamed S, Gagnon S, Leblanc D. Efficacy of articaine: A new amide local anesthetic. J Am Dent Assoc 2000;131:635–642.

79. Donaldson D, James-Perdok L, Craig B, Derkson G, Richardson A. A comparison of Ultracaine DS (articaine HCl) and Citanest forte (prilocaine HCl) in maxillary infiltration and mandibular nerve block. J Can Dent Assoc 1987;53:38–42.

80. Haas D, Harper D, Saso M, Young E. Comparison of articaine and prilocaine anesthesia by infiltration in maxillary and mandibular arches. Anesth Prog 1990;37:230–237.

81. Haas D, Harper D, Saso M, Young E. Lack of differential effect by Ultracaine (articaine) and Citanest (prilocaine) in infiltration anaesthesia. J Can Dent Assoc 1991;57:217–223.

82. Vahatalo K, Antila H, Lehtinen R. Articaine and lidocaine for maxillary infiltration anesthesia. Anesth Prog 1993;40:114–116.

83. Wright G, Weinberger S, Marti R, Plotzke O. The effectiveness of infiltration anesthesia in the mandibular primary molar region. Pediatr Dent 1991;13:278–283.

84. Claffey E, Reader A, Nusstein J, Beck M, Weaver J. Anesthetic efficacy of articaine for inferior alveolar nerve blocks in patients with irreversible pulpitis. J Endod 2004;30:568–571.

85. Tortamano IP, Siviero M, Costa CG, Buscariolo IA, Armonia PL. A comparison of the anesthetic efficacy of articaine and lidocaine in patients with irreversible pulpitis. J Endod 2009;35:165–168.

86. Tofoli GR, Ramacciato JC, de Oliveira PC, Volpato MC, Groppo FC, Ranali J. Comparison of effectiveness of 4% articaine associated with 1:100,000 or 1:200,000 epinephrine in inferior alveolar nerve block. Anesth Prog 2003;50:164–168.

87. Moore PA, Boynes SG, Hersh EV, et al. The anesthetic efficacy of 4 percent articaine 1:200,000 epinephrine: Two controlled clinical trials. J Am Dent Assoc 2006;137:1572–1581.

88. Brandt RG, Anderson PF, McDonald NJ, Sohn W, Peters MC. The pulpal anesthetic efficacy of articaine versus lidocaine in dentistry: A meta-analysis. J Am Dent Assoc 2011;142:493–504.

89. Kung J, McDonagh M, Sedgley CM. Does articaine provide an advantage over lidocaine in patients with symptomatic irreversible pulpitis? A systematic review and meta-analysis. J Endod 2015;41:1784–1794.

90. Davis W, Oakley J, Smith E. Comparison of the effectiveness of etidocaine and lidocaine as local anesthetic agents during oral surgery. Anesth Prog 1984;31:159–164.

91. Rosenquist J, Rosenquist K, Lee P. Comparison between lidocaine and bupivacaine as local anesthetics with diflunisal for postoperative pain control after lower third molar surgery. Anesth Prog 1988;35:1–4.

92. Dunsky JL, Moore PA. Long-acting local anesthetics: A comparison of bupivacaine and etidocaine in endodontics. J Endod 1984;10:457–460.

93. Moore PA, Dunsky JL. Bupivacaine anesthesia: A clinical trial for endodontic therapy. Oral Surg Oral Med Oral Pathol 1983;55:176–179.

94. Linden E, Abrams H, Matheny J, Kaplan A, Kopczyk R, Jasper S. A comparison of postoperative pain experience following periodontal surgery using two local anesthetic agents. J Periodontol 1986;57:637–642.

95. Crout RJ, Koraido G, Moore PA. A clinical trial of long-acting local anesthetics for periodontal surgery. Anesth Prog 1990;37:194–198.

96. Feldmann G, Nordenram A. Marcaine in oral surgery. A clinical comparative study with carbocaine. Acta Anaesthesiol Scand Suppl 1996;23:409–413.

97. Nespeca JA. Clinical trials with bupivacaine in oral surgery. Oral Surg Oral Med Oral Pathol 1976;42:301–307.

98. Pricco DF. An evaluation of bupivacaine for regional nerve block in oral surgery. J Oral Surg 1977;35:126–129.

99. Laskin JL, Wallace WR, DeLeo B. Use of bupivacaine hydrochloride in oral surgery—A clinical study. J Oral Surg 1977;35:25–29.

100. Trieger N, Gillen GH. Bupivacaine anesthesia and postoperative analgesia in oral surgery. Anesth Prog 1979;26:20–23.

101. Chapnick P, Baker G, Munroe CO. Bupivacaine anesthesia in oral surgery. J Can Dent Assoc 1980;46:441–443.

102. Danielsson K, Evers H, Holmlund A, Kjellman O, Nordenram A, Persso NE. Long-acting local anesthetics in oral surgery. Clinical evaluation of bupivacaine and etidocaine for mandibular nerve block. Int J Oral Maxillofac Surg 1986;15:119–126.

103. Rosenquist JB, Nystrom E. Long-acting analgesia or long-acting local anesthetic in controlling immediate postoperative pain after lower third molar surgery. Anesth Prog 1987;34:6–9.

104. Rosenquist J, Rosenquist K, Lee P. Comparison between lidocaine and bupivacaine as local anesthetics with diflunisal for postoperative pain control after lower third molar surgery. Anesth Prog 1988;35:1–4.

105. Tuffin JR, Cunliffe DR, Shaw SR. Do local analgesics injected at the time of third molar removal under general anaesthesia reduce significantly post-operative analgesic requirements? A double-blind controlled study. Br J Oral Maxillofac Surg 1989;27:27–32.

106. Bouloux GF, Punnia-Moorthy A. Bupivacaine versus lidocaine for third molar surgery: A double-blind, randomized, crossover study. J Oral Maxillofac Surg 1999;57:510–514.

107. Neal JA, Welch TB, Halliday RW. Analysis of the analgesic efficacy and cost-effective use of long-acting local anesthetics in outpatient third molar surgery. Oral Surg Oral Med Oral Pathol 1993;75:283–285.

108. Linden ET, Abrams H, Matheny J, Kaplan AL, Kopczyk RA, Jasper SJ. A comparison of postoperative pain experience following periodontal surgery using two local anesthetic agents. J Periodontol 1986;57:637–642.

109. Meechan JG, Blair GS. The effect of two different local anaesthetic solutions on pain experience following apicoectomy. Br Dent J 1993;175:410–413.

110. Kennedy M, Reader A, Beck M, Weaver J. Anesthetic efficacy of ropivacaine in maxillary anterior infiltration. Oral Surg Oral Med Oral Pathol Oral Radiol Endod 2001;91:406–412.

111. El-Sharrawy E, Yagiela J. Anesthetic efficacy of different ropivacaine concentrations for inferior alveolar nerve block. Anesth Prog 2006;53:3–7.

112. Branco FP, Ranali J, Ambrosano GM, Volpato MC. A double-blind comparison of 0.5% bupivacaine with 1:200,000 epinephrine and 0.5% levobupivacaine with 1:200,000 epinephrine for inferior alveolar nerve block. Oral Surg Oral Med Oral Pathol Oral Radiol Endod 2006;101:442–447.

113. Galindo A. pH-adjusted local anesthetics: Clinical experience. Reg Anesth 1983;8:35–36.

114. Al-Sultan AF. Effectiveness of pH adjusted lidocaine versus commercial lidocaine for maxillary infiltration anesthesia. Al-Rafidain Dent J 2004;4:34–39.

115. Al-Sultan AF, Fathie WK, Hamid RS. A clinical evaluation on the alkalization of local anesthetic solution in periapical surgery. Al-Rafidain Dent J 2006;6:71–77.

116. Whitcomb M, Drum M, Reader A, Nusstein J, Beck M. A prospective, randomized double-blind study of the anesthetic efficacy of sodium bicarbonate buffered 2% lidocaine with 1:100,000 epinephrine in inferior alveolar nerve blocks. Anesth Prog 2010;57:59–66.

117. Saatchi M, Khademi A, Baghaei B, Noormohammadi H. Effect of sodium bicarbonate-buffered lidocaine on the success of inferior alveolar nerve block for teeth with symptomatic irreversible pulpitis: A prospective, randomized double-blind study. J Endod 2015;41:33–35.

118. Schellenberg J, Drum M, Reader A, Nusstein J, Fowler S, Beck M. Effect of buffered 4% lidocaine on the success of the inferior alveolar nerve block in patients with symptomatic irreversible pulpitis: A prospective, randomized, double-blind study. J Endod 2015;41:791–796.

119. Shurtz R, Nusstein J, Reader A, Drum M, Fowler S, Beck M. Buffered 4% articaine as a primary buccal infiltration of the mandibular first molar: A prospective, randomized, double-blind study. J Endod 2015;41:1403–1407.

120. Balasco M, Drum M, Reader A, Nusstein J, Beck M. Buffered lidocaine for incision and drainage: A prospective, randomized double-blind study. J Endod 2013;39:1329–1334.

121. Harreld TK, Fowler S, Drum M, Reader A, Nusstein J, Beck M. Efficacy of a buffered 4% lidocaine formulation for incision and drainage: A prospective, randomized, double-blind study. J Endod 2015;41:1583–1588.

122. Kashyap VM, Desai R, Reddy PB, Menon S. Effect of alkalinisation of lignocaine for intraoral nerve block on pain during injection, and speed of onset of anaesthesia. Br J Oral Maxillofac Surg 2011;49(8):E72–E75.

123. Malamed SF, Tavana S, Falkel M. Faster onset and more comfortable injection with alkalinized 2% lidocaine with epinephrine 1:100,000. Compend Contin Educ Dent 2013;34:10–20.

124. Hobeich P, Simon S, Schneiderman E, He J. A prospective, randomized, double-blind comparison of the injection pain and anesthetic onset of 2% lidocaine with 1:100,000 epinephrine buffered with 5% and 10% sodium bicarbonate in maxillary infiltrations. J Endod 2013;39:597–599.

125. Wennberg E, Haljamäe H, Edwall G, Dhuner KG. Effects of commercial (pH approximately 3.5) and freshly prepared (pH approximately 6.5) lidocaine-adrenaline solutions on tissue pH. Acta Anaesthesiol Scand 1982;26:524–527.

126. Punnia-Moorthy A. Buffering capacity of normal and inflamed tissues following the injection of local anaesthetic solutions. Br J Anaesth 1988;61:154–159.

127. Gow-Gates GAE. Mandibular conduction anesthesia: A new technique using extraoral landmarks. Oral Surg Oral Med Oral Pathol 1973;36:321–328.

128. Malamed S. The Gow-Gates mandibular block: Evaluation after 4,275 cases. Oral Surg Oral Med Oral Pathol 1981;51:463–467.

129. Todorovic L, Stajcic Z, Petrovic V. Mandibular versus inferior alveolar dental anaesthesia: Clinical assessment of three different techniques. Int J Oral Maxillofac Surg 1986;15:733–738.

130. Montagnese TA, Reader A, Melfi R. A comparative study of the Gow-Gates technique and a standard technique for mandibular anesthesia. J Endod 1984;10:158–163.

131. Hung PC, Chang HH, Yang PJ, Kuo YS, Lan WH, Lin CP. Comparison of the Gow-Gates mandibular block and inferior alveolar nerve block using a standardized protocol. J Formos Med Assoc 2006;105:139–146.

132. Sisk AL. Evaluation of the Gow-Gates mandibular block for oral surgery. Anesth Prog 1985;32:143–146.

133. Akinosi J. A new approach to the mandibular nerve block. Br J Oral Surg 1977;15:83–87.

134. Vazirani SJ. Closed mouth mandibular nerve block: A new technique. Dent Dig 1960;66:10–13.

135. Sisk AL. Evaluation of the Akinosi mandibular block technique in oral surgery. J Oral Maxillofacial Surg 1986;44:113–115.

136. Yücel E, Hutchison IL. A comparative evaluation of the conventional and closed-mouth technique for inferior alveolar nerve block. Aust Dent J 1995;40:15–16.

137. Gonzalez M, Pena B, Caliz F, Marin SH, Diago P. A comparative study of direct mandibular block and the Akinosi technique. Med Oral 2003;8:143–149.

138. Jacobs S, Haas DA, Meechan JG, May S. Injection pain: Comparison of three mandibular block techniques and modulation by nitrous oxide/oxygen. J Am Dent Assoc 2003;134:869–876.

139. Robertson WD. Clinical evaluation of mandibular conduction anaesthesia. Gen Dent 1979;27:49–51.

140. Cruz EV, Quengua JB, Gutierrez IL, Abreu MA, Uy HG. A comparative study: Classical, Akinosi, and Gow-Gates techniques of mandibular nerve block. J Philipp Dent Assoc 1994;46(1):13–19.

141. Donkor P, Wong J, Punnia-Moorthy A. An evaluation of the closed mouth mandibular block technique. Int J Oral Maxillofac Surg 1990;19:216–219.

142. Monheim LM. Local Anesthesia and Pain Control in Dental Practice, ed 4. St Louis: Mosby, 1969:103.

143. Joyce AP, Donnelly JC. Evaluation of the effectiveness and comfort of incisive nerve anesthesia given inside or outside the mental foramen. J Endod 1993;19:409–411.

144. Whitworth J, Kanna MD, Corbett IP, Meechan JG. Influence of injection speed on the effectiveness of incisive/mental nerve block: A randomized, controlled, double-blind study in adult volunteers. J Endod 2007;33:1149–1154.

145. Batista da Silva C, Berto LA, Volpato MC, et al. Anesthetic efficacy of articaine and lidocaine for incisive/mental nerve block. J Endod 2010;36:438–441.

146. Jaber A, Whitworth JM, Corbett IP, Al-Baqshi B, Jauhar S, Meechan JG. Effect of massage on the efficacy of the mental and incisive nerve block. Anesth Prog 2013;60:15–20.

147. Phillips WH. Anatomic considerations in local anesthesia. J Oral Surg 1943;1:112–121.

148. Pampush TE. The mental foramen injection. Gen Dent 1982;30:506–507.

149. Northrop PM. Practical techniques in administration of local anesthetic agents. II. Questions and answers. J Am Dent Assoc 1949;38:444–449.

150. Dressman AS, Nusstein J, Drum M, Reader A. Anesthetic efficacy of a primary articaine infiltration and a repeat articaine infiltration in the incisive/mental nerve region of mandibular premolars: A prospective, randomized, single-blind study. J Endod 2013;39:313–318.

151. Yonchak T, Reader A, Beck M, Clark K, Meyers WJ. Anesthetic efficacy of infiltrations in mandibular anterior teeth. Anesth Prog 2001;48:55–60.

152. Meechan J, Ledvinka J. Pulpal anesthesia for mandibular central incisor teeth: A comparison of infiltration and intraligamentary injections. Int Endod J 2002;35:629–634.

153. Meechan JG, Kanaa MD, Corbett IP, Steen IN, Whitworth JM. Pulpal anesthesia for mandibular permanent first molar teeth: A double-blind randomized cross-over trial comparing buccal and buccal plus lingual infiltration injections in volunteers. Int Endod J 2006;39:764–769.

154. Nuzum FM, Drum M, Nusstein J, Reader A, Beck M. Anesthetic efficacy of articaine for a combination labial plus lingual infiltration versus a labial infiltration in the mandibular lateral incisor. J Endod 2010;36:952–956.

155. Jaber A, Whitworth JM, Corbett IP, Al-Basqshi B, Kanaa MD, Meechan JG. The efficacy of infiltration anaesthesia for adult mandibular incisors: A randomised double-blind cross-over trial comparing articaine and lidocaine buccal and buccal plus lingual infiltrations. Br Dent J 2010;209(9):E16.

156. Jung IY, Kim JH, Kim ES, Lee CY, Lee SJ. An evaluation of buccal infiltrations and inferior alveolar nerve blocks in pulpal anesthesia for mandibular first molars. J Endod 2008;34:11–13.

157. Corbett IP, Kanaa MD, Whitworth JM, Meechan JG. Articaine infiltration for anesthesia of mandibular first molars. J Endod 2008;34:514–518.

158. Pabst L, Nusstein J, Drum M, Reader A, Beck M. The efficacy of a repeated buccal infiltration of articaine in prolonging duration of pulpal anesthesia in the mandibular first molar. Anesth Prog 2009;56:128–134.

159. Meechan JG, Jaber AA, Corbett IP, Whitworth JM. Buccal versus lingual articaine infiltration for mandibular tooth anaesthesia: A randomized controlled trial. Int Endod J 2011;44:676–681.

160. McEntire M, Nusstein J, Drum M, Reader A, Beck M. Anesthetic efficacy of 4% articaine with 1:100,000 epinephrine versus 4% articaine with 1:200,000 epinephrine as primary buccal infiltration in the mandibular first molar. J Endod 2011;37:450–454.

161. Martin M, Nusstein J, Drum M, Reader A, Beck M. Anesthetic efficacy of 1.8 mL versus 3.6 mL of 4% articaine with 1:100,000 epinephrine as a primary buccal infiltration of the mandibular first molar. J Endod 2011;37:588–592.

162. Moore PA, Doll B, Delie RA, et al. Hemostatic and anesthetic efficacy of 4% articaine HCL with 1:200,000 epinephrine and 4% articaine HCL with 1:100,000 epinephrine when administered intraorally for periodontal surgery. J Periodontol 2007;78:247–253.

163. de Morais HH, Holanda Vasconcellos RJ, de Santana Santos T, Rocha NS, da Costa Araújo FA, de Carvalho RW. Clinical study of hemodynamic changes comparing 4% articaine hydrochloride with 1:100,000 and 1:200,000 epinephrine. Oral Surg Oral Med Oral Pathol Oral Radiol 2013;116(1):E14–22.

164. Saadoun AP, Malamed S. Intraseptal anesthesia in periodontal surgery. J Am Dent Assoc 1985;111: 249–256.

165. Woodmansey K. Intraseptal anesthesia: A review of a relevant injection technique. Gen Dent 2005;53:418420.

166. Brkovic BM, Savic BM, Andric M, Jurisic M, Todorovic L. Intraseptal vs. periodontal ligament anaesthesia for maxillary tooth extraction: Quality of local anaesthesia and haemodynamic response. Clin Oral Investig 2010;14:675–681.

167. Biocanin V, Brkovic B, Milicic B, Stojic D. Efficacy and safety of intraseptal and periodontal ligament anesthesia achieved by computer-controlled articaine + epinephrine delivery: A dose-finding study. Clin Oral Investig 2013;17:525–533.

168. Borodina OE, Petrkas AZh. Intraceptal anesthesia of lower and upper teeth [in Russian]. Stomatologiia (Mosk) 2009;88:19-20.

169. Doman SM. An audit of the use of intra-septal local anaesthesia in a dental practice in the South of England. Prim Dent Care 2011;18:67–71.

170. Marin MK. Intraseptal anesthesia in the general dental practice. Compendium 1987;8:204–206.

171. Bonar T, Nusstein J, Fowler S, Drum M, Reader A, Beck M. Anesthetic efficacy of articaine and lidocaine in a primary intraseptal injection. J Endod 2016;42(3):e11.

172. Yared GM, Dagher FB. Evaluation of lidocaine in human inferior alveolar nerve block. J Endod 1997;23:575–578.

173. Camarda AJ, Hochman MN, Franco L, Naseri L. A prospective clinical patient study evaluating the effect of increasing anesthetic volume on inferior alveolar nerve block success. Quintessence Int 2007;38:521–526.

174. Dagher FB, Yared GM, Machtou P. An evaluation of 2% lidocaine with different concentrations of epinephrine for inferior alveolar nerve block. J Endod 1997;23:178–180.

175. Looby J, Kirby C. Use of hyaluronidase with local anesthetic agents in dentistry. J Am Dent Assoc 1949;38:1–4.

176. Kirby CK, Eckenhoff JE, Looby JP. The use of hyaluronidase with local anesthetic agents in nerve block and infiltration anesthesia. Surgery 1949;25:101–104.

177. Courtney KR, Kendig JJ, Cohen EN. Frequency-dependent conduction block: The role of nerve impulse pattern in local anesthetic potency. Anesthesiology 1978;48:111–117.

178. Courtney KR. Structure-activity relations for frequency-dependent sodium channel block in nerve by local anesthetics. J Pharm Exp Ther 1980;213:114–119.

179. Fink BR, Cairns AM. Differential use-dependent (frequency-dependent) effects in single mammalian axons: Data and clinical considerations. Anesthesiology 1987;67:477–484.

180. Strichartz GR. The inhibition of sodium currents in myelinated nerve by quaternary derivatives of lidocaine. J Gen Physiol 1973;62:37–57.

181. Stevens MF, Klement W, Lipfert P. Conduction block in man is stimulation frequency dependent. Anaesthesist 1996;45:533–537.

182. Watson BV, Brown WF, Doherty TJ. Frequency-dependent conduction block in carpal tunnel syndrome. Muscle Nerve 2006;33:619–626.

183. Hutchison G, Halcomb T, Reader A, Drum M, Nusstein J, Beck M. A prospective, randomized single-blind study of the anesthetic efficacy of frequency-dependent conduction blockade of the inferior alveolar nerve. J Endod 2011;37:938–942.

184. Meyer RA, Jakubowski W. Use of tripelennamine and diphenhydramine as local anesthetics. J Am Dent Assoc 1964;69:112–117.

185. Welborn JF, Kane JP. Conduction anesthesia using diphenhydramine HCL. J Am Dent Assoc 1964;69:706–709.

186. Willett J, Reader A, Drum M, Nusstein J, Beck M. The anesthetic efficacy of diphenhydramine and the combination diphenhydramine/lidocaine for the inferior alveolar nerve block. J Endod 2008;34: 1446–1450.

187. Clause DW, Zach GA. Reaction to diphenhydramine hydrochloride (Benadryl) used as a local anesthetic. Gen Dent 1989;37:426–427.

188. Bigby J, Reader A, Nusstein J, Beck M. Anesthetic efficacy of lidocaine/meperidine for inferior alveolar nerve blocks in patients with irreversible pulpitis. J Endod 2007;33:7–10.

189. Takasugi Y, Furuya H, Moriya K, Okamoto Y. Clinical evaluation of inferior alveolar nerve block by injection into the pterygomandibular space anterior to the mandibular foramen. Anesth Prog 2000;47:125–129.

190. Crowley C. A Prospective, Randomized Study of the Anesthetic Efficacy of an Upright or Supine Position for Inferior Alveolar Nerve Blocks [thesis]. Columbus: The Ohio State University, 2016.

191. Rood JP. Inferior alveolar nerve blocks. The use of 5 per cent lignocaine. Br Dent J 1976;140:413–414.

192. Eldridge DJ, Rood JP. A double-blind trial of 5 per cent lignocaine solution. Br Dent J 1977;142:129–130.

193. Rood JP, Sowray JH. Clinical experience with 5% lignocaine solution. J Dent 1980;8:128–131.

194. Sandy J, Rood JP. Five percent lignocaine solution in children's dentistry. J Dent 1980;8:312–314.

195. Smith S, Reader A, Drum M, Nusstein J, Beck M. Anesthetic efficacy of a combination of 0.5 M mannitol plus 127.2 mg of lidocaine with 50 µg epinephrine in inferior alveolar nerve blocks: A prospective randomized, single-blind study. Anesth Prog 2013;60:3–10.

196. Frommer J, Mele F, Monroe C. The possible role of the mylohyoid nerve in mandibular posterior tooth sensation. J Am Dent Assoc 1972;85:113–117.

197. Wilson S, Johns P, Fuller P. The inferior alveolar and mylohyoid nerves: An anatomic study and relationship to local anesthesia of the anterior mandibular teeth. J Am Dent Assoc 1984;108:350–352.

198. Stein P, Brueckner J, Milliner M. Sensory innervation of mandibular teeth by the nerve to the mylohyoid: Implications in local anesthesia. Clin Anat 2007;20:591–595.

199. Bitner DP, Uzbelger Feldman D, Axx K, Albandar JM. Description and evaluation of an intraoral cervical plexus anesthetic technique. Clin Anat 2015;28:608–613.

200. Chanpong B, Tang R, Sawka A, Krebs C, Vaghadia H. Real-time ultrasonographic visualization for guided inferior alveolar nerve injection. Oral Surg Oral Med Oral Pathol Oral Radiol 2013;115:272–276.

201. Zeh DW, Katz RL. A new nerve stimulator for monitoring neuromuscular blockade and performing nerve blocks. Anesth Analg 1978;57:13–17.

202. Berns JM, Sadove MS. Mandibular block injection: A method of study using an injected radiopaque material. J Am Dent Assoc 1962;65:735–745.

203. Galbreath JC. Tracing the course of the mandibular block injection. Oral Surg Oral Med Oral Pathol 1970;30:571–582.

204. Ay S, Küçük D, Gümüş C, Kara MI. Distribution and absorption of local anesthetics in inferior alveolar nerve block: Evaluation by magnetic resonance imaging. J Oral Maxillofac Surg 2011;69:2722–2730.

205. Bremer G. Measurements of special significance in connection with anesthesia of the inferior alveolar nerve. Oral Surg 1952;5:966–988.

206. Menke RA, Gowgiel JM. Short-needle block anesthesia at the mandibular foramen. J Am Dent Assoc 1979;99:27–30.

207. Thangavelu K, Kannan R, Kumar NS, Rethish E, Sabitha S, Sayeeganesh N. Significance of localization of mandibular foramen in an inferior alveolar nerve block. J Nat Sci Biol Med 2012;3:156–160.

208. Cooley R, Robison S. Comparative evaluation of the 30-gauge dental needle. Oral Surg Oral Med Oral Pathol 1979;48:400–404.

209. Davidson M. Bevel-oriented mandibular injections: Needle deflection can be beneficial. Gen Dent 1989;37:410–412.

210. Hochman M, Friedman M. In vitro study of needle deflection: A linear insertion technique versus a bidirectional rotation insertion technique. Quintessence Int 2000;31:33–38.

211. Aldous J. Needle deflection: A factor in the administration of local anesthetics. J Am Dent Assoc 1968;77:602–604.

212. Robison S, Mayhew R, Cowan R, Hawley R. Comparative study of deflection characteristics and fragility of 25-, 27-, and 30-gauge short dental needles. J Am Dent Assoc 1984;109:920–924.

213. Jeske A, Boshart B. Deflection of conventional versus nondeflecting dental needles in vitro. Anesth Prog 1985;32:62–64.

214. Kennedy S, Reader A, Nusstein J, Beck M, Weaver J. The significance of needle deflection in success of the inferior alveolar nerve block in patients with irreversible pulpitis. J Endod 2003;29:630–633.

215. Rood J. The nerve supply of the mandibular incisor region. Br Dent J 1977;143:227–230.

216. Langlais RP, Broadus R, Glass BJ. Bifid mandibular canals in panoramic radiographs. J Am Dent Assoc 1985;110:923–926.

217. Kuribayashi A, Watanabe H, Imaizumi A, Tantanapornkul W, Katakami K, Kurabayahi T. Bifid mandibular canals: Cone beam computed tomography evaluation. Dentomaxillofac Radiol 2010;39:235–239.

218. Naitoh M, Hiraiwa H, Aimiya H, Ariji E. Observation of bifid mandibular canal using cone-beam computerized tomography. Int J Oral Maxillofac Implants 2009;24:155–159.

219. Lew K, Townsen G. Failure to obtain adequate anaesthesia associated with a bifid mandibular canal: A case report. Aust Dent J 2006;51:86–90.

220. de Jong RH. Local Anesthetics. St Louis: Mosby, 1994.

221. Strichartz G. Molecular mechanisms of nerve block by local anesthetics. Anesthesiology 1967;45:421–424.

222. Kanaa MD, Meechan JG, Corbett IP, Whitworth JM. Speed of injection influences efficacy of inferior alveolar nerve blocks: A double-blind randomized controlled trial in volunteers. J Endod 2006;32:919–923.

223. de Souza Melo MR, Sabey MJ, Lima CJ, de Almeida Souza LM, Groppo FC. The effect of 2 injection speeds on local anesthetic discomfort during inferior alveolar nerve blocks. Anesth Prog 2015;62:106–109.

224. McCartney M, Reader A, Beck M. Injection pain of the inferior alveolar nerve block in patients with irreversible pulpitis. Oral Surg Oral Med Oral Pathol Oral Radiol Endod 2007;104:571–575.

225. Popitz-Bergez FA, Leeson S, Strichartz GR, Thalhammer JG. Relation between functional deficit and intraneural local anesthetic during peripheral nerve block. A study in the rat sciatic nerve. Anesthesiology 1995;83:583–592.

226. Antonijevic I, Mousa S, Schafer M, Stein C. Perineural defect and peripheral opioid analgesia in inflammation. J Neurosci 1995;15:165–172.

227. Cohen H, Reader A, Drum M, Nusstein J, Beck M. Anesthetic efficacy of a combination of 0.9 M mannitol plus 68.8 mg of lidocaine with 50 µg epinephrine in inferior alveolar nerve blocks: A prospective randomized, single blind study. Anesth Prog 2013;60:145–152.

228. Younkin K, Reader A, Drum M, Nusstein J, Beck M. Anesthetic efficacy of a combination of 0.5 M mannitol plus 36.8 mg of lidocaine with 18.4 µg epinephrine in maxillary infiltration: A prospective, randomized, single-blind study. Anesth Prog 2014;61:63–68.

229. Fischer G, Riethmuller RH. Local Anesthesia in Dentistry, ed 2. Philadelphia: Lea & Febiger, 1914:90–91.

# Maxillary
# Anesthesia

**After reading this chapter, the practitioner should be able to:**

- Describe success, failure, onset, and duration of pulpal anesthesia using 2% lidocaine with 1:100,000 epinephrine.
- List alternative anesthetic solutions for infiltration injection in asymptomatic vital teeth.
- Discuss studies that have increased the duration of pulpal anesthesia for infiltrations.
- Describe alternate injection techniques.

Maxillary anesthesia is clinically more successful than mandibular anesthesia.[1] As a frame of reference, the most common injection for anesthetizing maxillary teeth is the infiltration injection. Descriptions of conventional techniques for maxillary anesthesia are available for review in numerous articles and textbooks.

# Maxillary Infiltration

## Success using lidocaine with epinephrine

Previous studies have evaluated the success of maxillary infiltrations using the electric pulp tester (EPT). Using a volume of 1.8 mL or less and various anesthetic formulations, pulpal anesthetic success (obtaining maximum output with an EPT) ranged from 62% to 100%.[2–20] In nerve block anesthesia, anesthetic success is defined as no patient response to EPT readings (two consecutive 80 readings) within 15 minutes and continuously sustaining the 80 reading for 60 minutes. For infiltration anesthesia, anesthetic success is defined as no patient response to two consecutive 80 readings with the EPT because pulpal anesthesia does not last for 60 minutes (see section on duration).

Malamed[21] recommends using 0.6 mL of anesthetic solution for local infiltration. Brunetto and coauthors[17] evaluated three volumes (0.6, 0.9, and 1.2 mL) of 2% lidocaine with 1:100,000 epinephrine infiltrated into the buccal vestibule of a maxillary canine. They re-

| Table 3-1 | Success rate using 1.8 mL of 2% lidocaine with 1:100,000 epinephrine for maxillary infiltration | |
|---|---|---|
| Tooth | Success rate[a] (%) | References |
| Central incisor | 87 | 22 |
| Lateral incisor | 90 | 12,14–16,18–20,22 |
| First premolar | 92 | 15 |
| First molar | 87 | 14–16,19,20,22 |

[a]Percentage of patients who have no response to two consecutive 80 readings with the EPT.

| Table 3-2 | Approximate onset of pulpal anesthesia for a maxillary infiltration using 1.8 mL of 2% lidocaine with 1:100,000 epinephrine | |
|---|---|---|
| Tooth | Time of onset[a] (min) | References |
| Lateral incisor | 3.6 | 12,14–16,18–20 |
| First premolar | 2.3 | 15 |
| First molar | 4.5 | 14–16,19,20 |

[a]Time of first of two consecutive 80 readings with the EPT.

ported a faster onset, greater success rate (no patient response to an 80 reading with the EPT), and longer duration when a volume of 1.2 mL was used versus 0.6 mL and 0.9 mL. However, the 1.2-mL volume did not provide pulpal anesthesia for 60 minutes.

Table 3-1 provides success rates for a labial or buccal infiltration using 1.8 mL of 2% lidocaine with 1:100,000 epinephrine in maxillary teeth. Pulpal anesthesia was not 100%. To confirm pulpal anesthesia, simply cold test the tooth under treatment.

**IN CONCLUSION,** *the infiltration injection of 1.8 mL of 2% lidocaine with 1:100,000 epinephrine may not always be 100% successful due to the individual variations in response to the drug administered, operator differences, and variations of anatomy as well as tooth position.*

## Onset of pulpal anesthesia

Table 3-2 provides onset times for the labial or buccal infiltration using 1.8 mL of 2% lidocaine with 1:100,000 epinephrine in various maxillary teeth. A number of authors have reported onset times of 2 to 5 minutes for maxillary infiltrations using lidocaine formulations.[2–20] Pulp testing the tooth with a cold refrigerant or an EPT will give the clinician a reliable indicator of onset of pulpal anesthesia.

**IN CONCLUSION,** *onset of pulpal anesthesia is usually within 5 minutes in the maxilla.*

## Duration of pulpal anesthesia

The potential problem with infiltration anesthesia in the maxilla is related to duration. The incidence of short duration of anesthesia (achieving an 80 reading and then losing this reading before 60 minutes) will range from about 66% in lateral incisors to 41% in first molars.[15,18–20] Table 3-3 provides approximate duration times for labial or buccal infiltration using 1.8 mL of 2% lidocaine with 1:100,000 epinephrine in various maxillary teeth.

Usually, duration of pulpal anesthesia in anterior teeth starts to decline around 30 to 35 minutes; in molars, the duration declines at around 45 to 50 minutes. This means that if a restorative procedure requires 60 minutes of pulpal anesthesia, the patient has the potential to experience pain.

**IN CONCLUSION,** *duration of pulpal anesthesia using an infiltration of 1.8 mL of 2% lidocaine with 1:100,000 epinephrine is around 30 to 35 minutes in anterior teeth and 45 to 50 minutes in molars.*

| Table 3-3 | Approximate duration of pulpal anesthesia for maxillary infiltration | | |
|---|---|---|---|
| | **Pulpal anesthesia (min)** | | |
| Local anesthetic agent (1.8 mL) | Lateral incisor | First molar | References |
| 2% lidocaine with 1:100,000 epinephrine | 30–35 | 45–50 | 12,14–16,18–20,22 |
| 2% lidocaine with 1:50,000 epinephrine | 45–50 | 50 | 19 |
| 2% mepivacaine with 1:20,000 levonordefrin | 30–35 | 45–50 | 22 |
| 3% mepivacaine plain (no vasoconstrictor) | 10–15 | 10–15 | 19 |
| 4% prilocaine with 1:200,000 epinephrine | 30–35 | 45–50 | 20 |
| 4% prilocaine plain (no vasoconstrictor) | 10–15 | 10–15 | 20 |
| 0.5% bupivacaine with 1:200,000 epinephrine | 10 | 25 | 14 |
| 4% articaine with 1:100,000 epinephrine | 30–35 | 45–50 | 16 |
| 4% articaine with 1:200,000 epinephrine | Not studied | Not studied | |

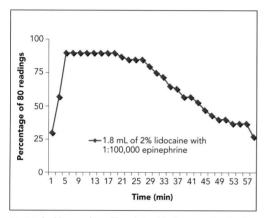

**Fig 3-1** Incidence of maxillary lateral incisor anesthesia. Results determined by lack of response to EPT at maximum reading (percentage of 80 readings) across 60 minutes. (Reprinted from Mikesell et al[15] with permission.)

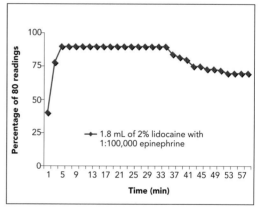

**Fig 3-2** Incidence of maxillary first premolar anesthesia. Results determined by lack of response to EPT at maximum reading (percentage of 80 readings) across 60 minutes. (Reprinted from Mikesell et al[15] with permission.)

## Time course of pulpal anesthesia

### *Maxillary lateral incisor*

Figure 3-1 depicts the time course for complete pulpal anesthesia for an asymptomatic lateral incisor as defined by the percentage of patients who do not respond to an 80 EPT reading across time for 60 minutes. The success rate is almost 90%. The duration of pulpal anesthesia is good until around 30 minutes, when a slow decline in pulpal anesthesia occurs.

### *Maxillary first premolar*

Figure 3-2 depicts the time course for complete pulpal anesthesia for an asymptomatic first premolar as defined by the percentage of patients who do not respond to an 80 EPT reading across time for 60 minutes. The success rate is similar to that for the lateral incisor, but the decline of pulpal anesthesia occurs around 37 minutes and is a little more gradual than in the lateral incisor.

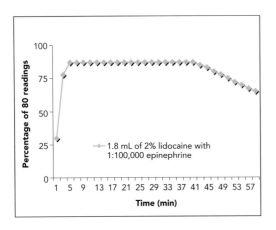

**Fig 3-3** Incidence of maxillary first molar anesthesia. Results determined by lack of response to EPT at maximum reading (percentage of 80 readings) across 60 minutes. (Reprinted from Mikesell et al[15] with permission.)

*Maxillary first molar*

Figure 3-3 depicts the time course for complete pulpal anesthesia for an asymptomatic first molar as defined by the percentage of patients who do not respond to an 80 EPT reading across time for 60 minutes. The success rate is similar to that for the lateral incisor and premolar, but the decline of pulpal anesthesia occurs after 45 minutes.

## Lip/cheek numbness or dead feeling of the teeth

Lip or cheek numbness signifies that the lip or cheek is numb—it does not guarantee pulpal anesthesia. In addition, the relationship of soft tissue anesthesia to duration of pulpal anesthesia is misleading. Soft tissue anesthesia lasts longer than pulpal anesthesia.[14,15,20]

Furthermore, when patients tap their teeth together following local anesthetic administration, they may feel that the teeth are anesthetized. Some clinicians take this as proof that clinical anesthesia has been obtained. However, when testing the teeth with a cold refrigerant or EPT, the clinician will find that the teeth are not always anesthetized.

**IN CONCLUSION,** *lip or cheek numbness or a dead feeling when tapping the teeth together does not always indicate pulpal anesthesia.*

# Alternate Anesthetic Solutions for Infiltration Injection

## Plain solutions: Mepivacaine and prilocaine

Solutions of 3% mepivacaine plain (Carbocaine, Cook-Waite) and 4% prilocaine plain (Citanest Plain, Dentsply) have been found to be equivalent to 2% lidocaine with 1:100,000 epinephrine for inferior alveolar nerve blocks (IANBs).[23] However, maxillary anesthesia is different. Mason and coauthors[19] and Katz and coauthors[20] reported a significant decline in pulpal anesthesia using a cartridge of 3% mepivacaine plain and 4% prilocaine plain formulations in the lateral incisor (Fig 3-4) with approximately 43% to 73% of the subjects having pulpal anesthesia at 20 minutes, 23% to 30% at 30 minutes, and 0% to 7% at 60 minutes.

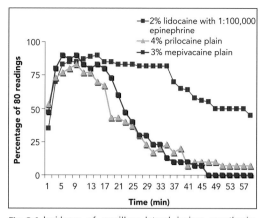

**Fig 3-4** Incidence of maxillary lateral incisor anesthesia: comparison of 3% mepivacaine, 4% prilocaine, and 2% lidocaine with 1:100,000 epinephrine. Results determined by lack of response to EPT at maximum reading (percentage of 80 readings) across 60 minutes. Both formulations without vasoconstrictors had a shorter duration of anesthesia than 2% lidocaine with 1:100,000 epinephrine. (Reprinted from Mason et al[19] with permission.)

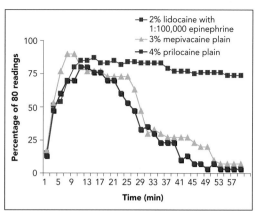

**Fig 3-5** Incidence of maxillary first molar anesthesia: comparison of 3% mepivacaine, 4% prilocaine, and 2% lidocaine with 1:100,000 epinephrine. Results determined by lack of response to EPT at maximum reading (percentage of 80 readings) across 60 minutes. Both formulations without vasoconstrictors had a shorter duration of anesthesia than 2% lidocaine with 1:100,000 epinephrine. (Reprinted from Mason et al[19] with permission.)

In the first molar, approximately 70% to 73% of the subjects had pulpal anesthesia at 20 minutes, 30% to 35% at 30 minutes, and only 7% to 20% at 47 minutes when using these formulations (Fig 3-5). The decline of pulpal anesthesia is more gradual in the first molar than in the lateral incisor. Generally, in the anterior and posterior teeth, these agents are indicated for procedures of short duration—10 to 15 minutes (see Table 3-3).

It must be remembered that these agents are generally not as safe as solutions with vasoconstrictors if large volumes are administered in an attempt to achieve anesthesia in the maxilla. Without the vasoconstrictor, these agents are rapidly absorbed systemically, resulting in excessive plasma concentrations and possible toxic reactions.[21,24]

**IN CONCLUSION,** *plain solutions of 3% mepivacaine and 4% prilocaine are indicated for procedures of short duration.*

## Prilocaine with epinephrine

Katz and coauthors[20] evaluated the anesthetic efficacy of 2% lidocaine with 1:100,000 epinephrine and 4% prilocaine with 1:200,000 epinephrine (Citanest Forte, Dentsply) in maxillary lateral incisors and first molars. They found that anesthetic success (no patient response to two consecutive 80 readings with the EPT) and onset of pulpal anesthesia were not significantly different between 2% lidocaine with 1:100,000 epinephrine and 4% prilocaine with 1:200,000 epinephrine for the lateral incisor and first molar. Neither anesthetic agent provided an hour of pulpal anesthesia (Figs 3-6 and 3-7).

**IN CONCLUSION,** *4% prilocaine with 1:200,000 epinephrine is similar to 2% lidocaine with 1:100,000 epinephrine for infiltration in the maxilla.*

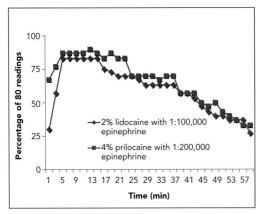

**Fig 3-6** Incidence of maxillary lateral incisor anesthesia: comparison of 4% prilocaine with 1:200,000 epinephrine to 2% lidocaine with 1:100,000 epinephrine. Results determined by lack of response to EPT at maximum reading (percentage of 80 readings) across 60 minutes. No significant difference between the two solutions was noted. (Reprinted from Katz et al[20] with permission.)

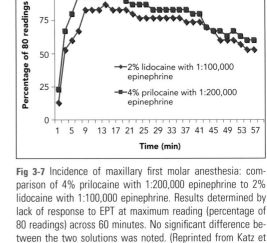

**Fig 3-7** Incidence of maxillary first molar anesthesia: comparison of 4% prilocaine with 1:200,000 epinephrine to 2% lidocaine with 1:100,000 epinephrine. Results determined by lack of response to EPT at maximum reading (percentage of 80 readings) across 60 minutes. No significant difference between the two solutions was noted. (Reprinted from Katz et al[20] with permission.)

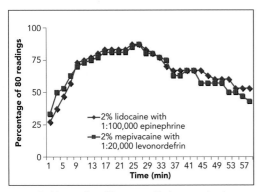

**Fig 3-8** Incidence of maxillary central incisor anesthesia: comparison of 2% mepivacaine with 1:20,000 levonordefrin and 2% lidocaine with 1:100,000 epinephrine. Results determined by lack of response to EPT at maximum reading (percentage of 80 readings) across 60 minutes. No significant difference between the two solutions was noted. (Reprinted from Lawaty et al[22] with permission.)

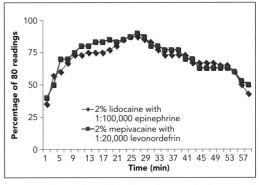

**Fig 3-9** Incidence of maxillary first molar anesthesia: comparison of 2% mepivacaine with 1:20,000 levonordefrin and 2% lidocaine with 1:100,000 epinephrine. Results determined by lack of response to EPT at maximum reading (percentage of 80 readings) across 60 minutes. No significant difference between the two solutions was noted. (Reprinted from Lawaty et al[22] with permission.)

## Mepivacaine with levonordefrin

Lawaty and coauthors[22] compared the anesthetic efficacy of 2% mepivacaine with 1:20,000 levonordefrin (Carbocaine) versus 2% lidocaine with 1:100,000 epinephrine in maxillary central incisors and first molars. They found that anesthetic success (no patient response to two consecutive 80 readings with the EPT) was not significantly different between 2% mepivacaine with 1:20,000 levonordefrin and 2% lidocaine with 1:100,000 epinephrine for the lateral incisor and first molar. However, neither anesthetic agent provided an hour of pulpal anesthesia (Figs 3-8 and 3-9).

**IN CONCLUSION,** *2% mepivacaine with 1:20,000 levonordefrin is similar to 2% lidocaine with 1:100,000 epinephrine for infiltration in the maxilla.*

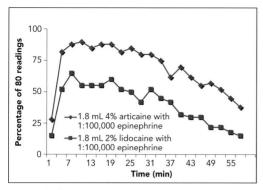

**Fig 3-10** Incidence of maxillary lateral incisor anesthesia: comparison of 4% articaine with 1:100,000 epinephrine and 2% lidocaine with 1:100,000 epinephrine. Results determined by lack of response to EPT at maximum reading (percentage of 80 readings) across 60 minutes. The articaine formulation had higher success rates. (Reprinted from Evans et al[16] with permission.)

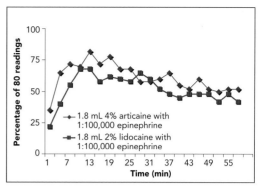

**Fig 3-11** Incidence of maxillary first molar anesthesia: comparison of 4% articaine with 1:100,000 epinephrine and 2% lidocaine with 1:100,000 epinephrine. Results determined by lack of response to EPT at maximum reading (percentage of 80 readings) across 60 minutes. No significant difference between the two solutions was noted. (Reprinted from Evans et al[16] with permission.)

## Articaine with epinephrine

Evans and coauthors[16] found that a maxillary infiltration of a cartridge of 4% articaine with 1:100,000 epinephrine (Septocaine, Septodont), when compared with a cartridge of 2% lidocaine with 1:100,000 epinephrine, statistically improved anesthetic success in the lateral incisor but not the first molar (Figs 3-10 and 3-11). They also found that one cartridge of 4% articaine with 1:100,000 epinephrine provided an onset of pulpal anesthesia around 3 to 4 minutes for maxillary infiltrations and was similar to a lidocaine solution for duration of pulpal anesthesia. Neither solution provided pulpal anesthesia for 1 hour.[16] Therefore, if an hour of pulpal anesthesia is required for the lateral incisor or first molar, neither solution provides the necessary duration when a cartridge of anesthetic solution is administered.

Injection pain was not significantly different between the articaine and lidocaine formulations.[16] The pain ratings of the needle insertion and placement were generally faint-to-weak pain. However, solution deposition values were higher than needle insertion and placement for both solutions. The pain ratings with both solutions were higher in the lateral incisor than the first molar. The articaine solution pain ratings were in the moderate range when compared with the lidocaine solution. Gross and coauthors[14] also found higher pain ratings for solution deposition in the maxillary lateral incisor when compared with the maxillary first molar. Therefore, the anterior region of the maxilla is a more sensitive area for dental injections.

Postoperative pain ratings were generally faint-to-weak pain.[16] The incidence of pain decreased over 3 days, which demonstrated that neither the articaine nor lidocaine formulations caused significant tissue damage. There were no reports of paresthesias. Haas and Lennon[25] indicated that paresthesias are rare and unlikely with infiltration anesthesia.

Three studies have found maxillary tooth extraction possible with just a buccal infiltration of articaine without a separate palatal injection.[26–28] However, with the use of magnetic resonance imaging and needle-stick stimulation, Ozeç and coauthors[29] could not establish the presence of, or an effect for, articaine in the palatal tissues after a buccal infiltration of 4% articaine with 1:200,000 or 1:100,000 epinephrine in molars and premolars.

**IN CONCLUSION,** *in anterior teeth, 4% articaine with 1:100,000 epinephrine may provide a higher success rate than 2% lidocaine with 1:100,000 epinephrine. There is no difference between the two anesthetic agents in the first molar.*

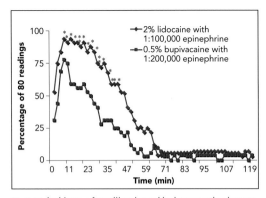

Fig 3-12 Incidence of maxillary lateral incisor anesthesia: comparison of 0.5% bupivacaine with 1:200,000 epinephrine and 2% lidocaine with 1:100,000 epinephrine. Results determined by lack of response to EPT at maximum reading (percentage of 80 readings) across 120 minutes. The asterisks indicate where the lidocaine solution was significantly better. (Reprinted from Gross et al[14] with permission.)

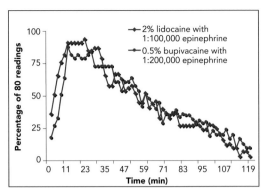

Fig 3-13 Incidence of maxillary first molar anesthesia: comparison of 0.5% bupivacaine with 1:200,000 epinephrine and 2% lidocaine with 1:100,000 epinephrine. Results determined by lack of response to EPT at maximum reading (percentage of 80 readings) across 120 minutes. No significant difference between the two solutions was noted. (Reprinted from Gross et al[14] with permission.)

## Bupivacaine with epinephrine

Success rates (no patient response to the EPT) of bupivacaine (Marcaine, Cook-Waite) range from 80% to 95% in the maxillary lateral incisor to 50% in the maxillary second premolars.[14,30–32] Gross and coauthors[14] determined the anesthetic efficacy of 1.8 mL of 0.5% bupivacaine with 1:200,000 epinephrine and 1.8 mL of 2% lidocaine with 1:100,000 epinephrine in maxillary lateral incisors and first molars. In maxillary lateral incisors, bupivacaine exhibited a significantly lower anesthetic success rate (no patient response to two consecutive 80 readings with the EPT) of 78% when compared with a 97% success rate with lidocaine. In maxillary first molars, bupivacaine's onset of pulpal anesthesia (7.7 minutes) was significantly slower than lidocaine (4.3 minutes). In the first molar, bupivacaine had a lower success rate than lidocaine (64% versus 82%), but there was no significant difference between the two solutions. Neither solution provided pulpal anesthesia for 1 hour (Figs 3-12 and 3-13). While bupivacaine provides long-acting anesthesia for the IANB, it does not provide prolonged pulpal anesthesia in maxillary infiltration injections.[14,30–33]

**IN CONCLUSION,** *1.8 mL of 0.5% bupivacaine with 1:200,000 epinephrine has a lower success rate than 1.8 mL of 2% lidocaine with 1:100,000 epinephrine in anterior teeth. In the first molar, there is no significant difference between the two agents. Neither agent provided pulpal anesthesia for an hour.*

### Soft tissue anesthesia

Gross and coauthors[14] used 1.8 mL of 0.5% bupivacaine with 1:200,000 epinephrine and 1.8 mL of 2% lidocaine with 1:100,000 epinephrine in maxillary lateral incisors and first molars. For the lateral incisor, they reported that the duration of lip numbness (177 minutes versus 128 minutes) and return to normal sensation (383 minutes versus 201 minutes) were significantly longer with a bupivacaine formulation compared with the lidocaine formulation, respectively. For the maxillary first molar, there was no statistically significant difference in duration of gingival numbness (135 minutes versus 116 minutes) and return to normal sensation (213 minutes versus 168 minutes) between the bupivacaine formulation and the lidocaine formulation, respectively. Other studies of maxillary infiltrations using bupivacaine with epinephrine have reported lip numbness durations of 250 to 384 minutes and numbness plus tingling durations of 512 to 548 minutes.[31,33–36]

While lip numbness lasts longer than pulpal anesthesia (see Table 3-3 and Figs 3-12 and 3-13), there is little advantage to having lip numbness for extended periods of time. Difficulty in eating and speaking and the possibility of soft tissue trauma are viewed as nuisances by the patient. Rosenquist and Nystrom[36] found that 34% of patients commented that the long-acting anesthesia produced by a bupivacaine solution was unpleasant. In a follow-up study, Rosenquist and coauthors[37] found that some patients were willing to sustain some pain after oral surgery if lip sensation was regained sooner.

**IN CONCLUSION,** *bupivacaine provides longer lip numbness when compared with lidocaine.*

## Prolonged postoperative analgesia

It is well known that a bupivacaine solution prolongs the postoperative analgesic period for IANB anesthesia.[37–41] In maxillary endodontic surgery, Meechan and Blair[42] found that a long-acting anesthetic used for infiltration anesthesia did not decrease postoperative pain or analgesic intake when compared with a lidocaine solution. The authors also found that the lidocaine solution provided better anesthesia and less hemorrhage than the long-acting anesthetic solution.

**IN CONCLUSION,** *while bupivacaine prolongs the postoperative analgesic period after an IANB, it may not extend the analgesic period in the maxilla.*

# Increasing the Duration of Pulpal Anesthesia for Infiltrations

## Increasing volume of solution

Mikesell and coauthors,[15] using 3.6 mL of 2% lidocaine with 1:100,000 epinephrine, reported that the incidence of anesthesia of short duration (ie, the patient had no response to two consecutive 80 readings, but lost the 80 reading and never regained it within a 60-minute period) was significantly decreased for the lateral incisor when compared with 1.8 mL of 2% lidocaine with 1:100,000 epinephrine. Approximately 97% of the subjects had pulpal anesthesia at 30 minutes, 72% at 45 minutes, and 50% at 60 minutes (Fig 3-14). However, 44% of the subjects still demonstrated anesthesia of short duration. Therefore, duration of pulpal anesthesia remains problematic in the lateral incisor even when 3.6 mL of 2% lidocaine with 1:100,000 epinephrine is administered.

In the premolars and first molars, anesthesia of short duration was reduced to 19% and 9%, respectively. Therefore, anesthesia achieved with a volume of 3.6 mL provides a longer duration than that achieved with a volume of 1.8 mL and offers better pulpal anesthesia after 49 minutes in posterior teeth (Figs 3-15 and 3-16). It is important to realize that even though pulpal anesthesia duration was prolonged with a volume of 3.6 mL, if an hour of pulpal anesthesia is required for the first premolar or first molar, 3.6 mL of 2% lidocaine with 1:100,000 epinephrine may not provide the necessary duration of pulpal anesthesia.

The pain of solution deposition was not different between the two volumes. However, with use of both volumes, there was a higher incidence of moderate pain in the lateral incisor when compared with the posterior teeth. This demonstrates again that the anterior maxilla is more sensitive than the posterior area.

**IN CONCLUSION,** *3.6 mL of 2% lidocaine with 1:100,000 epinephrine extends duration of pulpal anesthesia when compared with 1.8 mL of 2% lidocaine with 1:100,000 epinephrine in maxillary infiltrations. However, pulpal anesthesia does not last for 60 minutes.*

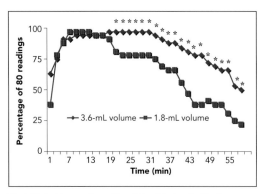

**Fig 3-14** Incidence of maxillary lateral incisor infiltration anesthesia: comparison of 1.8 mL and 3.6 mL of 2% lidocaine with 1:100,000 epinephrine. Results determined by lack of response to EPT at maximum reading (percentage of 80 readings) across 60 minutes. The higher volume was significantly better from the 21st minute until 59th minute *(asterisks)*. However, anesthesia did not last for 60 minutes. (Reprinted from Mikesell et al[15] with permission.)

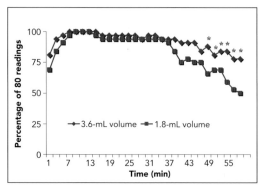

**Fig 3-15** Incidence of maxillary first premolar infiltration anesthesia: comparison of 1.8 mL and 3.6 mL of 2% lidocaine with 1:100,000 epinephrine. Results determined by lack of response to EPT at maximum reading (percentage of 80 readings) across 60 minutes. The higher volume was significantly better from the 49th minute until the 59th minute *(asterisks)*. However, anesthesia did not last for 60 minutes. (Reprinted from Mikesell et al[15] with permission.)

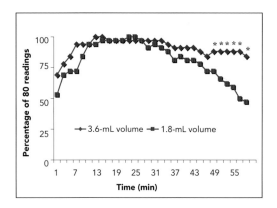

**Fig 3-16** Incidence of maxillary first molar infiltration anesthesia: comparison of 1.8 mL and 3.6 mL of 2% lidocaine with 1:100,000 epinephrine. Results determined by lack of response to EPT at maximum reading (percentage of 80 readings) across 60 minutes. The higher volume was significantly better from the 49th minute until the 59th minute *(asterisks)*. However, anesthesia did not last for 60 minutes. (Reprinted from Mikesell et al[15] with permission.)

## Increasing epinephrine concentration

Mason and coauthors[19] found that 1.8 mL of 2% lidocaine with 1:50,000 epinephrine significantly increased the duration of pulpal anesthesia when compared with 1.8 mL of 2% lidocaine with 1:100,000 epinephrine in maxillary lateral incisors. Approximately 97% of the subjects had pulpal anesthesia at 45 minutes and almost 80% at 60 minutes (Fig 3-17). The 1:50,000 epinephrine concentration in 1.8 mL of 2% lidocaine provided a longer duration than 3.6 mL of 2% lidocaine with 1:100,000 epinephrine (see Fig 3-14). However, duration of pulpal anesthesia was not 60 minutes. Pitt Ford and coauthors[9] also found that a higher epinephrine concentration increased duration in maxillary central incisors. Mason and coauthors[19] found that increasing the epinephrine concentration to 1:50,000 epinephrine was not significantly different than using a 1:100,000 epinephrine formulation in the maxillary first molar. Pulpal anesthesia started to decline for 2% lidocaine with 1:100,000 or 1:50,000 epinephrine after about 49 to 53 minutes (Fig 3-18). It is important to realize that if an hour of pulpal anesthesia is

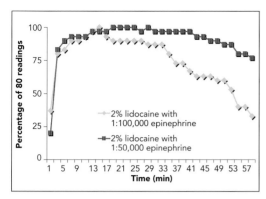

**Fig 3-17** Incidence of maxillary lateral incisor anesthesia: comparison of 2% lidocaine with 1:50,000 epinephrine and 2% lidocaine with 1:100,000 epinephrine. Results were determined by lack of response to EPT at maximum reading (percentage of 80 readings) across 60 minutes. The 2% lidocaine formulation with 1:50,000 epinephrine had a longer duration of anesthesia but did not last for 60 minutes. (Reprinted from Mason et al[19] with permission.)

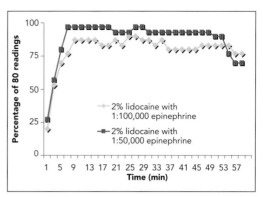

**Fig 3-18** Incidence of maxillary first molar anesthesia: comparison of 2% lidocaine with 1:50,000 epinephrine and 2% lidocaine with 1:100,000 epinephrine. Results determined by lack of response to EPT at maximum reading (percentage of 80 readings) across 60 minutes. No significant difference between the two solutions was noted. (Reprinted from Mason et al[19] with permission.)

required for the first molar, 1.8 mL of 2% lidocaine with either 1:100,000 or 1:50,000 epinephrine may not provide the necessary duration of pulpal anesthesia.

**IN CONCLUSION,** *for infiltrations in the maxilla, increasing the epinephrine concentration to 1:50,000 in a 2% lidocaine solution increases the duration of pulpal anesthesia in the lateral incisor but not in the first molar. However, duration of pulpal anesthesia is not 60 minutes in either tooth.*

## Repeating an infiltration after 30 minutes

Scott and coauthors[18] found that the repeated infiltration injection of a cartridge of 2% lidocaine with 1:100,000 epinephrine given 30 minutes after an initial infiltration of a cartridge of 2% lidocaine with 1:100,000 epinephrine significantly improved pulpal anesthesia from 37 minutes through 90 minutes in the maxillary lateral incisor (Fig 3-19). For the initial infiltration, approximately 78% of the subjects had pulpal anesthesia at 30 minutes. However, at 45 minutes, approximately 60% of the subjects had pulpal anesthesia, and at 60 minutes, only 33% had pulpal anesthesia. With the repeated infiltration, 90% of the subjects had pulpal anesthesia at 60 minutes. At 75 minutes, approximately 85% of the subjects had pulpal anesthesia, and at 90 minutes, 70% were anesthetized. The repeated infiltration was not painful.

This a very important finding. Knowing that standard infiltration anesthesia is of short duration and that repeating the infiltration at 30 minutes will provide pulpal anesthesia for 60 minutes or longer should be very helpful.

**IN CONCLUSION,** *giving a cartridge of 2% lidocaine with 1:100,000 epinephrine 30 minutes after giving an initial cartridge of the same anesthetic agent significantly improved pulpal anesthesia from 37 minutes through 90 minutes in the lateral incisor.*

### *Augmentation versus tachyphylaxis*

A drug's enhanced effectiveness when given repeatedly is referred to as *augmentation*, and *tachyphylaxis* is a declining effectiveness when a drug is given repeatedly.[43,44] Works by Scott and coauthors[18]

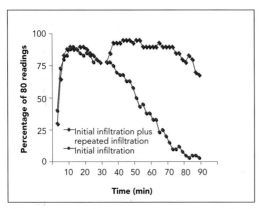

**Fig 3-19** Incidence of maxillary lateral incisor anesthesia: effect of a repeated infiltration injection of a cartridge of 2% lidocaine with 1:100,000 epinephrine given 30 minutes after an initial infiltration of a cartridge of 2% lidocaine with 1:100,000 epinephrine. Results determined by lack of response to EPT at maximum reading (percentage of 80 readings) across 90 minutes. The repeated infiltration significantly improved pulpal anesthesia from the 37th minutes through the 90 minute. (Reprinted from Scott et al[18] with permission.)

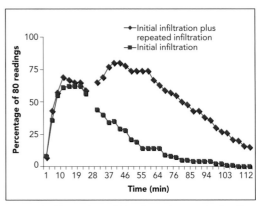

**Fig 3-20** Incidence of mandibular first molar anesthesia: effect of a repeated buccal infiltration injection of a cartridge of 4% articaine with 1:100,000 epinephrine given 25 minutes after an initial buccal infiltration of a cartridge of 4% articaine with 1:100,000 epinephrine. Results determined by lack of response to EPT at maximum reading (percentage of 80 readings) across 112 minutes. The repeated infiltration significantly improved pulpal anesthesia from the 28th through the 109th minute. (Reprinted from Pabst et al[45] with permission.)

and Pabst and coauthors[45] demonstrated a higher level of pulpal anesthesia after administration of a repeated infiltration (Figs 3-19 and 3-20). If the repeated infiltration provided the same effect as the initial infiltration, we would not necessarily expect a higher incidence of pulpal anesthesia. Therefore, it would seem that augmentation might be occurring. A prime consideration for whether augmentation or tachyphylaxis occurs is timing.[43,44] If an infiltration is given within a reasonable time as anesthesia wears off, augmentation is likely to occur.[43,44] However, if the infiltration is given some time after anesthesia wears off, tachyphylaxis frequently occurs.[43,44]

**IN CONCLUSION,** *a repeated infiltration just before pulpal anesthesia wears off (approximately 30 minutes) augments pulpal anesthesia.*

# Alternate Injection Techniques

## Posterior superior alveolar nerve block

The posterior superior alveolar (PSA) nerve block (Fig 3-21) has been advocated to anesthetize the first, second, and third molars.[46] The middle superior alveolar (MSA) nerve is thought to innervate the maxillary premolars and may play some role in pulpal innervation of the mesiobuccal root of the first molar.[46]

Pfeil and coauthors[47] measured the degree of pulpal anesthesia obtained with 1.8 mL and 3.6 mL of 2% lidocaine with 1:100,000 epinephrine for PSA nerve blocks. Anesthetic success (no patient response to two consecutive 80 readings with the EPT) for the 1.8 mL of 2% lidocaine with 1:100,000 epinephrine was 97% for the second molar and 77% for the first molar. Anesthetic success for the 3.6 mL of 2% lidocaine with 1:100,000 epinephrine was 100% for the second molar and 84% for the first molar (Figs 3-22 and 3-23). The differences were not statistically significant between the two an-

**Fig 3-21** Injection site for the PSA nerve block.

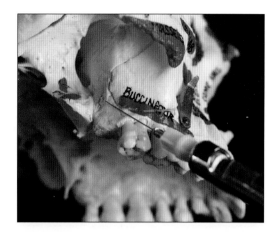

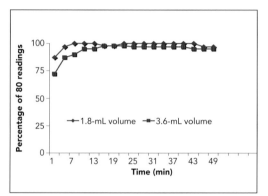

**Fig 3-22** Incidence of maxillary second molar anesthesia: comparison of the PSA nerve block using 1.8 mL and 3.6 mL of 2% lidocaine with 1:100,000 epinephrine. Results determined by lack of response to EPT at maximum reading (percentage of 80 readings) across 60 minutes. No significant difference between the two volumes was noted. (Reprinted from Pfeil et al[47] with permission.)

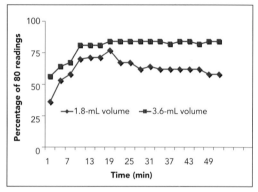

**Fig 3-23** Incidence of maxillary first molar anesthesia: comparison of the PSA nerve block using 1.8 mL and 3.6 mL of 2% lidocaine with 1:100,000 epinephrine. Results determined by lack of response to EPT at maximum reading (percentage of 80 readings) across 60 minutes. The 3.6-mL volume prolonged the duration of anesthesia. (Reprinted from Pfeil et al[47] with permission.)

esthetic volumes. Anesthetic success for the premolars for both volumes was in the low-to-moderate range and would not provide predictable pulpal anesthesia. For the first molar, the 3.6-mL volume of the lidocaine formulation provided a statistically longer duration of pulpal anesthesia than the 1.8-mL volume. The pain of depositing a 3.6-mL volume of a lidocaine solution was not statistically higher than the pain of depositing a 1.8-mL volume.

Loetscher and coauthors[46] evaluated pulpal anesthesia in an experimental study using 30 subjects, 1.2 mL of 2% lidocaine with 1:100,000 epinephrine, and dry ice (ie, solid carbon dioxide). They found that the PSA nerve block successfully anesthetized 88% of first molars. If a separate first molar infiltration of 0.6 mL of 2% lidocaine with 1:100,000 epinephrine was added to the PSA nerve block, 92% of the first molars were anesthetized. The second molars were successfully anesthetized with just the PSA nerve block alone.

Generally, the PSA nerve block will provide pulpal anesthesia for the second molars.[46,47] To ensure patient comfort for the first molar, an additional buccal infiltration injection after the PSA block may be needed.

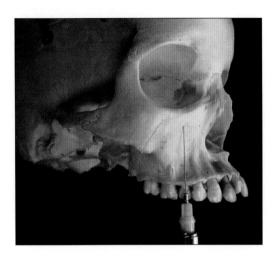

**Fig 3-24** The needle path for the intraoral infraorbital nerve block is parallel to the long axis of the second premolar until it approximates the infraorbital foramen. (Reprinted from Karkut et al[49] with permission.)

**IN CONCLUSION,** *because of the success rate of infiltration in the molars (see section on maxillary infiltrations), the PSA nerve block is not advocated for routine restorative procedures.*

## Intraoral infraorbital nerve block

Malamed[21] describes the maxillary infraorbital nerve block as an effective method of achieving profound pulpal anesthesia from the maxillary central incisor through the canine. He states that the pulps of the premolars and the mesiobuccal root of the first molar will also be anesthetized in about 72% of patients.[21]

Berberich and coauthors[48] compared the anesthetic efficacy of a cartridge of 2% lidocaine with 1:100,000 epinephrine, a cartridge of 2% lidocaine with 1:50,000 epinephrine, and a cartridge of 3% mepivacaine in the intraoral infraorbital nerve block (Fig 3-24). They reported that the intraoral infraorbital nerve block resulted in profound soft tissue anesthesia but was ineffective in providing profound pulpal anesthesia (no patient response to two consecutive 80 readings with the EPT) of the maxillary central incisor, lateral incisor, and first molar (Fig 3-25). Corbett and coauthors[50] found similar results using 1 mL of 2% lidocaine with 1:80,000 epinephrine. Successful pulpal anesthesia of the canine and first and second premolars ranged from 75% to 92% using 2% lidocaine with 1:100,000 and 1:50,000 epinephrine. However, pulpal anesthesia did not last for 60 minutes (see Fig 3-25). The use of 3% mepivacaine provided a shorter duration of anesthesia than the lidocaine formulations with epinephrine in the canines and premolars. For pulpal anesthesia, this injection technique is similar to an infiltration injection over the premolars.

**IN CONCLUSION,** *the intraoral infraorbital nerve block does not provide effective pulpal anesthesia for the central incisor, lateral incisor, or first molar. It is somewhat effective for the canine and premolars, but pulpal anesthesia does not last for 60 minutes. A plain solution of 3% mepivacaine results in an even shorter duration of pulpal anesthesia. Because of the success rate of the infiltration in the maxillary teeth (see section on maxillary infiltrations), the intraoral infraorbital nerve block is not advocated for routine restorative procedures.*

## Extraoral infraorbital nerve block

Karkut and coauthors[49] compared the local anesthetic efficacy of the extraoral infraorbital nerve block (Fig 3-26) with the intraoral infraorbital nerve block (see Fig 3-24) using a cartridge of 2% lidocaine

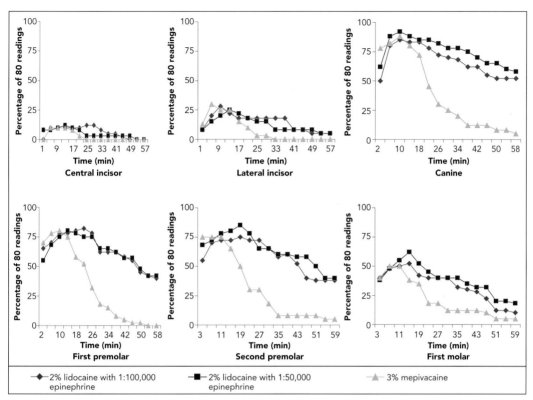

**Fig 3-25** Incidence of maxillary anesthesia from the central incisor to the first molar for the intraoral infraorbital nerve block: comparison of 2% lidocaine with 1:50,000 epinephrine, 3% mepivacaine, and 2% lidocaine with 1:100,000 epinephrine. Results determined by lack of response to EPT at maximum reading (percentage of 80 readings) across 60 minutes. The intraoral infraorbital nerve block was ineffective in providing profound pulpal anesthesia of the maxillary central incisor, lateral incisor, and first molar. Successful pulpal anesthesia of the canine and first and second premolars ranged from 75% to 92% using the lidocaine formulations. The 3% mepivacaine formulation provided a shorter duration of anesthesia than the lidocaine formulations with epinephrine in the canines and premolars. (Reprinted from Berberich et al[48] with permission.)

with 1:100,000 epinephrine. They reported that the extraoral and intraoral infraorbital nerve blocks were effective in providing soft tissue anesthesia but were ineffective in providing profound pulpal anesthesia (no patient response to two consecutive 80 readings with the EPT) of the maxillary central incisor (15% success) and lateral incisor (22% success) (Fig 3-27). Successful pulpal anesthesia for both nerve blocks was 92% for the canine, 80% to 90% for the first and second premolars, and 65% to 70% for the first molar, with no significant differences between the two nerve blocks (see Fig 3-27). Pulpal anesthesia did not last for an hour for any of the teeth. Needle insertion pain and postoperative sequelae were more common with the extraoral infraorbital nerve block.

**IN CONCLUSION,** *the extraoral infraorbital nerve block does not provide effective pulpal anesthesia for the central incisor, lateral incisor, or first molar. It is somewhat effective for the canine and premolars, but pulpal anesthesia does not last for 60 minutes. Because of the success rate of the infiltration in the maxillary teeth (see section on maxillary infiltrations), the extraoral infraorbital nerve block is not advocated for routine restorative procedures.*

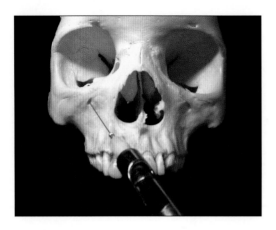

**Fig 3-26** The needle path for the extraoral infraorbital nerve block would be backward, upward, and outward to penetrate the infraorbital canal. (Reprinted from Karkut et al[49] with permission.)

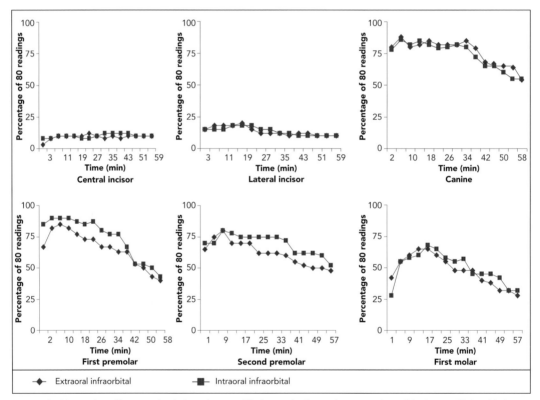

Extraoral infraorbital

Intraoral infraorbital

**Fig 3-27** Incidence of maxillary anesthesia from the central incisor to the first molar: comparison of the intraoral infraorbital nerve block to the extraoral infraorbital nerve block. Results determined by lack of response to EPT at maximum reading (percentage of 80 readings) across 60 minutes. Both nerve blocks were ineffective in providing profound pulpal anesthesia of the maxillary central incisor, lateral incisor, and first molar. No significant difference between the two techniques was noted. Successful pulpal anesthesia of the canine for both nerve blocks was 92%; success of the first and second premolars ranged from 80% to 90%. (Reprinted from Karkut et al[49] with permission.)

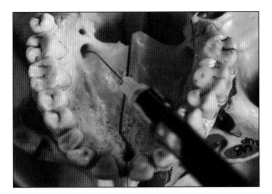

Fig 3-28 The greater palatine approach to the second division nerve block must negotiate the greater palatine canal to the pterygopalatine fossa.

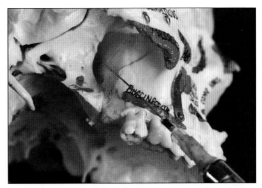

Fig 3-29 The high tuberosity approach to the second division nerve block places the needle around the posterior maxilla until the needle enters the pterygopalatine fossa.

## Second division nerve block

Malamed[21] described the second division nerve block as an effective method of achieving profound anesthesia in the hemimaxilla. This nerve block has been described using two intraoral techniques[51–62]: (1) the greater palatine approach, which involves negotiating the greater palatine canal to the pterygopalatine fossa (Fig 3-28); and (2) the high tuberosity approach, which places the needle around the posterior maxilla until the needle enters the pterygopalatine fossa (Fig 3-29).

Broering and coauthors[63] compared the anesthetic efficacy of the greater palatine second division nerve block and the high tuberosity second division nerve block technique using 3.6 mL of 2% lidocaine with 1:100,000 epinephrine. They reported that both techniques resulted in a high success rate (95% to 100%) of pulpal anesthesia (no patient response to two consecutive 80 readings with the EPT) for first and second molars (Fig 3-30). Around 70% to 80% of the second premolars were anesthetized with both techniques. Both techniques were ineffective for profound pulpal anesthesia of the anterior teeth and first premolars. The high tuberosity approach is preferred over the greater palatine technique because the success rates are similar and it is less painful.[63]

**IN CONCLUSION,** *a second division nerve block does not provide pulpal anesthesia for the central incisor, lateral incisor, canine, or first premolar. The blocks are effective for pulpal anesthesia of the molars. Because of the success rate of the infiltration over the molars (see section on maxillary infiltration), the second division nerve block is not advocated for routine restorative procedures.*

### *High tuberosity second division nerve block using 3% mepivacaine*

Forloine and coauthors[64] compared the anesthetic efficacy of 3.6 mL of 2% lidocaine with 1:100,000 epinephrine and 3.6 mL of 3% mepivacaine in the high tuberosity second division nerve block. They found that the high tuberosity approach to the second division nerve block, with both anesthetic formulations, resulted in a high success rate (92% to 98%) for the first and second molars (Fig 3-31). Approximately 76% to 78% of the second premolars were anesthetized with both anesthetic formulations. Both anesthetic formulations were ineffective for the anterior teeth and first premolars. The use of 3% mepivacaine provided a significantly shorter duration of pulpal anesthesia than 2% lidocaine with 1:100,000 epinephrine in the molars and premolars (see Fig 3-31).

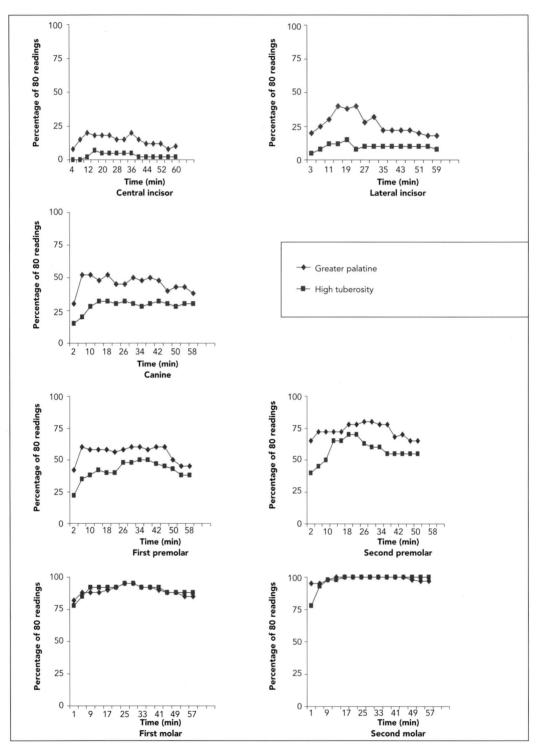

**Fig 3-30** Incidence of maxillary anesthesia from the central incisor to the second molar: comparison of the greater palatine technique and the high tuberosity technique for the second division nerve block. Results determined by lack of response to EPT at maximum reading (percentage of 80 readings) across 60 minutes. The two techniques were similar. The first and second molars had the highest success rates. The anterior teeth were not effectively anesthetized. (Reprinted from Broering et al[63] with permission.)

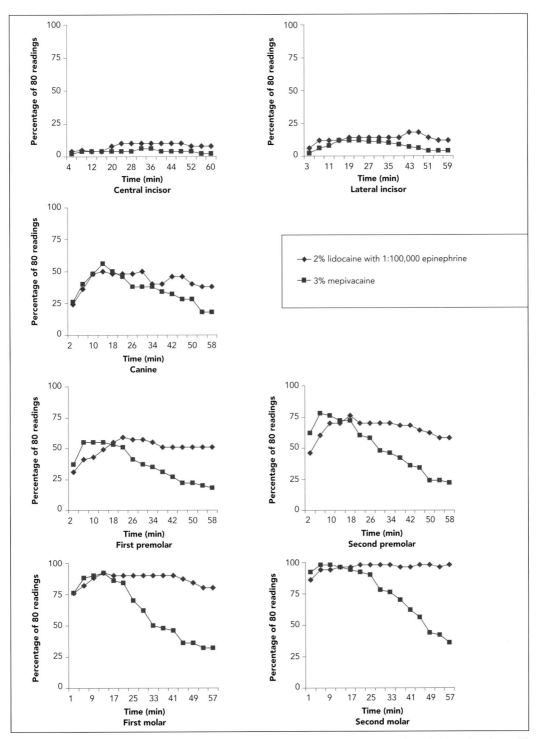

**Fig 3-31** Incidence of maxillary anesthesia from the central incisor to the second molar: comparison of 3% mepivacaine to 2% lidocaine with 1:100,000 epinephrine for the high tuberosity approach to the second division nerve block. Results determined by lack of response to EPT at maximum reading (percentage of 80 readings) across 60 minutes. Using 2% lidocaine with 1:100,000 epinephrine, the first and second molars had the highest success rates. The anterior teeth were not effectively anesthetized. The 3% mepivacaine solution provided a significantly shorter duration of pulpal anesthesia. (Reprinted from Forloine et al[64] with permission.)

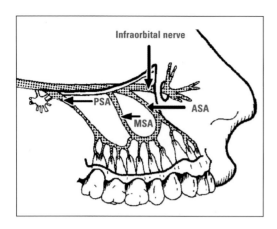

**Fig 3-32** Maxillary division of the trigeminal nerve showing the infraorbital nerve, ASA nerve, PSA nerve, and MSA nerve. (Reprinted from Lee et al[67] with permission.)

**IN CONCLUSION,** *3% mepivacaine provided a shorter duration of pulpal anesthesia when compared with 2% lidocaine with 1:100,000 epinephrine. Because of the success rate of the infiltration in the molars (see section on maxillary infiltration), the second division nerve block is not advocated for routine restorative procedures.*

## Palatal–anterior superior alveolar nerve block

Traditionally, maxillary anterior teeth have been anesthetized by administering an infiltration injection near the apex of the target tooth. A site-specific injection for anesthetizing anterior maxillary teeth has been introduced: the palatal–anterior superior alveolar (P–ASA) injection.[65,66] The P–ASA injection uses a palatal injection into the incisive canal and derives its name from the injection's ability to supposedly anesthetize both the right and left anterior superior alveolar (ASA) nerves (Fig 3-32). Friedman and Hochman[65,66] state that bilateral pulpal anesthesia of the maxillary incisors and usually the canines will be achieved with the P–ASA injection of 0.9 to 1.4 mL of anesthetic solution with an expected duration of approximately 60 minutes.

Burns and coauthors[68] compared the anesthetic efficacy of 2% lidocaine with 1:100,000 epinephrine and 3% mepivacaine using the CompuDent (Milestone Scientific) computer-controlled local anesthetic delivery (CCLAD) system—formerly known as the *Wand*—to administer the P–ASA injection. The results indicated that 3% mepivacaine would generally be less effective than 2% lidocaine with 1:100,000 epinephrine in the P–ASA technique. The 2% lidocaine with epinephrine solution resulted in successful pulpal anesthesia from 32% to 58% of the time and would not clinically ensure predictable pulpal anesthesia for the maxillary incisors and canines (Fig 3-33).

Regarding the pain of needle insertion for the P–ASA injection, Nusstein and coauthors[69] found that 30% to 43% of the subjects reported moderate-to-severe pain. For needle placement into the incisive canal, 54% to 58% of the subjects reported moderate-to-severe pain. For anesthetic solution deposition, 8% to 12% of the subjects reported moderate pain. Regarding postoperative pain after numbness wore off on the day of the injection, 12% to 18% of the subjects reported moderate pain, and 2% reported severe pain. Postoperative problems were relatively minor, with approximately 12% to 18% of the subjects having experienced temporary numbness/paresthesia of the incisive papilla and 20% to 28% having had incisive papilla swelling or soreness.

**IN CONCLUSION,** *the P–ASA nerve block has the potential to be a painful injection and does not provide predictable pulpal anesthesia for the maxillary incisors and canines.*

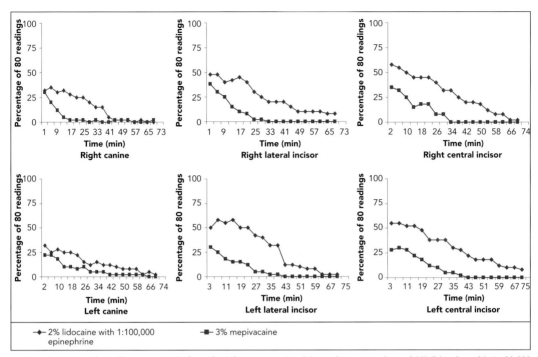

**Fig 3-33** Incidence of maxillary anesthesia from the left canine to the right canine: comparison of 2% lidocaine with 1:100,000 epinephrine and 3% mepivacaine plain for the P–ASA injection technique. Results determined by lack of response to EPT at maximum reading (percentage of 80 readings) across 72 minutes. The modest-to-low success rates of the lidocaine and mepivacaine solutions would not ensure predictable pulpal anesthesia of the maxillary incisors and canines. (Reprinted from Burns et al[68] with permission.)

## Anterior middle superior alveolar nerve block

Another technique has been introduced for anesthetizing maxillary teeth: the anterior middle superior alveolar (AMSA) nerve block injection.[66,70,71] The AMSA injection site is located palatally at a point that bisects the premolars and is approximately halfway between the midpalatine raphe and the crest of the free gingival margin (Fig 3-34). The AMSA nerve block derives its name from the injection's ability to supposedly anesthetize both the ASA and MSA nerves[66,70,71] (see Fig 3-32). Friedman and Hochman[66,70,71] state that pulpal anesthesia of the maxillary central and lateral incisors, canines, and first and second premolars will be achieved with the AMSA injection of 0.6 to 1.4 mL of anesthetic solution with an expected duration of approximately 45 to 60 minutes. A bilateral AMSA injection supposedly anesthetizes 10 maxillary teeth extending from the second premolar on one side to the second premolar on the opposite side.[71]

Lee and coauthors[67] found that the AMSA injection using the CompuDent CCLAD system and 1.4 mL of 2% lidocaine with 1:100,000 epinephrine was more successful than the conventional syringe technique using the same amount of lidocaine with epinephrine. The authors found anesthetic success rates (no patient response to two consecutive 80 readings with the EPT) of 42% to 55% for the second premolar, 20% to 42% for the first premolar, 32% to 52% for the canine, 42% to 58% for the lateral incisor, and 30% to 35% for the central incisor. The modest-to-low success rates, slow onset, and declining duration of pulpal anesthesia over 60 minutes would not ensure predictable pulpal anesthesia from the second premolar to the central incisor (Fig 3-35). Velasco and coauthors[72] found a success rate (no patient response to two consecutive 80 readings with the EPT) of 66% for the second

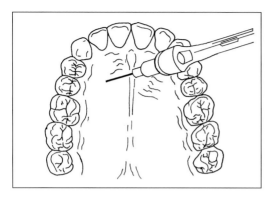

**Fig 3-34** Palatal injection site for the AMSA injection. (Reprinted from Lee et al[67] with permission.)

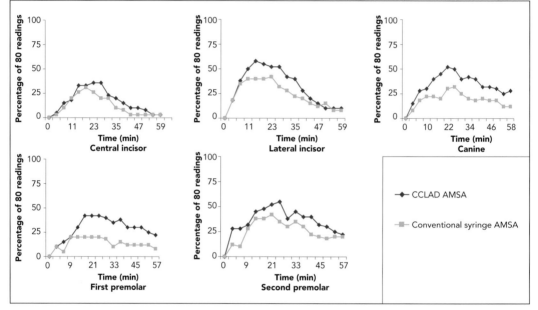

**Fig 3-35** Incidence of maxillary anesthesia from the second premolar to the central incisor: comparison of the AMSA injection using the CompuDent CCLAD system versus a conventional syringe. Results determined by lack of response to EPT at maximum reading (percentage of 80 readings) across 60 minutes. The CompuDent system was more successful, but the modest-to-low success rates, slow onset, and declining duration of pulpal anesthesia would not ensure predictable pulpal anesthesia from the second premolar to the central incisor. (Reprinted from Lee et al[67] with permission.)

premolar, 40% for the first premolar, 60% for the canine, 23% for the lateral incisor, and 17% for the central incisor. Corbett and coauthors[50] found a higher success rate for this injection using 1 mL of 2% lidocaine with 1:80,000 epinephrine. However, the success rates would not provide predictable pulpal anesthesia from the second premolar to the central incisor. The graphs of Fukayama and coauthors[73] on AMSA injection showed similar results. In a preliminary study, de Souza Tolentino and coauthors[74] found the AMSA injection similar to supraperiosteal injection techniques for subgingival scaling and root planing. However, they felt more clinical trials should be performed.

Nusstein and coauthors[75] studied the pain of the AMSA injection. Comparison of the CompuDent CCLAD system and the conventional syringe technique resulted in the following respective pain ratings: 38% and 32% moderate pain and 0% and 2% severe pain on needle insertion; 25% and 40% moderate pain and 0% and 2% severe pain on solution deposition. The AMSA injection using the CompuDent CCLAD system resulted in statistically lower pain ratings upon anesthetic solution deposition. Yenisey[76] also found lower pain scores for needle insertion and solution deposition using a CCLAD system for the AMSA technique compared with conventional injections. However, the AMSA, using either a CCLAD system or a conventional syringe, has the potential to be a painful injection. The incidence of postinjection pain and sequelae was low with both techniques.

**IN CONCLUSION,** *the AMSA nerve block has the potential to be a painful injection and would not ensure predictable pulpal anesthesia from the second premolar to the central incisor.*

## Tetracaine nasal spray for maxillary anesthesia

Ciancio and coauthors[77] evaluated tetracaine/oxymetazoline nasal spray for anesthesia of maxillary teeth. The authors found that the combination nasal spray was adequate for a number of maxillary dental procedures. Kovanaze Nasal Spray (St. Renatus) was recently cleared by the United States Food and Drug Administration for dental use. It is used for restorative procedures on the premolars and anterior teeth as well as the maxillary primary teeth in children who weigh 88 pounds or more.

**IN CONCLUSION,** *further research is needed to confirm the efficacy of the combination of tetracaine/oxymetazoline nasal spray for anesthesia of maxillary teeth.*

## Addition of mannitol to lidocaine for maxillary infiltrations

Younkin and coauthors[78] determined the anesthetic efficacy of lidocaine with epinephrine compared to lidocaine with epinephrine plus 0.5 M mannitol in maxillary lateral incisor infiltrations. The authors concluded that adding 0.5 M mannitol to lidocaine with epinephrine was not significantly more effective in achieving a greater percentage of total pulpal anesthesia than a lidocaine formulation without mannitol in the maxillary lateral incisor (Fig 3-36). The addition of mannitol to lidocaine increases IANB success, but the addition of mannitol is only effective with nerve block and not with maxillary infiltration.

**IN CONCLUSION,** *the addition of mannitol to lidocaine in maxillary infiltration anesthesia does not increase success.*

## Buccal and palatal infiltration of the first molar

Guglielmo and coauthors[79] evaluated the anesthetic efficacy of a combination palatal (using 0.5 mL of 2% lidocaine with 1:100,000 epinephrine) and buccal infiltration (using 1.8 mL of 2% lidocaine with 1:100,000 epinephrine) compared with a buccal infiltration alone in the maxillary first molar. They reported that the anesthetic success rates (no patient response to two consecutive 80 readings with the EPT) were 88% for the buccal infiltration and 95% for the buccal plus palatal infiltration. The difference was not statistically significant. The buccal plus palatal infiltration significantly increased the incidence of pulpal anesthesia from 21 through 57 minutes. While there was an increased incidence of pulpal anesthesia with the combination buccal plus palatal infiltration, anesthesia was not provided for 60 minutes (Fig 3-37). A palatal infiltration may be helpful as a supplemental injection when the buccal infiltration is not totally effective.

**IN CONCLUSION,** *the combination buccal plus palatal infiltration increased the incidence of pulpal anesthesia over just a buccal infiltration in the first molar.*

## Soft tissue anesthesia of the palate

Meechan and coauthors[80] found that a greater palatine nerve block and a palatal infiltration next to the second premolar provided similar soft tissue anesthesia.

**IN CONCLUSION,** *a greater palatine nerve block and a palatal infiltration next to the second premolar provide similar soft tissue anesthesia.*

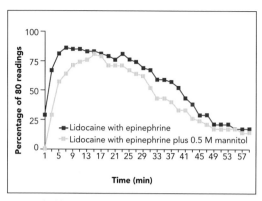

Fig 3-36 Incidence of lateral incisor anesthesia as determined by lack of response to EPT at maximum reading (percentage of 80 readings), at each postinjection time interval, for the two anesthetic formulations. Adding 0.5 M mannitol to a lidocaine with epinephrine formulation was not significantly more effective in achieving a greater percentage of total pulpal anesthesia than a lidocaine formulation without mannitol for maxillary anterior infiltration. (Reprinted from Younkin et al[78] with permission.)

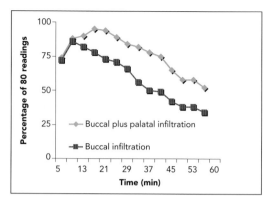

Fig 3-37 Incidence of maxillary first molar anesthesia: comparison of combination palatal and buccal infiltration with a buccal infiltration using 2% lidocaine with 1:100,000 epinephrine. Results determined by lack of response to EPT at maximum reading (percentage of 80 readings) across 60 minutes. The combination palatal and buccal infiltration increased pulpal anesthesia, but anesthesia did not last an hour. (Reprinted from Guglielmo et al[79] with permission.)

## Administering palatal anesthesia

Palatal anesthesia is necessary for the rubber dam clamp and for matrix bands. Various methods have been used to administer palatal anesthesia. For palatal injections using the CompuDent CCLAD system, Johnson and Primosch[81] compared infiltration pain with a topical anesthetic, pressure anesthesia with a cotton-tipped applicator, a combination of both methods, and neither method in the palate. They found no difference among the various site preparation methods used. Nusstein and coauthors[75] found that the CompuDent CCLAD system was less painful for solution deposition than using a standard syringe.

An anecdotal method for anesthetizing the palatal tissue has been proposed. After a labial or buccal infiltration of anesthetic solution, infiltrations of the labial or buccal papillae are given after the infiltration has taken effect. After a few minutes, the lingual papillae are infiltrated. After waiting for a few minutes, the area of infiltration may be enlarged to include more of the palate (if needed, for example, for surgery). While time-consuming, this method may be less painful than a direct palatal infiltration. This method needs to be studied to see if the pain of palatal infiltration can be decreased compared with other common approaches.

**IN CONCLUSION,** *palatal infiltration has the potential to be painful. Further research is needed to decrease the pain of palatal infiltration.*

# Final Thoughts

We covered a lot of good information in this chapter. If we think back to our youth in college, we seemed to learn and understand information at a sustained and rapid pace—remember calculus and organic chemistry (Figs 3-38 and 3-39)? Perhaps, as we grow older, information comes at a slower pace, allowing us to absorb the important points. I think time is nature's way of keeping everything from happening all at once.

**Fig 3-38** Sample equations in calculus.

$$\frac{d}{dx}\int_a^x f\,(t)dt = f(x) \text{ and } \int_a^b F'(x)dx = F(b) - F(a)$$

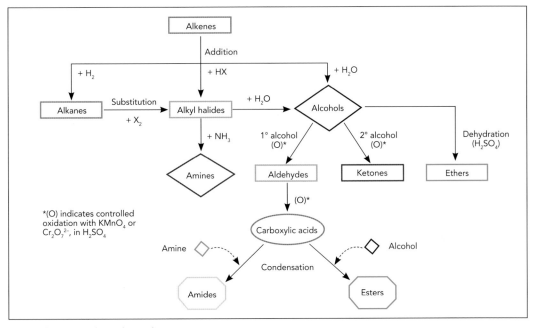

**Fig 3-39** Flow chart of organic reactions.

# References

1. Kaufman E, Weinstein P, Milgrom P. Difficulties in achieving local anesthesia. J Am Dent Assoc 1984;108:205–208.
2. Bjorn H, Huldt S. The efficiency of xylocaine as a dental terminal anesthetic as compared to that of procaine. Svensk Tandl Tidskr 1947;40:831–852.
3. Petersen JK, Luck H, Kristensen F, Mikkelsen L. A comparison of four commonly used local analgesics. Int J Oral Surg 1977;6:51–59.
4. Nordenram A, Danielsson K. Local anesthesia in elderly patients. An experimental study of oral infiltration anaesthesia. Swed Dent J 1990;14:19–24.
5. Haas DA, Harper DG, Saso MA, Young ER. Lack of differential effect by Ultracaine (articaine) and Citanest (prilocaine) in infiltration anesthesia. J Can Dent Assoc 1991;57:217–223.
6. Haas DA, Harper DG, Saso MA, Young ER. Comparison of articaine and prilocaine anesthesia by infiltration in maxillary and mandibular arches. Anesth Prog 1990;37:230–237.
7. Knöll-Kohler E, Förtsch G. Pulpal anesthesia dependent on epinephrine dose in 2% lidocaine: A randomized controlled double-blind crossover study. Oral Surg Oral Med Oral Pathol Oral Radiol Endod 1992;73:537–540.
8. Vahatalo K, Antila H, Lehtinen R. Articaine and lidocaine for maxillary infiltration anesthesia. Anesth Prog 1993;40:114–116.
9. Pitt Ford TR, Seare MA, McDonald F. Action of adrenaline on the effect of dental local anaesthetic solutions. Endod Dent Traumatol 1993;9:31–35.
10. Premdas CE, Pitt Ford TR. Effect of palatal injections on pulpal blood flow in premolars. Endod Dent Traumatol 1995;11:274–278.
11. Chng HS, Pitt Ford TR, McDonald F. Effects of prilocaine local anesthetic solutions on pulpal blood flow in maxillary canines. Endod Dent Traumatol 1996;12:89–95.
12. Nusstein J, Wood M, Reader A, Beck M, Weaver J. Comparison of the degree of pulpal anesthesia achieved with the intraosseous injection and infiltration injection using 2% lidocaine with 1:100,000 epinephrine. Gen Dent 2005;53:50–53.
13. Costa CG, Tortamano IP, Rocha RG, Francishone CE, Tortamano N. Onset and duration periods of articaine and lidocaine on maxillary infiltration. Quintessence Int 2005;36:197–201.
14. Gross R, McCartney M, Reader A, Beck M. A prospective, randomized, double-blind comparison of bupivacaine and lidocaine for maxillary infiltrations. J Endod 2007;33:1021–1024.

15. Mikesell A, Drum M, Reader A, Beck M. Anesthetic efficacy of 1.8 mL and 3.6 mL of 2% lidocaine with 1:100,000 epinephrine for maxillary infiltrations. J Endod 2008;34:121–125.

16. Evans G, Nusstein J, Drum M, Reader A, Beck M. A prospective, randomized double-blind comparison of articaine and lidocaine for maxillary infiltrations. J Endod 2008;34:389–393.

17. Brunetto PC, Ranali J, Ambrosano GMB, et al. Anesthetic efficacy of 3 volumes of lidocaine with epinephrine in maxillary infiltration anesthesia. Anesth Prog 2008;55:29–34.

18. Scott J, Drum M, Reader A, Nusstein J, Beck M. The efficacy of a repeated infiltration in prolonging duration of pulpal anesthesia in maxillary lateral incisors. J Am Dent Assoc 2009;140:318–324.

19. Mason R, Drum M, Reader A, Nusstein J, Beck M. A prospective, randomized, double-blind comparison of 2% lidocaine with 1:100,000 and 1:50,000 epinephrine and 3% mepivacaine for maxillary infiltrations. J Endod 2009;35:1173–1177.

20. Katz S, Drum M, Reader A, Nusstein J, Beck M. A prospective, randomized, double-blind comparison of 2% lidocaine with 1:100,000 epinephrine, 4% prilocaine with 1:200,000 epinephrine and 4% prilocaine for maxillary infiltrations. Anesth Prog 2010;57:45–51.

21. Malamed S. Handbook of Local Anesthesia, ed 5. St Louis: Mosby, 2004.

22. Lawaty I, Drum M, Reader A, Nusstein J. A prospective, randomized, double-blind comparison of 2% mepivacaine with 1:20,000 levonordefrin versus 2% lidocaine with 1:100,000 epinephrine for maxillary infiltrations. Anesth Prog 2010;57:139–144.

23. McLean C, Reader A, Beck M, Meyers WJ. An evaluation of 4% prilocaine and 3% mepivacaine compared with 2% lidocaine (1:100,000 epinephrine) for inferior alveolar nerve block. J Endod 1993;19:146–150.

24. Chin KL, Yagiela JA, Quinn CL, Henderson KR, Duperon DF. Serum concentrations after intraoral injection in young children. J Calif Dent Assoc 2003;31:757–764.

25. Haas DA, Lennon D. A 21-year retrospective study of reports of paresthesia following local anesthetic administration. J Can Dent Assoc 1995;61:319–320,323–326,329–330.

26. Peng M, Zhu ZM, Yang XM. Feasibility of permanent maxillary tooth removal using articaine anesthesia without palatal injection [in Chinese]. Hua Xi Kou Qiang Yi Xue Za Zhi 2008;26:416–418.

27. Uckan S, Dayangac E, Araz K. Is permanent maxillary tooth removal without palatal injection possible? Oral Surg Oral Med Oral Pathol Oral Radiol Endod 2006;102:733–735.

28. Fan S, Chen W, Yang Z, Huang Z. Comparison of the efficiencies of permanent maxillary tooth removal performed with a single buccal infiltration versus routine buccal and palatal injection. Oral Surg Oral Med Oral Pathol Oral Radiol Endod 2009;107:359–363.

29. Ozeç I, Taşdemir U, Gümüş C, Solak O. Is it possible to anesthetize palatal tissues with buccal 4% articaine injection? J Oral Maxillofac Surg 2010;68:1032–1037.

30. Danielsson K, Evers H, Nordenram A. Long-acting local anesthetics in oral surgery: An experimental evaluation of bupivacaine and etidocaine for oral infiltration anesthesia. Anesth Prog 1985;32:65–68.

31. Kennedy M, Reader A, Beck M, Weaver J. Anesthetic efficacy of ropivacaine in maxillary anterior infiltration. Oral Surg Oral Med Oral Pathol Oral Radiol Endod 2001;91:406–412.

32. Teplitsky P, Hablichek C, Kushneriuk J. A comparison of bupivacaine to lidocaine with respect to duration in the maxilla and mandible. J Can Dent Assoc 1987;53:475–478.

33. Branco FP, Ranali J, Ambrosano GM, Volpato MC. A double-blind comparison of 0.5% bupivacaine with 1:200,000 epinephrine and 0.5% levobupivacaine with 1:200,000 epinephrine for the inferior alveolar nerve block. Oral Surg Oral Med Oral Pathol Oral Radiol Endod 2006;101:442–447.

34. Pricco DF. Clinical trials of bupivacaine anesthesia and postoperative analgesia in oral surgery. J Oral Surg 1977;35:26–29.

35. Dunsky J, Moore P. Long-acting local anesthetics: A comparison of bupivacaine and etidocaine hydrochloride in endodontics. J Endod 1984;10:457–460.

36. Rosenquist JB, Nystrom E. Long-acting analgesia or long-acting local anesthetic in controlling immediate postoperative pain after lower third molar surgery. Anesth Prog 1987;34:6–9.

37. Rosenquist J, Rosenquist K, Lee P. Comparison between lidocaine and bupivacaine as local anesthetics with diflunisal for postoperative pain control after lower third molar surgery. Anesth Prog 1988;35:1–4.

38. Tuffin JR, Cunliffe DR, Shaw SR. Do local analgesics injected at the time of third molar removal under general anaesthesia reduce significantly post-operative analgesic requirements? A double-blind controlled study. Br J Oral Maxillofac Surg 1989;27:27–32.

39. Moore P, Dunsky J. Bupivacaine anesthesia—A clinical trial for endodontic therapy. Oral Surg Oral Med Oral Pathol 1983;55:176–179.

40. Neal JA, Welch TB, Halliday RW. Analysis of the analgesic efficacy and cost-effective use of long-acting local anesthetics in outpatient third molar surgery. Oral Surg Oral Med Oral Pathol 1993;75:283–285.

41. Fernandez C, Reader A, Beck M, Nusstein J. A prospective, randomized, double-blind comparison of bupivacaine and lidocaine for inferior alveolar nerve blocks. J Endod 2005;31:499–503.

42. Meechan JG, Blair GS. The effect of two different local anaesthetic solutions on pain experience following apicoectomy. Br Dent J 1993;175:410–413.

43. De Jong RH. Local Anesthetics. St Louis: Mosby, 1994:243–244.

44. Choi RH, Birknes JK, Popitz-Bergez FA, Kissin I, Strichartz GR. Pharmacokinetic nature of tachyphylaxis to lidocaine: Peripheral nerve blocks and infiltration anesthesia in rats. Life Sci 1997;61:177–184.

45. Pabst L, Nusstein J, Drum M, Reader A, Beck M. The efficacy of a repeated buccal infiltration of articaine in prolonging duration of pulpal anesthesia in the mandibular first molar. Anesth Prog 2009;56:128–134.

46. Loetscher C, Melton D, Walton R. Injection regimen for anesthesia of the maxillary first molar. J Am Dent Assoc 1988;117:337–340.

47. Pfeil L, Drum M, Reader A, Gilles J, Nusstein J. Anesthetic efficacy of 1.8 milliters and 3.6 milliters of 2% lidocaine with 1:100,000 epinephrine for posterior superior alveolar nerve blocks. J Endod 2010;36:598–601.

48. Berberich G, Reader A, Drum M, Nusstein J, Beck M. A prospective, randomized, double-blind comparison of the anesthetic efficacy of 2% lidocaine with 1:100,000 and 1:50,000 epinephrine and 3% mepivacaine in the intraoral, infraorbital nerve block. J Endod 2009;35:1498–1504.

49. Karkut B, Reader A, Drum M, Nusstein J, Beck M. A comparison of the local anesthetic efficacy of the extraoral versus the intraoral infraorbital nerve block. J Am Dent Assoc 2010;141:185–192.

50. Corbett IP, Jaber AA, Whitworth JM, Meechan JG. A comparison of the anterior middle superior alveolar nerve block and infraorbital nerve block for anesthesia of maxillary anterior teeth. J Am Dent Assoc 2010;141:1442–1448.

51. Bennett CR. Monheim's Local Anesthesia and Pain Control in Dental Practice, ed 3. St Louis: Mosby, 1983:3–6,34–53,91–97.

52. Baddour H, Hubbard A, Tilson H. Maxillary nerve block use prior to awake intubation. Anesth Prog 1979;26:43–45.

53. Cohn S. The advantages of the greater palatine foramen nerve block. J Endod 1986;14:268–269.

54. Mercuri L. Intraoral second division nerve block. Oral Surg Oral Med Oral Pathol 1979;47:109–113.

55. Johnson L. Regional nerve blocks in general dentistry. Gen Dent 1982;30:414–418.

56. Poore T, Carney F. Maxillary nerve block: A useful technique. Oral Surg Oral Med Oral Pathol 1973;31:749–755.

57. Stebbins H, Burch R. Intraoral and extraoral injections. J Oral Surg Anesth Hosp Dent Serv 1961;19:21–29.

58. Topazian R, Simon G. Extraoral mandibular and maxillary block techniques. Oral Surg Oral Med Oral Pathol 1962;15:296–300.

59. Adriani J. Labat's Regional Anesthesia Techniques and Clinical Applications, ed 4. St Louis: Warren H. Green, 1985:145–153.

60. Cook W. The second division block via the pterygopalatine canal. Mod Dent 1951;18:11–22.

61. Priman J, Etter L. Significance of variations of the skull in blocking the maxillary nerve—Anatomical and radiological study. Anesthesiology 1961;31:41–48.

62. Malamed S, Trieger N. Intraoral maxillary nerve block: An anatomical and clinical study. Anesth Prog 1979;30:44–48.

63. Broering R, Reader A, Drum M, Nusstein J, Beck M. A prospective, randomized comparison of the anesthetic efficacy of the greater palatine and high tuberosity second division nerve blocks. J Endod 2009;35:1337–1342.

64. Forloine A, Drum M, Reader A, Nusstein J, Beck M. A prospective, randomized, double-blind comparison of the anesthetic efficacy of two percent lidocaine with 1:100,000 epinephrine and three percent mepivacaine in the maxillary high tuberosity second division nerve block. J Endod 2010;36:1770–1777.

65. Friedman M, Hochman M. P-ASA block injection: A new palatal technique to anesthetize maxillary anterior teeth. J Esthet Dent 1999;11:63–71.

66. Friedman M, Hochman M. Using AMSA and P-ASA nerve blocks for esthetic restorative dentistry. Gen Dent 2001;49:506–511.

67. Lee S, Reader A, Nusstein J, Beck M, Weaver J. Anesthetic efficacy of the anterior middle superior alveolar (AMSA) injection. Anesth Prog 2004;51:80–89.

68. Burns Y, Reader A, Nusstein J, Beck M, Weaver J. Anesthetic efficacy of the palatal anterior superior alveolar (P-ASA) injection. J Am Dent Assoc 2004;135:1269–1276.

69. Nusstein J, Burns Y, Reader A, Beck M, Weaver J. Injection pain and postinjection pain of the palatal–anterior superior alveolar injection, administered with the Wand Plus system, comparing 2% lidocaine with 1:100,000 epinephrine to 3% mepivacaine. Oral Surg Oral Med Oral Pathol Oral Radiol Endod 2004;97:164–172.

70. Friedman M, Hochman M. A 21st century computerized injection system for local pain control. Compend Contin Educ Dent 1997;18:995–1000.

71. Friedman M, Hochman M. The AMSA injection: A new concept for local anesthesia of maxillary teeth using a computer-controlled injection system. Quintessence Int 1998;29:297–303.

72. Velasco I, Soto R. Anterior and middle superior alveolar nerve block for anesthesia of maxillary teeth using conventional syringe. Dent Res J (Isfahan) 2012;9:535–540.

73. Fukayama H, Yoshikawa F, Kohase H, Umino M, Suzuki N. Efficacy of anterior and middle superior alveolar (AMSA) anesthesia using a new injection system: The Wand. Quintessence Int 2003;34:537–541.

74. de Souza Tolentino L, Barbisan Souza A, Girardi AA, Romito GA, Araújo MG. The anesthetic effect of anterior middle superior alveolar technique (AMSA). Anesth Prog 2015;62:153–158.

75. Nusstein J, Lee S, Reader A, Beck M, Weaver J. Injection pain and postinjection pain of the anterior middle superior alveolar injection administered with the Wand or conventional syringe. Oral Surg Oral Med Oral Pathol Endod 2004;98:124–131.

76. Yenisey M. Comparison of the pain levels of computer-controlled and conventional anesthesia techniques in prosthodontic treatment. J Appl Oral Sci 2009;17:414–420.

77. Ciancio SG, Hutcheson MC, Ayoub F, et al. Safety and efficacy of a novel nasal spray for maxillary dental anesthesia. J Dent Res 2013;92(7 suppl):43S–48S.

78. Younkin K, Reader A, Drum M, Nusstein J, Beck M. Anesthetic efficacy of a combination of 0.5 M mannitol plus 36.8 mg of lidocaine with 18.4 µg epinephrine in maxillary infiltration: A prospective, randomized, single-blind study. Anesth Prog 2014;61:63–68.

79. Guglielmo A, Drum M, Reader A, Nusstein J. Anethetic efficacy of a combination palatal and buccal infiltration of the maxillary first molar. J Endod 2011;37:460–462.

80. Meechan JG, Day PF, McMillian AS. Local anesthesia in the palate: A comparison of techniques and solutions. Anesth Prog 2000;47:139–142.

81. Johnson J, Primosch RE. Influence of site preparation methods on the pain reported during palatal infiltration using the Wand Local Anesthetic System. Am J Dent 2003;16:165–169.

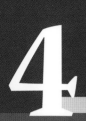

# Supplemental Anesthesia

**After reading this chapter, the practitioner should be able to:**

- Describe supplemental infiltration injections, indications, and success rates.
- Discuss primary and supplemental intraligamentary injections, indications, and success rates.
- Summarize primary and supplemental intraosseous injections, indications, and success rates.

Supplemental injections are essential when anesthesia from conventional injections is inadequate and the pain is too severe for the dentist to proceed. There are three such supplemental techniques: *(1)* infiltration injections, *(2)* intraligamentary injections, and *(3)* intraosseous injections.

If the patient has profound lip numbness and experiences pain on restorative or endodontic treatment, repeating the inferior alveolar nerve block (IANB) does not help the problem. Remember Walter's Law: If you're already in a hole, it's no use to keep digging.

Clinicians may think that another injection is helpful because the patient sometimes achieves pulpal anesthesia after the second injection. However, the second injection does not provide additional anesthesia; the patient may just be experiencing slow onset of pulpal anesthesia that finally registers after the second injection has been administered.

## Supplemental Infiltration Injections

Generally, infiltration injections have not been successful when added to the IANB. The finding that articaine infiltration is superior to lidocaine infiltration has changed how we look at supplemental infiltrations after the IANB. Additionally, repeated infiltrations in the maxilla have not been advocated in the past because we did not know that the initial infiltration would not provide anesthesia for 60 minutes.

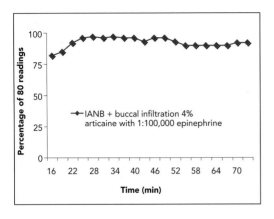

**Fig 4-1** Incidence of mandibular first molar anesthesia for a combination IANB plus a buccal infiltration of 4% articaine with 1:100,000 epinephrine. Results were determined by lack of response to an EPT at maximum reading (percentage of 80 readings) across 75 minutes. The articaine infiltration resulted in a fairly high incidence of pulpal anesthesia through the 50th minute. (Reprinted from Haase et al[1] with permission.)

## Mandibular first molar infiltration of an articaine formulation following an IANB

Haase and coauthors[1] found that 4% articaine with 1:100,000 epinephrine resulted in a higher success rate (88%) than 2% lidocaine with 1:100,000 epinephrine (71% success rate) when combined with the IANB (no patient response to two consecutive 80 readings with the electric pulp tester [EPT] within 10 minutes and sustaining the 80 reading through the 60th minute). For the 4% articaine formulation, pulpal anesthesia reached a plateau following the infiltration and maintained a fairly high percentage of 80 readings through the 50th minute (Fig 4-1). Therefore, for dental procedures requiring profound pulpal anesthesia, high success rates will be obtained at least through the 50th minute. Kanaa and coauthors[2] also found that the IANB supplemented with a buccal articaine infiltration was more successful (92% success rate) than an IANB alone (56% success rate) (no patient response to two consecutive 80 readings with the EPT).

The pain of the buccal infiltration was in the faint-to-weak range for needle insertion, needle placement, and solution deposition. Postoperative pain was also in the faint-to-weak range. The only postoperative complication was slight swelling and bruising (3% to 6% incidence).

It may be prudent for the clinician to wait for signs of lip numbness before giving the buccal infiltration. Without an effective block, buccal infiltration alone will not be completely successful and will have a short duration.[3,4] An additional consideration is that buccal infiltration of a full-cartridge of anesthetic in the vicinity of the mandibular first molar produces mental nerve anesthesia in some patients. This is a result of movement of the anesthetic solution anteriorly.[3] The numbness would preclude the ability to assess the IANB with the symptom of lip numbness.

Regarding the second molar, the relatively thick mandibular bone in the second molar region may hinder anesthetic diffusion if articaine is used as a supplemental infiltration following an IANB.

For the premolars, further investigation is required to determine the success of a buccal infiltration of articaine over the premolars following an IANB. There is some evidence that it should be successful.[1–4]

**IN CONCLUSION,** *adding a buccal infiltration of a cartridge of articaine for the first molar following an IANB should be successful for pulpal anesthesia.*

## Mandibular infiltrations of articaine for anterior teeth

Nuzum and coauthors[5] found that the labial infiltration of a cartridge of 4% articaine with 1:100,000 epinephrine plus a supplemental lingual infiltration of a cartridge of 4% articaine with 1:100,000 epi-

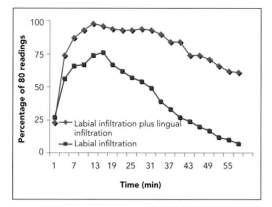

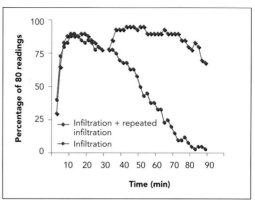

**Fig 4-2** Incidence of mandibular lateral incisor anesthesia: comparison of using articaine for a combination labial and lingual infiltration versus a labial infiltration alone. Results were determined by lack of response to an EPT at maximum reading (percentage of 80 readings) across 60 minutes. The labial plus lingual infiltration significantly improved anesthesia but did not provide anesthesia for an hour. (Reprinted from Nuzum et al[5] with permission.)

**Fig 4-3** Incidence of maxillary lateral incisor anesthesia: comparison of a repeated infiltration injection of a cartridge of 2% lidocaine with 1:100,000 epinephrine given 30 minutes after an initial infiltration of a cartridge of 2% lidocaine with 1:100,000 epinephrine versus the initial infiltration alone. Results were determined by lack of response to an EPT at maximum reading (percentage of 80 readings) across 90 minutes. The repeated infiltration significantly improved pulpal anesthesia from the 37th minute through the 90th minute. (Reprinted from Scott et al[7] with permission.)

nephrine significantly improved the success rate (no patient response to two consecutive 80 readings with the EPT) to 98% when compared with a labial infiltration of a cartridge of the same articaine formulation (76% success) (Fig 4-2). Jaber and coauthors[6] found that 4% articaine was more effective than 2% lidocaine (both with 1:100,000 epinephrine) in anesthetizing mandibular incisors after labial or labial plus lingual infiltrations. However, neither solution sustained anesthesia for 45 minutes. Therefore, it may be indicated to add additional articaine on the labial to extend the duration of pulpal anesthesia.

Another option would be to administer an IANB and then add articaine infiltrations in the anterior teeth to increase success.

**IN CONCLUSION,** *labial and lingual infiltrations of articaine in anterior teeth will be successful initially but will not last for 60 minutes. Adding articaine infiltrations following an IANB should increase success in anterior teeth.*

## Repeated infiltration to increase anesthesia duration in maxillary teeth

Scott and coauthors[7] found that the repeated labial infiltration injection of a cartridge of 2% lidocaine with 1:100,000 epinephrine given 30 minutes after an initial labial infiltration of a cartridge of 2% lidocaine with 1:100,000 epinephrine significantly improved pulpal anesthesia from 37 minutes through 90 minutes in the maxillary lateral incisor (Fig 4-3). For the initial infiltration, approximately 78% of the subjects had pulpal anesthesia at 30 minutes. However, at 45 minutes, approximately 60% of the subjects had pulpal anesthesia. At 60 minutes, only 33% had pulpal anesthesia. With the repeated infiltration, 90% of the subjects had pulpal anesthesia at 60 minutes. At 75 minutes, approximately 85% of the subjects had pulpal anesthesia, and 70% percent were anesthetized at 90 minutes. The repeated infiltration was not painful.

The repeated infiltration can be applied to any of the maxillary teeth. Clinically, we know that infiltrations will not provide pulpal anesthesia for an hour. Therefore, a repeated infiltration should be very helpful in prolonging the duration of pulpal anesthesia. This is a very important finding.

**IN CONCLUSION,** *giving a repeated infiltration of a cartridge of 2% lidocaine with 1:100,000 epinephrine at 30 minutes will significantly improve the duration of pulpal anesthesia.*

# Intraligamentary Injection

## Technique using a standard syringe or a pressure syringe

A 30-gauge ultrashort needle or a 27- or 25-gauge short needle is placed on a standard syringe or pressure syringe. Different needle gauges (25, 27, or 30) have been shown to be equally effective for the intraligamentary injection.[8,9] The needle is inserted into the mesial gingival sulcus at a 30-degree angle to the long axis of the tooth with the bevel facing away from the tooth and toward the alveolar bone. The needle is supported by the fingers or hemostat (if an ultrashort needle is not used) and is positioned with maximum penetration (wedged between the root and crestal bone). For a conventional syringe, heavy pressure is *slowly* applied on the syringe handle for approximately 10 to 20 seconds. For a pressure syringe, the trigger is *slowly* squeezed once or twice with resistance. Back pressure is important. If there is no back pressure—that is, if the anesthetic solution readily flows out of the sulcus—the needle needs to be repositioned and the technique repeated until back pressure is attained. The injection is then repeated on the distal surface. Only a small volume (approximately 0.2 mL) of anesthetic is deposited on each surface. However, when using the CompuDent (Milestone Scientific) computer-assisted local anesthetic delivery (CCLAD) unit—formerly known as the *Wand*— 0.7 mL of anesthetic solution can be delivered on each surface.

Special ligamental syringes are not more effective than a standard syringe.[8,10,11] However, the CompuDent CCLAD system increases the duration of pulpal anesthesia.[12]

## CompuDent CCLAD technology

The CompuDent CCLAD system can be used to administer an intraligamentary injection. The CompuDent accommodates a standard local anesthetic cartridge that is linked by sterile microtubing to a disposable, penlike handpiece with a Leur-Lok needle attached to the end (Fig 4-4a). The device is activated by a foot control that automates the infusion of local anesthetic solution at a controlled rate. A slow or fast flow rate may be initiated and maintained by a foot pedal control. The fast rate delivers 1.4 mL of solution in 45 seconds. The slow rate delivers 1.4 mL of solution in approximately 4 minutes and 45 seconds. The slow rate is used for the intraligamentary injection.

### Intraligamentary injection technique

A cartridge of 2% lidocaine with 1:100,000 epinephrine is placed into the plastic barrel of the CCLAD handpiece assembly, which is then placed into the cartridge holder socket with a quarter turn in a counterclockwise direction (Fig 4-4b). The cap is removed from the needle, and the foot pedal is depressed once to activate the purge cycle to remove air from the plastic tubing and fill the line with anesthetic solution.

The intraligamentary injection is administered with a 27-gauge ½-inch needle attached to the disposable tubing and handpiece assembly. The plastic handle can be shortened by breaking off the portion of the handle near the needle assembly for ease of placement, particularly in posterior teeth (Fig 4-4c). The injection is performed by inserting the needle in the gingival sulcus at the mesiobuccal line angle of the tooth with the needle directed at an approximately 30-degree angle to the long axis of the tooth in the buccolingual plane. The needle is placed into the sulcus with the bevel facing away from

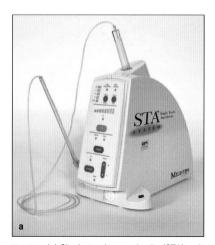

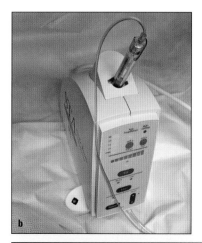

**Fig 4-4** *(a)* Single-tooth anesthesia (STA) unit or CCLAD, formerly referred to as the *Wand*. The handpiece assembly and microtubing are also shown. (Courtesy of Milestone Scientific.) *(b)* The handpiece assembly is placed into the cartridge holder socket with a quarter turn in a counterclockwise direction. *(c)* The plastic handle can be shortened by breaking off the portion of the handle near the needle assembly for ease of placement, particularly in posterior teeth.

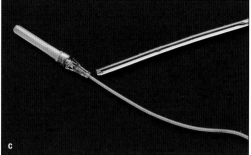

the tooth and toward the alveolar bone. The needle is advanced with firm pressure until it cannot be advanced any farther. The CCLAD unit is activated at a slow rate (by partially depressing the foot pedal) for 8 seconds. Then by removing the foot from the foot pedal, the anesthesia delivery unit is activated on cruise control (continuous flow of anesthetic solution at the slow rate). Audible chimes from the machine and indicator lights on the front of the unit will allow monitoring of volume of anesthetic solution delivered (see Fig 4-4a). Approximately 1 drop of anesthetic solution is delivered every other second on the slow setting. Once 0.7 mL of the anesthetic solution is delivered as shown by the indicator lights, the injection is stopped by lightly tapping the foot pedal once. The time to administer 0.7 mL of anesthetic solution will be approximately 2 minutes and 22 seconds. The injection is then repeated on the distal aspect of the tooth using the same technique and sequence of steps listed above. The total amount of anesthetic solution delivered on the mesial and distal of the tooth is approximately 1.4 mL.

## Single-tooth anesthesia technology

The STA Single Tooth Anesthesia System (Milestone Scientific) device uses dynamic pressure-sensing (DPS) technology that allows continuous feedback during the intraligamentary injection[13] (see Fig 4-4a). Lights on the STA unit give audible and visual indicators that indicate the correct pressures involved to deliver the anesthetic solution by intraligamentary injection. Therefore, the STA unit transforms a blind intraligamentary injection with a syringe into an accurate pressure-sensing injection. The use of the term *single-tooth anesthesia* basically means that the device can be used to anesthetize a single tooth during an appointment. It does not imply that adjacent teeth will not be anesthetized, because they will be. However, no published studies on permanent teeth have been performed to evaluate this new technology.

**IN CONCLUSION,** *the STA device needs to be studied.*

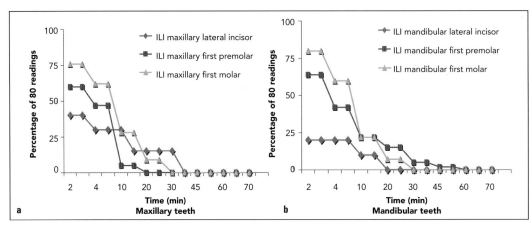

**Fig 4-5** Primary intraligamentary injection (ILI) using 2% lidocaine with 1:100,000 epinephrine in maxillary *(a)* and mandibular *(b)* teeth. Results were determined by lack of response to an EPT at maximum reading (percentage of 80 readings) across 70 minutes. The success rates were highest in the maxillary first molar (75%), mandibular first molar (79%), and first premolars (63%). The maxillary and mandibular lateral incisors had the lowest success rates (39% and 18%, respectively). (Reprinted from White et al[20] with permission.)

## Success rates

### Standard primary injection

The success of the primary intraligamentary injection in achieving pulpal anesthesia has been reported to be 18% to 100% using a conventional syringe or high-pressure syringe.[9–12,14–28] White and coauthors[20] and Schleder and coauthors[21] administered a primary intraligamentary injection using 2% lidocaine with 1:100,000 epinephrine to maxillary and mandibular teeth. The success rates (no patient response to an 80 reading with the EPT) were highest in the maxillary first molar (75%), mandibular first molar (79%), and first premolars (63%) (Fig 4-5). The maxillary and mandibular lateral incisors had the lowest success rates (39% and 18%, respectively). Therefore, the primary intraligamentary injection is not completely successful for pulpal anesthesia. The duration of pulpal anesthesia declines rapidly after the first 10 minutes (see Fig 4-5). The primary intraligamentary injection will not be successful in mandibular anterior teeth.[20,26]

**IN CONCLUSION,** *the primary intraligamentary injection will not be successful in mandibular anterior teeth. In molars and premolars, the primary intraligamentary injection is not completely successful for pulpal anesthesia, and the duration declines rapidly after the first 10 minutes.*

### Primary injection using the CompuDent CCLAD system

Berlin and coauthors[12] compared the anesthetic efficacy of the primary intraligamentary injection of 1.4 mL of 4% articaine with 1:100,000 epinephrine and 1.4 mL of 2% lidocaine with 1:100,000 epinephrine in the mandibular first molar administered with the CompuDent CCLAD system. Successful pulpal anesthesia was obtained 86% of the time with the articaine solution and 74% of the time with the lidocaine solution. There was no significant difference between the articaine and lidocaine solutions (Fig 4-6). The success rate using the CCLAD system for intraligamentary injections was similar to the success rate reported in previous experimental studies with a high-pressure syringe. However, the duration of pulpal anesthesia was longer (around 20 minutes) than reported in previous experimental studies using the high-pressure syringe because more anesthetic solution could be delivered with the CCLAD (see Figs 4-5 and 4-6).

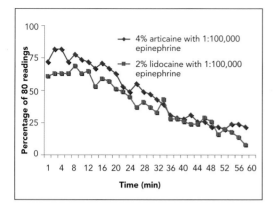

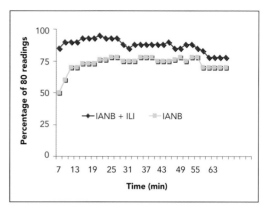

**Fig 4-6** Incidence of mandibular first molar anesthesia: comparison of primary intraligamentary injection of articaine versus lidocaine. Results were determined by lack of response to an EPT at maximum reading (percentage of 80 readings) across 60 minutes. No significant difference between the two solutions was noted. (Reprinted from Berlin et al[12] with permission.)

**Fig 4-7** Incidence of mandibular first molar anesthesia for a combination IANB plus an intraligamentary injection (ILI). Results were determined by lack of response to an EPT at maximum reading (percentage of 80 readings) across 67 minutes. Adding a supplemental intraligamentary injection to an IANB significantly increased pulpal anesthesia for 23 minutes. (Reprinted from Childers et al[24] with permission.)

For needle insertion, moderate pain was reported 14% to 27% of the time, with 0% to 4% of patients reporting severe pain. For solution deposition, moderate pain was reported 8% to 18% of the time, with no reports of severe pain. Regarding heart rate changes, neither anesthetic solution resulted in a significant increase in heart rate over baseline readings. One day postinjection, there was a 20% to 31% incidence of moderate-to-severe pain. The moderate-to-severe pain ratings decreased over the next 2 days.

**IN CONCLUSION,** *for the primary intraligamentary injection of the first molar with the CompuDent system, success was similar for articaine and lidocaine formulations. However, pulpal anesthesia was not completely successful (74% to 86%). The duration of pulpal anesthesia was longer (around 20 minutes) than with a pressure syringe (around 10 minutes).*

## Primary intraligamentary injection versus IANB

Dumbrigue and coauthors[25] compared the effectiveness of a primary intraligamentary injection versus the IANB in extraction of mandibular teeth. Fifty percent of the teeth were removed without discomfort using the intraligamentary technique and 86% using the IANB. Oztas and coauthors[29] found that pain during treatment was higher when the primary intraligamentary injection was used when compared with the IANB in children.

**IN CONCLUSION,** *the IANB was more successful than a primary intraligamentary injection.*

## Supplemental injection

Childers and coauthors[24] found that when the intraligamentary injection using 2% lidocaine with 1:100,000 epinephrine was given following the IANB, the incidence of pulpal anesthesia for the first molar was increased for the first 23 minutes (Fig 4-7).

**IN CONCLUSION,** *adding a supplemental intraligamentary injection of 2% lidocaine with 1:100,000 epinephrine following an IANB increased pulpal anesthesia for 23 minutes.*

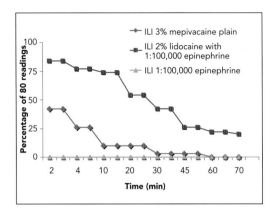

**Fig 4-8** Primary intraligamentary injection (ILI) using 2% lidocaine with 1:100,000 epinephrine, 3% mepivacaine plain, and 1:100,000 epinephrine. Results were determined by lack of response to an EPT at maximum reading (percentage of 80 readings) across 70 minutes. A plain solution of 3% mepivacaine was not effective, and the injection of a vasoconstrictor (1:100,000 epinephrine) alone did not result in pulpal anesthesia. (Reprinted from Schleder et al[21] with permission.)

## Considerations

### *Mechanism of action*

The intraligamentary injection forces anesthetic solutions through the cribriform plate into the marrow spaces around the tooth.[30–33] Therefore, it is an intraosseous injection. The primary route is not via the periodontal ligament. Studies have shown that the most important factor for anesthetic success is injecting under strong back pressure.[8–12,14–26] Back pressure is necessary for success, but the mechanism of action is not a pressure anesthesia[31,33] like the intrapulpal injection.[34,35]

    **IN CONCLUSION,** *the intraligamentary injection should be considered an intraosseous injection.*

### *Anesthetic solutions*

The presence of a vasoconstrictor significantly increases the efficacy of the injection[12,19,21,23,36–38] (Fig 4-8). A plain solution of 3% mepivacaine is not effective for intraligamentary injections.[21] The injection of just a vasoconstrictor (1:100,000 epinephrine) alone does not result in pulpal anesthesia.[21] Anesthetic solutions with reduced vasoconstrictor concentrations (bupivacaine or etidocaine with 1:200,000 epinephrine) are not very effective with this technique.[18,36,37] Articaine (4% articaine with 1:100,000 epinephrine) is similar to lidocaine (2% lidocaine with 1:100,000 epinephrine)[12] (see Fig 4-6).

    **IN CONCLUSION,** *anesthetic solutions without vasoconstrictors or with reduced vasoconstrictor concentrations are not effective for pulpal anesthesia with the intraligamentary injection.*

### *Amount of solution delivered*

Usually, about 0.2 mL of solution is deposited with each mesial and distal injection using a traditional or pressure syringe. However, the exact amount is not always known because some of the anesthetic solution will escape from the sulcus during the injection. More anesthetic solution can be deposited with the CompuDent CCLAD system.

    **IN CONCLUSION,** *only a small amount of anesthetic solution is given with the intraligamentary technique using a traditional syringe or pressure syringe, which accounts for the short duration of pulpal anesthesia.*

### *Intraligamentary injection discomfort*

**Primary injection**

As a primary injection, List and coauthors,[39] D'Souza and coauthors,[11] and Meechan and Ledvinka[26] reported low pain ratings with the injection. In asymptomatic subjects, Schleder and coauthors,[21] White and coauthors,[20] and Moore and coauthors,[19] using intraligamentary pressure syringes, and Nusstein and coauthors,[40] using the CompuDent CCLAD system, reported an approximately 32% incidence of moderate pain with needle insertion in various maxillary and mandibular teeth. Solution deposition re-

| Table 4-1 | Approximate duration of pulpal anesthesia of local anesthetic agents for primary intraligamentary anesthesia[a] | | | |
|---|---|---|---|---|
| | Approximate pulpal anesthesia duration | | | |
| | Premolars | | First molars | |
| Local anesthetic agent | Mandibular | Maxillary | Mandibular | Maxillary |
| 2% lidocaine with 1:100,000 epinephrine | 10 min[b] | 10 min[b] | 10 min[b] | 10 min[b] |
| 2% lidocaine with 1:50,000 epinephrine | Not indicated; epinephrine concentration may be too high | | | |
| 2% mepivacaine with 1:20,000 levonordefrin | Not studied; should be similar to 2% lidocaine with 1:100,000 epinephrine | | | |
| 3% mepivacaine plain | Not indicated; formulations without vasoconstrictors are not effective[18,21,37,38] | | | |
| 4% prilocaine with 1:200,000 epinephrine | Not studied | Not studied | Not studied | Not studied |
| 4% prilocaine plain | Not indicated; formulations without vasoconstrictors are not effective[18,21,36,37] | | | |
| 0.5% bupivacaine with 1:200,000 epinephrine | Not indicated; formulations with reduced vasoconstrictors are not effective[18,36,37] | | | |
| 4% articaine with 1:100,000 epinephrine | Not studied | Not studied | 20 min[c] | Not studied |
| 4% articaine with 1:200,000 epinephrine | Not studied | Not studied | Not studied | Not studied |

[a]Intraligamentary anesthesia is not indicated in mandibular anterior teeth because of low success rates or in maxillary anterior teeth because of painful injection.
[b]White and coauthors[20] and Schleder and coauthors[21] using a pressure syringe and a total of approximately 0.4 mL of formulation.
[c]Berlin and coauthors[12] using the CompuDent CCLAD unit and 1.4 mL of 4% articaine with 1:100,000 epinephrine.

sulted in an incidence of moderate pain of approximately 14%. Generally, the clinician should be aware that moderate pain may be experienced when using the intraligamentary injection. In maxillary lateral incisors, the intraligamentary injection can be very painful (52% moderate pain and 17% severe pain).[20] Because of this pain, we recommend that an infiltration be used in maxillary anterior teeth rather than a primary intraligamentary injection. Meechan and Thomason[41] found that a eutectic mixture of local anesthetic (EMLA) cream reduced the discomfort associated with intraligamentary injections.

**IN CONCLUSION,** *the primary intraligamentary injection has the potential to be painful. It should not be used in maxillary anterior teeth because of the high incidence of moderate-to-severe pain.*

### Supplemental injection
When administered as a supplemental injection following an IANB to anesthetize pain-free vital teeth, low moderate-to-severe pain ratings (3%) have been reported for needle insertion and solution deposition.[24]

**IN CONCLUSION,** *the supplemental intraligamentary injection has a low potential to be painful in asymptomatic patients.*

## Onset of anesthesia
The onset of anesthesia is immediate.[8,10,12,19–21] Therefore, there is no waiting period for the onset of anesthesia. If anesthesia is still not adequate, reinjection is indicated.

**IN CONCLUSION,** *onset is immediate.*

## Duration
### Primary injection
Table 4-1 lists pulpal anesthesia duration of various local anesthetic agents for a primary intraligamentary injection.

As a primary injection, experimental studies with the EPT have shown the duration of profound pulpal anesthesia to be approximately 10 minutes using standard or pressure syringes.[19–21]

Pulpal anesthesia is longer (approximately 20 minutes) when the CompuDent CCLAD system is used.[12]

**IN CONCLUSION,** *the duration of pulpal anesthesia declines rapidly after the first 10 minutes as a primary injection. If using the CompuDent system, duration will be approximately 20 minutes.*

**Supplemental injection**

When used as a supplemental technique following an IANB with a pressure syringe and 2% lidocaine with 1:100,000 epinephrine in pain-free teeth, the duration of pulpal anesthetic effect was approximately 23 minutes[24] (see Fig 4-7).

**IN CONCLUSION,** *the duration of pulpal anesthesia is approximately 23 minutes as a supplemental intraligamentary injection.*

## Postoperative discomfort

When used as a primary intraligamentary technique, postinjection pain has been reported in the majority of subjects.[11,20,21] D'Souza and coauthors[11] found that only a few subjects reported moderate pain, while Schleder and coauthors[21] and White and coauthors,[20] using a pressure syringe, reported an approximately 87% incidence of moderate pain. Nusstein and coauthors,[40] using the CompuDent CCLAD system, found that approximately 31% of the subjects reported moderate pain. Most of this discomfort occurs the first day after injection, and the duration of discomfort averages 14 hours to 3 days.[11,20,21,40] D'Souza and coworkers[11] found that the discomfort was related to damage from the insertion of the needle and not from the pressure of depositing the solution. Additionally, about 37% of patients will report that their tooth feels high in occlusion.[20,21,40] There is no difference in postoperative discomfort between articaine and lidocaine formulations when using the CompuDent CCLAD system.[40]

**IN CONCLUSION,** *there is a potential for moderate postoperative pain following a primary intraligamentary injection.*

## Risk of avulsion

Nelson[42] reported on the avulsion of a tooth following intraligamentary injections in a letter to the editor, which offers no scientific validation. No clinical or experimental study has reported avulsion or loosening of teeth with this technique.[19–21] Therefore, avulsion should not be a concern when using the intraligamentary injection technique.

**IN CONCLUSION,** *avulsion should not occur with the intraligamentary technique.*

## Selective anesthesia of pulpally involved teeth

Although it has been reported that the intraligamentary injection can be used in the differential diagnosis of pulpally involved teeth,[43,44] experimental studies have demonstrated that adjacent teeth also become anesthetized with the intraligamentary injection of a single tooth.[19–21]

**IN CONCLUSION,** *the intraligamentary injection should not be used for the differential diagnosis of pulpally involved teeth.*

## Systemic effects

Smith and Pashley[45] found that intraligamentary injections of epinephrine-containing solutions caused cardiovascular responses similar to an intravenous injection when using a high-pressure syringe in dogs. Cannell and coauthors[46] found that the intraligamentary injections of epinephrine-containing anesthetic solutions did not significantly change heart rate, rhythm, amplitude, or blood pressure when using a high-pressure syringe in human volunteers. An experimental study by Nusstein and coauthors[40] compared the heart rate changes of the primary intraligamentary injection of 1.4 mL of

4% articaine with 1:100,000 epinephrine and 1.4 mL of 2% lidocaine with 1:100,000 epinephrine administered with a CCLAD system in the mandibular first molar. They found that the readings during and after the intraligamentary injection were statistically the same as at baseline. Therefore, these results would support the human study by Cannell and coauthors[46] that reported that intraligamentary injections do not cause significant changes in heart rate.

IN CONCLUSION, *intraligamentary injections do not cause significant changes in heart rate.*

## Safety of the periodontium

Clinical and animal studies have shown the relative safety of this injection technique.[10,19–21,40,47–53] Minor damage is created, but only at the site of needle penetration, and this subsequently undergoes repair. In rare instances, periodontal abscesses and deep pocket formation have occurred after intraligamentary injections.[20,24] Therefore, there is a risk of periodontal abscess formation and bone loss when using the intraligamentary technique. While it is uncommon, the clinician should be aware of this complication.

Histologic areas of root resorption following intraligamentary injections have also been reported.[54,55] It is likely that these would heal with time.[55]

Cromley and Adams[56] found that the intraligamentary injection was safe in the presence of mild-to-moderate gingival inflammation or incipient periodontitis.

IN CONCLUSION, *generally intraligamentary injections are safe, but there have been reports of periodontal abscesses and bone loss.*

## Safety of the pulp

Clinical and animal studies have shown no effect on the pulp following intraligamentary injections.[19–21,55,57,58] However, there are marked physiologic changes in the pulp with a rapid and prolonged decrease in blood flow caused by the epinephrine.[38] Kim[38] felt that the use of the intraligamentary injection during restorative procedures would result in the accumulation of inflammatory mediators and that these would not be effectively removed (due to the decrease in blood flow). Plamondon and coworkers[59] studied the pulpal effects of combined cavity preparation and intraligamentary injections. They found that the intraligamentary injection with an anesthetic solution containing a vasoconstrictor, in conjunction with a deep cavity preparation, did not produce a more severe reaction than the controls (cavity preparation only). The depth of the cavity preparation was the most important factor. Therefore, it seems very unlikely that the intraligamentary injection would cause pulpal necrosis.

IN CONCLUSION, *intraligamentary injections are safe for the pulp.*

## Safety in primary teeth

Brännstrom and coworkers[60] have shown that the intraligamentary injection of primary teeth may cause enamel hypoplasia of the developing permanent teeth. However, the effect was not due to the injection itself but to the anesthetic agents used. That is, the cytotoxic anesthetic agents bound to the enamel matrix in the developing tooth germ. The same effect would seemingly be produced by an infiltration injection next to the developing tooth.

IN CONCLUSION, *the recommendation that intraligamentary injections be used with great care in primary teeth close to developing permanent teeth may not be correct.*

# Precautions

Do not use intraligamentary injections in painful necrotic teeth with periapical radiolucencies or teeth exhibiting cellulitis or abscess formation. This would be very painful and would likely not provide profound anesthesia.

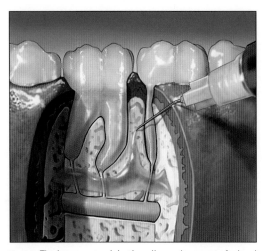

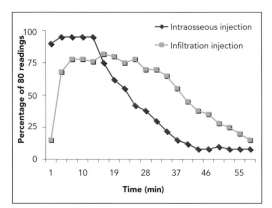

**Fig 4-10** Incidence of maxillary lateral incisor anesthesia: comparison of an intraosseous technique and an infiltration using 1.8 mL of 2% lidocaine with 1:100,000 epinephrine. Results were determined by lack of response to an EPT at maximum reading (percentage of 80 readings) across 60 minutes. The intraosseous technique had a quicker onset and a shorter duration of anesthesia. (Reprinted from Nusstein et al[62] with permission.)

**Fig 4-9** The intraosseous injection allows placement of a local anesthetic solution directly into the cancellous bone adjacent to the tooth to be anesthetized. (Reprinted from Reader[61] with permission.)

Patients with a clinical manifestation of bisphosphonate-related osteonecrosis of the jaw (ONJ) should not receive intraligamentary injections. Although not studied, patients taking oral bisphosphonates may be able to receive intraligamentary injections. Further information is needed.

# Intraosseous Anesthesia

The intraosseous injection allows placement of a local anesthetic solution directly into the cancellous bone adjacent to the tooth to be anesthetized (Fig 4-9).

## How similar are infiltration and intraosseous injections?

Nusstein and coauthors[62] compared infiltration and intraosseous injections in the maxillary lateral incisor using 1.8 mL of 2% lidocaine with 1:100,000 epinephrine. The two techniques were similar except that the intraosseous technique had a quicker onset and a shorter duration of anesthesia (Fig 4-10). Beneito-Brotons and coauthors[63] and Peñarrocha-Oltra[64] and coauthors also showed a faster onset and shorter duration with intraosseous anesthesia. The differences are explained as follows. The anesthetic solution is present in the cancellous bone with the intraosseous injection initially and is then depleted by absorption into the general circulation. The anesthetic solution with the infiltration injection is deposited in the soft tissues and then passes through the barriers of the periosteum and cortical bone. The soft tissue reservoir of local anesthetic solution with the infiltration injection allows a more favorable infusion of anesthetic solution over time.

**IN CONCLUSION,** *intraosseous anesthesia has a quicker onset and a shorter duration of anesthesia than infiltration anesthesia.*

## What do we tell patients when administering intraosseous anesthesia?

An example of an explanation of intraosseous anesthesia *when using a solution with a vasoconstrictor* would be, "Your tooth isn't as numb as we would like. Therefore, we are going to give additional numbing solution next to your tooth. You will feel some vibrations and possibly your heart may beat a little faster." We should not say, "We are going to drill through your gum and bone and then give you a shot of the anesthetic." For the IANB, we do not give detailed description such as, "We are going to go through the mucosal surface, then some tissue and possibly muscle, then hit the bone, and possibly the nerve." We simply say, "We are going to get you comfortable by numbing your tooth."

**IN CONCLUSION,** *communication about the intraosseous injection should be no different than what is said when administering other local anesthesia.*

## Intraosseous injection systems

There are two intraosseous systems that have been extensively studied clinically—the Stabident system (Fairfax Dental) and the X-Tip system (Dentsply Maillefer). Three other anesthetic systems have been available—the Anesto system (Innovadontics), the Comfort Control Syringe (Dentsply), and the IntraFlow (Pro-Dex), which is no longer marketed.

Note: Videos and information on the various systems are available at the manufacturer websites.

### Stabident system

The Stabident system is composed of a slow-speed handpiece–driven perforator and a solid 27-gauge wire with a beveled end that drills a small hole through the cortical plate (Fig 4-11a). The anesthetic solution is delivered to cancellous bone through the 27-gauge ultrashort injector needle placed into the hole made by the perforator (Fig 4-11b).

#### Technique

With the patient in a reclining position, the area of perforation and injection is on a horizontal line of the buccal gingival margins of the adjacent teeth and a vertical line that passes through the interdental papilla distal to the tooth to be injected (Fig 4-11c). A point approximately 2 mm below the intersection of these lines is selected as the perforation site. The soft tissue is first anesthetized by infiltration. Five minutes after the infiltration injection, pressure is applied at the determined perforation site with a periodontal probe. If the patient feels pain, an additional amount of anesthetic solution is administered. Once soft tissue anesthesia is achieved, the perforator is placed through the gingiva perpendicular to the cortical plate (Fig 4-11d). With the point gently resting against bone, the handpiece is activated at full speed while pushing the perforator with light pressure against bone and then slightly withdrawing the perforator and then pushing it against the bone. This action is continued until a "breakthrough" into the cancellous bone is achieved (taking approximately 2 to 5 seconds) or the perforator is placed to length. However, in mandibular anterior teeth, the perforator should not be inserted to full length because it may go through the lingual surface.

Clinical tip: A sterile endodontic rubber stopper can be placed on the injector needle to provide a better seal with the mucosal tissue. The needle can be bent at the hub to a 60- to 80-degree angle to allow for ease of insertion in posterior teeth. The needle is precisely aligned with and inserted into the perforation (Fig 4-11e).

Clinical tip: Watch the angle and pathway of the perforator. Then, without taking your eyes away from the target site, have the assistant hand the syringe to you and place the needle in the same pathway as the perforator. If the needle will not enter the perforation site, reperforate the same site and try again. Sometimes placing a periodontal probe into the perforator hole makes it easier to visualize the angle of needle entry.

Once the needle fully enters the perforation, a full cartridge of anesthetic solution is *slowly* delivered over a 1- to 2-minute time period with light pressure. If back pressure is encountered, the needle is rotated approximately a quarter turn and deposition is reattempted. If this attempt is unsuccessful, the needle should be removed and checked for blockage. If the needle is not blocked, it is reinserted, or the site is opened with a new perforator and the injection is repeated. In some cases, all efforts fail and a new perforation at another site is needed.

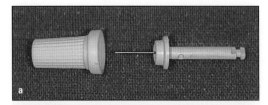 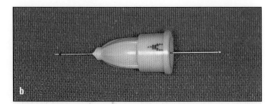

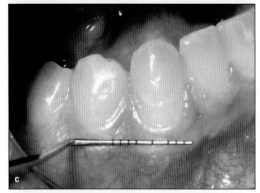 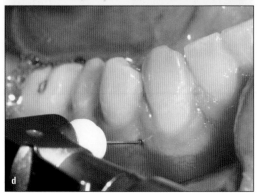

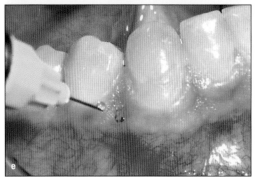

**Fig 4-11** *(a)* Stabident perforator, a solid 27-gauge wire with a beveled end that is placed in a slow-speed handpiece. *(b)* The 27-gauge ultrashort Stabident injector needle is placed into the hole made by the perforator. *(c)* The area of perforation and injection for the Stabident system is approximately 2 mm below a horizontal line of the buccal gingival margins of the adjacent teeth and a vertical line that passes through the interdental papilla distal to the tooth to be injected. *(d)* The Stabident perforator is placed through the gingiva perpendicular to the cortical plate. *(e)* The Stabident perforator needle is precisely aligned with and inserted into the perforation.

**Perforations**

Stabident perforations were rated as easy (could be completed in less than 5 seconds using only light pressure) 76% of the time.[65] The subjective feeling the operator experiences during a difficult perforation (a perforation that requires moderate pressure or takes longer than 5 seconds to penetrate the cortical bone) is that the bone is more dense or thicker than normal. The incidence of a difficult perforation with the Stabident perforator is around 24%.

**IN CONCLUSION,** *easy perforations will occur the majority of the time with the Stabident system.*

## X-Tip system

The X-Tip anesthesia delivery system consists of a device that separates into two parts: the drill and guide sleeve component (Fig 4-12a). The drill (a special hollow needle) leads the guide sleeve through the cortical plate, where it is separated and withdrawn. The remaining guide sleeve is designed to accept a 27-gauge needle to inject the anesthetic solution (Fig 4-12b). The guide sleeve is removed after the intraosseous injection is complete.

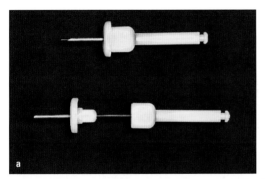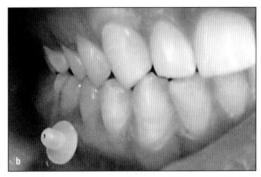

**Fig 4-12** *(a)* The X-Tip anesthesia delivery system consists of an X-Tip *(top)* that separates *(bottom)* into the drill (ie, a special hollow needle) and the guide sleeve component. *(b)* Anesthetic solution is injected through the X-Tip guide sleeve.

## Technique

With the patient in a reclining position, the area of perforation is determined as explained for the Stabident system. If the site is in alveolar mucosa, the site is approximately 3 to 7 mm inferior to the Stabident perforation site. The following describes use of the X-Tip system if the site is in alveolar mucosa.

The alveolar mucosal soft tissue adjacent to the determined perforation site is anesthetized by infiltration. Five minutes after the infiltration injection, pressure is applied at the determined perforation site with a periodontal probe. If the patient feels pain, an additional amount of anesthetic solution is administered. The guide sleeve of the X-Tip system is secured against the drill via finger pressure as the red protective covering is withdrawn. The alveolar mucosa is pulled taut using the fingers of the other hand to minimize engaging the mucosal tissue during rotation of the perforator. The perforator is pushed through the alveolar mucosa until the X-Tip contacts bone. With the drill held at a 90-degree angle to the bone, the slow-speed handpiece is activated at full speed while pushing the perforator lightly against bone and then slightly withdrawing the perforator and then pushing it against bone. This action is continued until a "breakthrough" feeling is observed or the perforator is placed to length. However, in mandibular anterior teeth, the perforator should not be inserted to full length because it may go through the lingual surface. The handpiece is always activated while the perforator is within bone to prevent lodging or breakage that might occur if the perforator is allowed to stop rotating. The drill is then withdrawn from the guide sleeve, leaving the guide sleeve in place (see Fig 4-12b).

Clinical tip: A sterile endodontic rubber stopper can be placed on the injector needle to provide a better seal with the guide sleeve. Before inserting the 27-gauge X-Tip needle into the guide sleeve, the needle can be bent at the hub to a 60- to 80-degree angle to allow for ease of insertion in posterior teeth.

A standard syringe is held in a pen-grip fashion, the needle is inserted into the guide sleeve to its hub, and the anesthetic solution is delivered *slowly* over a 1- to 2-minute time period with light pressure. If back pressure (greater than light finger pressure on the syringe handle to deliver the solution) is encountered on solution deposition, the needle is rotated approximately a quarter turn and deposition is reattempted. If not successful, the needle is removed and checked for blockage. If blocked, select a new needle and syringe. If not blocked, reinsert the needle through the guide sleeve and deposit the solution. In some cases, the solution cannot be deposited. If this is the case, remove the guide sleeve and choose another perforation site. Upon completion of solution deposition, the guide sleeve is removed using a hemostat. The guide sleeve can be left in place if the clinician anticipates that additional anesthetic is needed during the appointment.

**Perforations**

For the X-Tip perforation, 78% of the perforations were rated as easy.[65] There were no differences between the Stabident and X-Tip systems. Therefore, even though the X-Tip perforation is performed in a more apical location, the two systems are clinically comparable for ease of perforation.

   **IN CONCLUSION,** *easy perforations will occur the majority of the time with the X-Tip system.*

**Guide sleeve removal**

Guide sleeve removal with the X-Tip system was rated as easy (removal within 5 seconds) 68% of the time.[65] Difficult removal (requiring more than 5 seconds) occurred 32% of the time. Although difficult removal is based on time, it is worth mentioning that guide sleeve removal required both effort and time in approximately 12% to 17% of patients.[65] In a few patients, the guide sleeve may separate from the plastic sheath, leaving the 3-mm metal segment projecting from the bone. It can be removed with hemostats or Stieglitz forceps.

   **IN CONCLUSION,** *easy guide sleeve removal will occur the majority of the time with the X-Tip system.*

## Anesto system

Anesto gained FDA clearance in 2010. The system consists of a handpiece that drills through the cortical bone and a lever arm that delivers the local anesthetic (Fig 4-13a).

**Technique**

Open the protective covering of the intraosseous needle and screw the needle onto the needle clamping device (Fig 4-13b). Insert the anesthetic cartridge in the needle clamping device (Fig 4-13c). Using the locking knob, slide the plunger to the furthest back position and rotate the locking knob clockwise (Fig 4-13d). Withdraw the retention sleeve of the handpiece and insert the needle cartridge assembly (Fig 4-13e). Fit the handpiece onto the motor. Activate the press button and fit the needle changer onto the protective cap of the injection needle. Remove the protective cap (Fig 4-13f).

   Once the penetration site is selected and anesthesia administered, place the needle through the mucosa and start the drill by stepping on the rheostat. Apply firm pressure to the handpiece and advance the rotating perforator through the cortical plate. Generally, this takes 2 to 5 seconds but may take longer. Once the perforation is accomplished, stop the motor and rotate the locking knob counterclockwise. Press the dosage lever with gentle finger pressure. If the anesthetic solution is not being delivered (dosage lever does not depress), rotate the needle and assembly head after activation of the motor. If still blocked, remove the needle by activating the motor and try another perforation site after adding another needle and cartridge of anesthetic. Once the desired anesthetic dosage has been delivered, start the motor by stepping on the foot pedal. The needle will begin rotating again and can be withdrawn in a single, smooth motion.

   It is sometimes difficult to administer intraosseous anesthesia in molars with the Anesto system because of the straight-line access required with this device.

## Comfort Control Syringe

The Comfort Control Syringe is an electronic delivery system for local anesthesia and has five different injection rates that are preprogrammed into the system (Fig 4-14). The problem is that the presettings may not allow enough anesthetic solution to be delivered for certain types of injections. No objective studies have evaluated the Comfort Control Syringe system in clinical dentistry.

## IntraFlow system

The IntraFlow system combines a slow-speed handpiece with an anesthetic cartridge dispenser system and a rotating needle/drill (Fig 4-15). The anesthetic solution is delivered after the cortical bone is perforated. This system is no longer marketed.

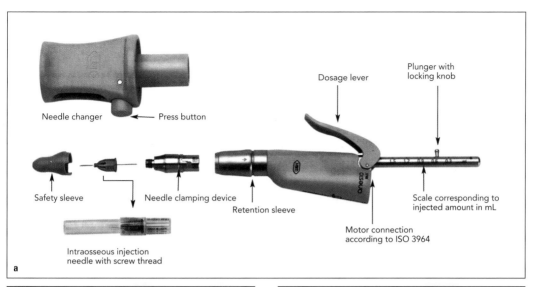

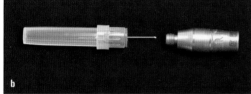

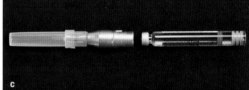

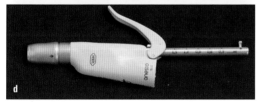

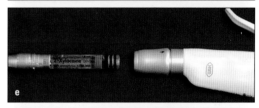

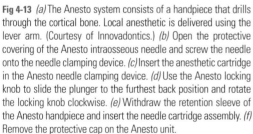

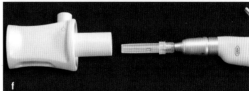

**Fig 4-13** *(a)* The Anesto system consists of a handpiece that drills through the cortical bone. Local anesthetic is delivered using the lever arm. (Courtesy of Innovadontics.) *(b)* Open the protective covering of the Anesto intraosseous needle and screw the needle onto the needle clamping device. *(c)* Insert the anesthetic cartridge in the Anesto needle clamping device. *(d)* Use the Anesto locking knob to slide the plunger to the furthest back position and rotate the locking knob clockwise. *(e)* Withdraw the retention sleeve of the Anesto handpiece and insert the needle cartridge assembly. *(f)* Remove the protective cap on the Anesto unit.

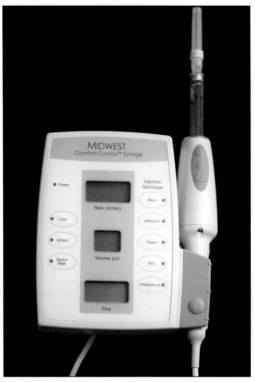

**Fig 4-14** The Comfort Control Syringe is an electronic delivery system for local anesthesia and has five different injection rates that are preprogrammed into the system.

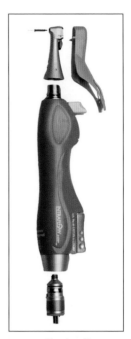

**Fig 4-15** The IntraFlow system combines a slow-speed handpiece with an anesthetic cartridge dispenser system and a rotating needle/drill. It is no longer marketed. (Courtesy of Pro-Dex.)

## Intraosseous needles

Dentsply-MPL Technologies has also introduced intraosseous needles. However, it is questionable if the short injector part of the needle would penetrate through the cortical bone in posterior teeth. Needle bending and clogging may also present problems with these needles.

## Considerations

### Drilling into tooth with perforation

This should not be a major concern because quite a bit of pressure and time is required when encountering a tooth root. The tactile difference between bone and tooth should be easily detected. Once this resistance is noticed, and the perforator is not advancing, withdraw the perforator and select another site. There should be little consequence to making a small superficial hole in the surface of the tooth. It should heal over time.

**IN CONCLUSION,** *drilling into a root should not be a great concern because a large amount of pressure is needed to drill into a root.*

### Pulp safety

Clinical studies have shown no effect on the pulp following intraosseous injections.[65–67] All pulps tested at normal baseline levels at follow-up visits.

## Leakage of anesthetic solution from first perforation when a new perforation is needed

In cases where a new perforation is needed because the initial procedure was not successful in delivering anesthetic solution intraosseously, the injection of the anesthetic solution at the new site sometimes causes the solution to flow from the first perforation site. To counteract this, simply place a gloved finger over the first perforation site to keep the anesthetic solution from flowing out of the hole—just like the little Dutch boy at the dike.

**IN CONCLUSION,** *if leakage of anesthetic solution occurs from the first perforation site, cover it with a gloved finger.*

## Lip numbness

The manufacturers of Stabident and X-Tip state that there is a lack of lip anesthesia when the intraosseous injection is given.[68,69] Gallatin and coauthors[65] found that lip numbness subjectively occurred in 100% of the Stabident injections and in 94% of the X-Tip injections when the intraosseous injection using 2% lidocaine with 1:100,000 epinephrine was given at a site distal to the mandibular first molar. Replogle and coauthors[66] and Coggins and coauthors[67] also reported lip anesthesia when using 1.8 mL of 2% lidocaine with 1:100,000 epinephrine in a primary Stabident injection of the mandibular first molar. Lip numbness is most likely related to the initial intramedullary deposition with extravasation of local anesthetic solution from the mental foramen. It is probably not related to numbing the inferior alveolar nerve within the bone. A preliminary study demonstrated with computer tomography that a Stabident injection of 1.4 mL of a mixture of lidocaine with a radiologic contrast medium distal to the mandibular first molars in dogs showed considerable extravasation of solution from the mental foramen (Klein U, Matamoros A, Hamilton S, Johnson N, unpublished data, 2000). This effect probably occurs in humans as well and accounts for the lip numbness (mental nerve anesthesia).

**IN CONCLUSION,** *for the mandibular first molar, the intraosseous injections will usually result in lip numbness.*

## Pain of perforation and solution deposition

When using the Stabident or X-Tip system as a primary method in asymptomatic subjects, Coggins and coauthors,[67] Replogle and coauthors,[66] and Gallatin and coauthors[65] reported an approximately 23% incidence of moderate pain for perforation in various maxillary and mandibular teeth. Needle insertion resulted in approximately a 9% incidence of moderate pain. Solution deposition resulted in approximately a 21% incidence of moderate pain. Generally, the clinician should be aware that moderate pain may be experienced when using the intraosseous injection technique.

As a supplemental technique in asymptomatic patients, only 3% of the patients will have pain with perforation and needle insertion.[70–72] Approximately 17% may have moderate pain during solution deposition.[70–72]

**IN CONCLUSION,** *the primary intraosseous injection has the potential to be painful approximately 23% of the time. There is less potential for pain when the intraosseous injection is used as a supplemental technique.*

## Perforator separation and breakage

In about 1% of uses of the Stabident and X-Tip systems, the metal perforators separate from the plastic shank during use.[62,65–67,70–75] The metal perforator is easily removed with a hemostat. The separation usually occurs during a difficult perforation (eg, dense cortical bone), and it is likely that the metal is heated excessively due to friction with the bone, causing the plastic hub to melt slightly.

No perforator breakage (ie, metal perforator breaking into parts) has been reported in numerous studies.[62,65–67,70–75] However, if this does occur clinically because of sudden movement of the patient,

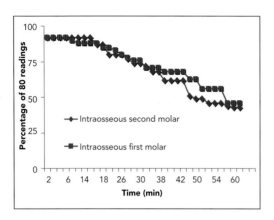

**Fig 4-16** When a distal intraosseous injection is given on the first molar, the second molar obtains equally successful pulpal anesthesia as the first molar.

a simple surgical flap can be reflected and the section of the perforator removed. If the clinician does not feel comfortable performing the procedure, referral to an endodontist is indicated.

**IN CONCLUSION,** *perforator separation and breakage are very rare.*

## Optimal injection site selection

### Location

It is important to remember that a site *distal* to the tooth to be anesthetized will result in the best anesthesia. This recommendation is based on the numerous studies that show the greatest anesthetic effect for a distal injection.[62,65–67,70–75] An exception to this rule would be in maxillary and mandibular second molars in which a *mesial* site should be selected. The recommendation for the mesial injection of the second molars is based on the numerous studies that have demonstrated that the second molar obtains equally successful pulpal anesthesia as the first molar when a distal injection is given on the first molar[62,65–67,70–75] (Fig 4-16).

**IN CONCLUSION,** *the optimal injection site is distal to the tooth to be anesthetized, except for the second molars, where a mesial site should be selected.*

### Attached gingiva or alveolar mucosa

Both the Stabident and X-Tip intraosseous systems instruct the user to locate the perforation site in attached gingiva. The gingival site allows the perforation to be made through a minimal thickness of cortical bone and is generally equidistant between adjacent root structures. However, because the guide sleeve remains in place with the X-Tip system, two studies have successfully used it in alveolar mucosa at a more apical location.[65,76] The X-Tip system has a definite clinical advantage over the Stabident system because the X-Tip perforation may be made at an apical location in unattached gingiva. If the Stabident system is used apically in alveolar mucosa, it is almost impossible to find the hole to deliver the anesthetic solution. Therefore, the clinician may want to consider using the X-Tip in an apical location in specific clinical situations. For example, when periodontal pocketing does not allow perforation into cancellous bone through the more coronal attached gingiva (Fig 4-17a) or there is a lack of interproximal space (roots are too close together) (Fig 4-17b), the X-Tip system can be used to achieve pulpal anesthesia. Furthermore, if the Stabident system fails, the clinician may want to consider using the X-Tip apically to achieve pulpal anesthesia.

**IN CONCLUSION,** *the X-Tip system can be used successfully in alveolar mucosa at a more apical location.*

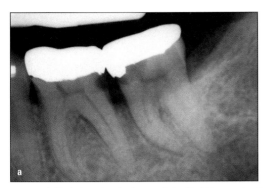 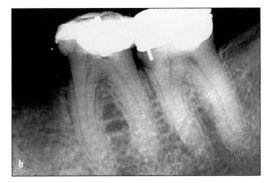

**Fig 4-17** *(a)* Periodontal pocketing precludes Stabident perforation into cancellous bone through the more coronal attached gingiva. *(b)* Lack of interproximal space (roots are too close together) precludes Stabident perforation.

**Fig 4-18** Incidence of mandibular first molar anesthesia: comparison of a primary intraosseous injection (IO) using the Stabident technique and the X-Tip technique. Results were determined by lack of response to an EPT at maximum reading (percentage of 80 readings) across 60 minutes. No significant difference between the two techniques was noted. (Reprinted from Gallatin et al[65] with permission.)

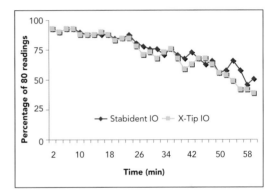

## *Success of a primary injection using lidocaine with epinephrine*

Using a cartridge of 2% lidocaine with 1:100,000 epinephrine, Coggins and coauthors[67] found success rates (no patient response to two consecutive 80 readings with the EPT) of 93% for the maxillary first molar, 90% for the maxillary lateral incisor, 75% for the mandibular first molar, and 78% for the mandibular lateral incisor. Replogle and coauthors[66] reported a similar success rate for the mandibular first molar using a lidocaine formulation. However, Gallatin and coauthors[65] found success rates (no patient response to two consecutive 80 readings with the EPT) of 93% for the mandibular first molar when using the Stabident and X-Tip systems with a cartridge of 2% lidocaine with 1:100,000 epinephrine (Fig 4-18). The higher success rate in the study by Gallatin and coauthors[65] may be related to back pressure occurring in the earlier studies by Coggins and coauthors[67] and Replogle and coauthors.[66] Inadvertently, backflow into the oral cavity may have been included as failure of pulpal anesthesia in these early studies. When compared with the primary intraligamentary injection, the intraosseous injection has a higher success rate and longer duration of pulpal anesthesia (see Figs 4-6 and 4-18). Gallatin and coauthors[65] also found no difference in success between the Stabident and X-Tip systems (see Fig 4-18). Chamberlain and coauthors[77] found that 95% of patients were successfully anesthetized for restorative procedures when using the Stabident system. Sixou and Barbosa-Rogier[78] found a clinical success rate of 92% in children and adolescents using an intraosseous system.

   **IN CONCLUSION,** *high success rates in the mandibular first molar (93%) have been reported when the intraosseous injection is used as a primary injection.*

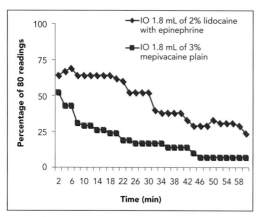

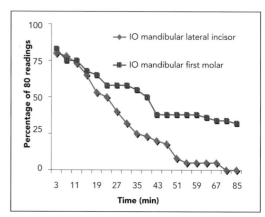

**Fig 4-19** Incidence of mandibular first molar anesthesia: comparison of a primary intraosseous injection (IO) using 1.8 mL of 3% mepivacaine and 1.8 mL of 2% lidocaine with 1:100,000 epinephrine. Results were determined by lack of response to an EPT at maximum reading (percentage of 80 readings) across 60 minutes. The 3% mepivacaine formulation was less successful. (Reprinted from Replogle et al[66] with permission.)

**Fig 4-20** Incidence of mandibular first molar and lateral incisor anesthesia using a primary intraosseous injection (IO) using 1.8 mL of 2% lidocaine with 1:100,000 epinephrine. Results were determined by lack of response to an EPT at maximum reading (percentage of 80 readings) across 60 minutes. The lateral incisor has a more rapid decline of pulpal anesthesia when compared with the first molar. (Reprinted from Coggins et al[67] with permission.)

## Success of a primary injection using mepivacaine

Replogle and coauthors[66] using a primary intraosseous injection found a 45% success rate (no patient response to two consecutive 80 readings with the EPT) for a 3% mepivacaine solution (1.8 mL) compared with a 74% success rate for 2% lidocaine with 1:100,000 epinephrine (1.8 mL) in mandibular first molars (Fig 4-19). Therefore, 3% mepivacaine is not as successful as 2% lidocaine with 1:100,000 epinephrine.

**IN CONCLUSION,** *the success rate is lower (45%) when using 3% mepivacaine plain as a primary intraosseous injection.*

## Duration of a primary intraosseous injection

With a primary intraosseous injection of anesthetic solutions with vasoconstrictors, duration of pulpal anesthesia declines steadily over an hour[65-67] (see Fig 4-18). The duration of useful pulpal anesthesia is approximately 20 to 30 minutes. When compared with the mandibular first molar, the mandibular lateral incisor has a more rapid decline of pulpal anesthesia (Fig 4-20). There is a shorter duration of pulpal anesthesia with 3% mepivacaine or solutions with reduced vasoconstrictor concentrations (eg, 1.5% etidocaine with 1:200,000 epinephrine) when compared with 2% lidocaine with 1:100,000 epinephrine[66,79] (see Fig 4-19). In general, the duration of pulpal anesthesia of 20 to 30 minutes is a drawback to using the technique as a primary injection technique.

**IN CONCLUSION,** *duration is approximately 20 to 30 minutes using 2% lidocaine with 1:100,000 epinephrine. Duration is shorter with 3% mepivacaine.*

## Success of a supplemental injection following an IANB in asymptomatic patients

The supplemental intraosseous injection of 1.8 mL of 2% lidocaine with 1:100,000 epinephrine following an IANB will provide a quick onset and a high incidence of pulpal anesthesia for approximately 60 minutes[70] (Fig 4-21). This is an important finding. Clinicians will appreciate the immediate onset and the duration of pulpal anesthesia.

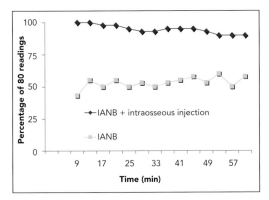

Fig 4-21 Incidence of mandibular first molar anesthesia for a combination IANB plus an intraosseous injection using 1.8 mL of 2% lidocaine with 1:100,000 epinephrine. Results were determined by lack of response to an EPT at maximum reading (percentage of 80 readings) across 60 minutes. Adding a supplemental intraosseous injection to an IANB will provide a quick onset and a high incidence of pulpal anesthesia for approximately 60 minutes. (Reprinted from Dunbar et al[70] with permission.)

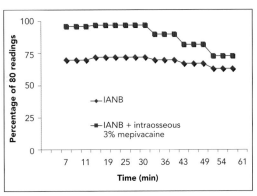

Fig 4-22 Incidence of mandibular first molar anesthesia for a combination IANB plus an intraosseous injection using 1.8 mL of 3% mepivacaine plain. Results were determined by lack of response to an EPT at maximum reading (percentage of 80 readings) across 60 minutes. Using 3% mepivacaine for a supplemental intraosseous injection results in a short duration of pulpal anesthesia (around 30 minutes). (Reprinted from Gallatin et al[75] with permission.)

Clinical tip: It may be prudent for the clinician to wait for signs of lip numbness before giving the intraosseous injection because without an effective IANB, intraosseous anesthesia alone may not be completely successful and would have a short duration.[65–67]

**IN CONCLUSION,** *the supplemental intraosseous injection of 1.8 mL of 2% lidocaine with 1:100,000 epinephrine following an IANB will provide a quick onset and a high incidence of pulpal anesthesia for approximately 60 minutes.*

## Onset of anesthesia

The onset of anesthesia is immediate.[62,65–67,70–75,80] Therefore, there is no waiting period for onset of anesthesia.

## Duration of a supplemental intraosseous injection in asymptomatic patients

With a supplemental intraosseous injection following an IANB in asymptomatic patients, duration of pulpal anesthesia is very good (around 60 minutes) when using a cartridge of a local anesthetic solution with a vasoconstrictor[70,73,74] (see Fig 4-21).

Using half a cartridge of 2% lidocaine with 1:100,000 epinephrine for a supplemental intraosseous injection following an IANB results in a shorter duration of pulpal anesthesia.[71]

A solution of 3% mepivacaine will result in a shorter anesthetic duration—around 30 minutes[75] (Fig 4-22).

Generally, the advantage of using the intraosseous injection (full cartridge with a vasoconstrictor) as a supplemental technique following an IANB is that onset is immediate and duration of pulpal anesthesia is an hour. This result is priceless.

**IN CONCLUSION,** *duration of pulpal anesthesia using a cartridge of 2% lidocaine with 1:100,000 epinephrine for a supplemental intraosseous injection following an IANB is approximately 60 minutes. Duration of pulpal anesthesia using a plain solution of 3% mepivacaine is approximately 30 minutes.*

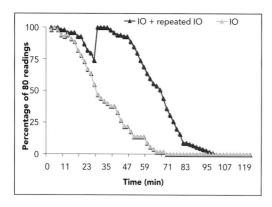

**Fig 4-23** Incidence of mandibular first molar anesthesia for a primary intraosseous injection (IO) and repeated intraosseous injection 30 minutes after the initial intraosseous injection using 1.4 mL of 2% lidocaine with 1:100,000 epinephrine. Results were determined by lack of response to an EPT at maximum reading (percentage of 80 readings) across 120 minutes. The repeated intraosseous injection provided an additional 15 to 20 minutes of anesthesia. (Reprinted from Jensen et al[82] with permission.)

## Success of a supplemental injection for extractions

In a clinical study of extractions of mandibular molars, Prohić and coauthors[81] found that the success of the IANB alone was 74%. After administration of supplemental intraosseous anesthesia using 2% lidocaine with epinephrine following an IANB, the success rate was increased to 95%.

**IN CONCLUSION,** *the supplemental intraosseous injection is also valuable for extractions.*

## The key to success with an intraosseous injection

The key to success with the intraosseous injection is flow of the anesthetic into the cancellous space. If anesthetic solution flows out of the perforation site into the oral cavity, no anesthetic effect will be realized. Reperforation or choosing another perforation site would be a good choice to gain access to the cancellous bone.

In less than 10% of intraosseous injections, constricted cancellous spaces may limit the distribution of the anesthetic solution around the apices of the teeth.[62,65–67,70–75,80] Therefore, failure may result even when the anesthetic solution is delivered intraosseously.

**IN CONCLUSION,** *the anesthetic solution must flow into the cancellous bone.*

## Repeating the intraosseous injection

Jensen and coauthors[82] found that repeating the intraosseous injection (1.4 mL of 2% lidocaine with 1:100,000 epinephrine) 30 minutes after the initial primary intraosseous injection provided an additional 15 to 20 minutes of pulpal anesthesia (Fig 4-23). This was similar to the duration of pulpal anesthesia with the initial intraosseous injection.

Reitz and coauthors[83] found that the repeated intraosseous injection of half a cartridge of 2% lidocaine with 1:100,000 epinephrine given 30 minutes following a combination IANB plus an intraosseous injection did not significantly increase pulpal anesthesia in mandibular second premolars. Apparently, half a cartridge of 2% lidocaine with 1:100,000 epinephrine is not as useful as a full cartridge or 1.4 mL.

**IN CONCLUSION,** *repeating the intraosseous injection of 1.4 mL of 2% lidocaine with 1:100,000 epinephrine 30 minutes after the initial primary intraosseous injection provides an additional 15 to 20 minutes of pulpal anesthesia.*

## Systemic effects with the intraosseous injection

### Heart rate

Various authors have reported a subjective transient increase in heart rate (46% to 93% of the time) with the Stabident or X-Tip intraosseous injection of epinephrine- and levonordefrin-containing solu-

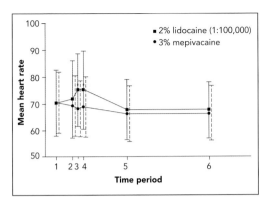

**Fig 4-24** Mean heart rate values (± standard deviations) for patients receiving primary intraosseous injections using 2% lidocaine with 1:100,000 epinephrine and 3% mepivacaine. Significant differences were found at time periods 3 and 4 with the lidocaine solution. In most patients, the heart rate returned to baseline readings within 4 minutes (time period 5). (Reprinted from Replogle et al[84] with permission.)

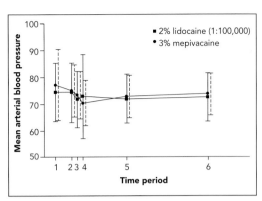

**Fig 4-25** Mean arterial blood pressure (± standard deviations) for patients receiving primary intraosseous injections using 2% lidocaine with 1:100,000 epinephrine and 3% mepivacaine. No significant differences between the two anesthetic formulations were noted. (Reprinted from Replogle et al[84] with permission.)

tions.[65,67,70–76,80,84] Replogle and coauthors[84] reported electrocardiogram recordings showing that 67% of their subjects objectively had an increased heart rate with the Stabident intraosseous injection of 1.8 mL of 2% lidocaine with 1:100,000 epinephrine. The mean increase was 28 beats per minute. Chamberlain and coauthors[77] found that the Stabident intraosseous injection of 2% lidocaine with 1:100,000 epinephrine resulted in a mean heart rate increase of 12 beats per minute. Guglielmo and coauthors[73] reported that the supplemental Stabident intraosseous injection of 1.8 mL of either 2% lidocaine with 1:100,000 epinephrine or 2% mepivacaine with 1:20,000 levonordefrin resulted in a mean increase in heart rate of 23 to 24 beats per minute (measured with a pulse oximeter) in 80% of the subjects. Stabile and coauthors[74] found that the supplemental intraosseous injection of 1.8 mL of 1.5% etidocaine with 1:200,000 epinephrine resulted in a mean increase in heart rate of 32 beats per minute (measured with a pulse oximeter) in 90% of the subjects. Bigby and coauthors[80] found a pulse rate increase of 32 beats per minute using 4% articaine with 1:100,000 epinephrine. Wood and coauthors[85] found that a transient heart rate increase (measured with a pulse oximeter) will occur with the intraosseous injection but not with the infiltration injection of 1.8 mL of 2% lidocaine with 1:100,000 epinephrine in the maxillary anterior region. Verma and coauthors[86] found a 96% incidence of subjective/objective increase in heart rate with intraosseous injection. Zarei and coauthors[87] found a transient increase (9 to 10 beats per minute) in heart rate with intraosseous injection.

Generally, all these studies showed that the heart rate returned to baseline readings within 4 minutes (Fig 4-24). Therefore, injection of anesthetic solutions containing vasoconstrictors, using either the Stabident or X-Tip system, will result in a transient heart rate increase. No significant change in diastolic, systolic, or mean arterial blood pressure will be observed with the intraosseous injection of 2% lidocaine with 1:100,000 epinephrine[77,84] (Fig 4-25).

**IN CONCLUSION,** *injection of anesthetic solutions containing vasoconstrictors, using either the Stabident or X-Tip system, will result in a short-lived heart rate increase.*

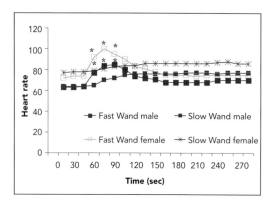

**Fig 4-26** Slowing the rate of the intraosseous solution deposition of 2% lidocaine with 1:100,000 epinephrine with the slow rate of the CompuDent (Wand) CCLAD system significantly reduced the heart rate increase *(asterisks)* when compared with a fast rate of solution deposition. (Reprinted from Susi et al[88] with permission.)

### Reducing heart rate increase by slowing solution deposition

Slowing the rate of the intraosseous solution deposition of 2% lidocaine with 1:100,000 epinephrine by utilizing the slow rate (4 minutes and 45 seconds) of the CompuDent CCLAD system significantly reduced the heart rate increase (only 10 to 12 beats per minute) when compared with a fast rate (45 seconds), which resulted in a heart rate increase of 25 beats per minute[88] (Fig 4-26).

**IN CONCLUSION,** *a slow rate of anesthetic solution deposition (4 minutes and 45 seconds) decreased the heart rate effect of an intraosseous injection.*

### Clinical significance of heart rate increase

While the heart rate increase with the Stabident or X-Tip intraosseous injection of 2% lidocaine with 1:100,000 epinephrine would likely be noticed by the patient, it would not be clinically significant in most healthy patients.[84] The heart rate increase and duration with the intraosseous injection are less than recommended for aerobic conditioning (eg, for a 25-year-old, a heart rate of 136 to 166 beats per minute would be maintained for 20 minutes).[84] However, the patient should be informed of an increase in heart rate to lessen anxiety.

**IN CONCLUSION,** *the heart rate increase from the intraosseous injection would not be clinically significant in most healthy patients.*

## Epinephrine sensitivity

After receiving epinephrine-containing solutions in standard infiltrations and nerve blocks, some patients may overreact to the effects of epinephrine. They may continue to focus on the uncomfortable feeling that their heart is beating fast, causing concern for the practitioner. While these effects are transient, some sensitive patients subsequently refuse to receive epinephrine and may even claim that they are allergic. Because the heart rate effects of an intraosseous injection of epinephrine-containing solutions generally occur more often than they do with infiltrations and nerve blocks, we recommend that dental practitioners choose 3% mepivacaine for these patients.

**IN CONCLUSION,** *a plain solution of 3% mepivacaine should be used in patients sensitive to epinephrine.*

## Medical conditions as contraindications to vasoconstrictors

Vasoconstrictors are contraindicated for intraosseous anesthesia in patients with untreated hyperthyroidism and pheochromocytoma.[89] In addition, Malamed[89] stated that vasoconstrictors should be avoided in patients with high blood pressure (higher than 200 mm Hg systolic or 115 mm Hg diastolic), cardiac dysrhythmias, unstable angina, or severe cardiovascular disease. However, these conditions are contraindications to even routine dental treatment. Therefore, the contraindication to epinephrine or levonordefrin is not the crucial issue in these patients. Rather, it is the safety of performing any dental treatment at all.

**IN CONCLUSION,** *serious medical conditions are contraindications to routine dental treatment.*

## Drug therapies as contraindications to vasoconstrictors

Please review the discussion of vasoconstrictors and drug interaction in chapter 1.

In general, the recommendations on drug interactions state that minimum dosages of epinephrine should be used with frequent aspiration and a slow rate of injection. Because many of these recommendations may not apply to intraosseous injections, epinephrine-containing solutions should not be used intraosseously in patients receiving treatment with certain medications (see chapter 1). A plain solution of 3% mepivacaine would be a good choice for these patients.

**IN CONCLUSION,** *for intraosseous anesthesia in patients taking some systemic medications, a plain solution of 3% mepivacaine should be used.*

## Mepivacaine in medically compromised patients

There will be no significant increase in heart rate when 3% mepivacaine is used for intraosseous anesthesia.[75,84] Thus, in those patients whose medical conditions or drug therapies suggest caution in administering epinephrine or levonordefrin-containing solutions, 3% mepivacaine would be an excellent alternative for supplemental intraosseous injections.[75,84]

**IN CONCLUSION,** *in medically compromised patients, 3% mepivacaine can be used for supplemental intraosseous anesthesia.*

## Long-acting anesthetic agents

In an attempt to increase the duration of pulpal anesthesia with intraosseous injections, some clinicians may use long-acting anesthetic agents. Bupivacaine (Marcaine, Cook-Waite) is a long-acting anesthetic agent but only for IANBs. Long-acting anesthetic agents are not long-acting for intraosseous and maxillary infiltration anesthesia.[74,79,90,91] It is important to realize that bupivacaine has cardiotoxic effects[92] and is basically equivalent to 2% lidocaine with epinephrine in terms of efficacy, duration, and heart rate effects for intraosseous anesthesia. Therefore, bupivacaine offers no clinical advantage.

**IN CONCLUSION,** *long-acting anesthetics offer no advantage over 2% lidocaine with 1:100,000 epinephrine for intraosseous anesthesia.*

## Plasma levels of lidocaine

Some authors have cautioned that administration of an overly large volume of local anesthetic with an intraosseous injection could lead to overdose reactions.[93] Wood and coauthors[85] found that the venous plasma levels of lidocaine were the same for maxillary anterior intraosseous and infiltration injections when using human subjects and 1.8 mL of 2% lidocaine with 1:100,000 epinephrine (Fig 4-27). While there is a short-lived effect on the heart rate due to the vasoconstrictor, the plasma concentration of lidocaine delivered with the intraosseous injection is no more than that delivered with an infiltration. Therefore, the intraosseous technique should not be considered an intravascular injection. Additionally, if it were an intravascular injection, little or no anesthetic effect would be demonstrated. That is, all the local anesthetic solution would be carried into the vascular system with none left for pulpal anesthesia. Obviously, clinical and experimental studies have demonstrated clinical anesthesia with intraosseous techniques.[64–67,70–75,79,80] The same precautions for the maximum amount of lidocaine given for an infiltration injection would also apply to an intraosseous injection.

**IN CONCLUSION,** *plasma levels of lidocaine are the same for intraosseous and infiltration anesthesia.*

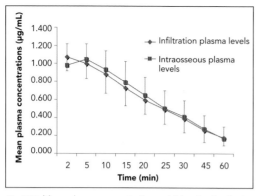

**Fig 4-27** Mean plasma concentrations of lidocaine for the intraosseous and infiltration injection techniques. No significant differences were seen between the two techniques at any time period. (Reprinted from Wood et al[85] with permission.)

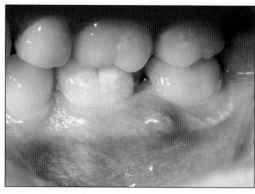

**Fig 4-28** Postoperative swelling at an intraosseous perforation site.

## Postoperative effects

### Discomfort

As a primary and supplemental technique with the Stabident system, approximately 12% of patients will report moderate postoperative pain.[66,67,71,73,94] Postoperative discomfort with the Stabident intraosseous injection is less than that reported for the intraligamentary injection (approximately 31% to 87% incidence of moderate pain).[20,21]

Gallatin and coauthors[94] found that significantly more males experienced postoperative pain with the X-Tip system than with the Stabident system. They felt this was related to denser and more mineralized bone in the posterior mandible in males and the fact that the diameter of the X-Tip perforating system is larger than the diameter of the Stabident perforator, resulting in more frictional heat during perforation.

**IN CONCLUSION,** *approximately 12% of patients will report moderate postoperative pain after receiving an intraosseous injection. This is less than that reported for the intraligamentary injection.*

### Problems

For the Stabident system, less than 5% of patients will develop swelling or exudate at the site of perforation[66,67,71,73,94] (Fig 4-28). Gallatin and coauthors[94] found that the X-Tip system may have a slightly higher incidence of postoperative swelling clinically. With both systems, the swelling and exudate may be present for weeks after the injection but will usually resolve with time.[66,67,71,73,94] These slow-healing perforation sites may be due to overheating of the bone caused by pressure during perforation. Over the last 10 years, anecdotal reports conveyed to the authors from clinicians who use intraosseous anesthesia routinely for endodontic therapy have outlined a very rare occurrence of nonhealing sites that required a minor surgical procedure (curettage) for resolution. Recently, Woodmansey and coauthors[95] wrote a case report in which osteonecrosis supposedly occurred due to intraosseous anesthesia. However, this case report did not confirm that intraosseous anesthesia caused osteonecrosis. Basically, an inexperienced dental student performed the intraosseous injection and separated a portion of an X-Tip perforator. Judging from the photographs in the article, the intraosseous injection was coronal to the ideal site. Following separation, gingival surgery with bone removal was performed.

Follow-up appointments were very poor over a long period of time, and eventually the first and second molars were extracted. The patient also was HIV-positive and was on medications for the condition. This may have contributed to poor bone healing. A number of well-controlled studies using experienced operators have not reported osteonecrosis.[66,67,71,73,94]

With both the Stabident and X-Tip systems, approximately 5% to 15% of patients will report that their tooth "feels high" when chewing for a few days.[66,67,71,73,94] This feeling is most likely an increased awareness to biting that results from soreness in the area caused by damage from perforation or inflammation of the bone. The incidence with the intraosseous injection is lower than that reported with the intraligamentary injection (37% incidence).[20,21]

**IN CONCLUSION,** *less than 5% of patients will develop swelling or exudate at the site of perforations. Generally, these sites heal with time.*

## Precautions

Do not use intraosseous injections in painful teeth with necrotic pulps and periapical radiolucencies or teeth exhibiting cellulitis or abscess formation. This would be very painful and would likely not provide profound anesthesia.

In addition, patients with clinical manifestations of bisphosphonate-related ONJ should not receive intraosseous injections. Although it has not been studied, patients taking oral bisphosphonates may be able to receive intraosseous injections. Further information is needed.

# Final Thoughts

There is good information on supplemental anesthesia. A lot of this information was not available until a few years ago. Supplemental injections should lead the clinician to successful pulpal anesthesia.

We should be eager to try new ideas but cautious in adapting new methods that do not have good research to support them. Remember: Never run a marathon in a new pair of shoes. You run the risk of suffering the agony of "de feet."

# References

1. Haase A, Reader A, Nusstein J, Beck M, Drum M. Comparing anesthetic efficacy of articaine versus lidocaine as a supplemental buccal infiltration of the mandibular first molar after an inferior alveolar nerve block. J Am Dent Assoc 2008;139:1228–1235.
2. Kanaa MD, Whitworth JM, Corbett IP, Meechan JG. Articaine buccal infiltration enhances the effectiveness of lidocaine inferior alveolar nerve block. Int Endod J 2009;42:238–246.
3. Robertson D, Nusstein J, Reader A, Beck M, McCartney M. The anesthetic efficacy of articaine in buccal infiltration of mandibular posterior teeth. J Am Dent Assoc 2007;138:1104–1112.
4. Pabst L, Nusstein J, Drum M, Reader A, Beck M. The efficacy of a repeated buccal infiltration of articaine in prolonging duration of pulpal anesthesia in the mandibular first molar. Anesth Prog 2009;56:128–134.
5. Nuzum FM, Drum M, Nusstein J, Reader A, Beck M. Anesthetic efficacy of articaine for a combination labial plus lingual infiltration versus a labial infiltration in the mandibular lateral incisor. J Endod 2010;36:952–956.
6. Jaber A, Whitworth JM, Corbett IP, Al-Basqshi B, Kanaa MD, Meechan JG. The efficacy of infiltration anaesthesia for adult mandibular incisors: A randomised double-blind cross-over trial comparing articaine and lidocaine buccal and buccal plus lingual infiltrations. Br Dent J 2010;209(9):E16.
7. Scott J, Drum M, Reader A, Nusstein J, Beck M. The efficacy of a repeated infiltration in prolonging duration of pulpal anesthesia in maxillary lateral incisors. J Am Dent Assoc 2009;140:318–324.
8. Walton RE, Abbott BJ. Periodontal ligament injection: A clinical evaluation. J Am Dent Assoc 1981;103:571–575.
9. Malamed SF. The periodontal ligament (PDL) injection: An alternative to inferior alveolar nerve block. Oral Surg Oral Med Oral Pathol 1982;53:117–121.
10. Smith GN, Walton RE, Abbott BJ. Clinical evaluation of periodontal ligament anesthesia using a pressure syringe. J Am Dent Assoc 1983;107:953–956.
11. D'Souza JE, Walton RE, Peterson LC. Periodontal ligament injection: An evaluation of the extent of anesthesia and postinjection discomfort. J Am Dent Assoc 1987;114:341–344.

12. Berlin J, Nusstein J, Reader A, Beck M, Weaver J. Efficacy of articaine and lidocaine in a primary intra-ligamentary injection administered with a computer-controlled local anesthetic delivery system. Oral Surg Oral Med Oral Pathol Oral Radiol Endod 2005;99: 361–366.

13. Hochman M. Single-tooth anesthesia: Pressure-sensing technology provides innovative advancement in the field of dental local anesthesia. Compendium 2007;28:186–193.

14. Kaufman E, Galili D, Garfunkel AA. Intraligamentary anesthesia: A clinical study. J Prosthet Dent 1983;49:337–339.

15. Khedari AJ. Alternative to mandibular block injections through interligamentary anesthesia. Quintessence Int 1982;2:231–237.

16. Ricciardi A. Periodontal anesthesia for all dental procedures: A seven year clinical study. CDS Rev 1984;77(6):24–28.

17. Kaufman E, LeResche L, Sommers E, Dworkin SF, Truelove EL. Intraligamentary anesthesia: A double-blind comparative study. J Am Dent Assoc 1986;108:175–178.

18. Johnson GK, Hlava GL, Kalkwarf KL. A comparison of periodontal intraligamental anesthesia using etidocaine HCL and lidocaine HCL. Anesth Prog 1985;32:202–205.

19. Moore KD, Reader A, Meyers WJ, Beck M, Weaver J. A comparison of the periodontal ligament injection using 2% lidocaine with 1:100,000 epinephrine and saline in human mandibular premolars. Anesth Prog 1987;34:181–186.

20. White JJ, Reader A, Beck M, Meyers WJ. The periodontal ligament injection: A comparison of the efficacy in human maxillary and mandibular teeth. J Endod 1988;14:508–514.

21. Schleder JR, Reader A, Beck M, Meyers WJ. The periodontal ligament injection: A comparison of 2% lidocaine, 3% mepivacaine, and 1:100,000 epinephrine to 2% lidocaine with 1:100,000 epinephrine in human mandibular premolars. J Endod 1988;14:397–404.

22. Edwards RW, Head TW. A clinical trial of intraligamentary anesthesia. J Dent Res 1989;68:1210–1213.

23. McLean ME, Wayman BE, Mayhew RB. Duration of anesthesia using the periodontal ligament injection: A comparison of bupivacaine to lidocaine. Anesth Pain Control Dent 1992;4:207–213.

24. Childers M, Reader A, Nist R, Beck M, Meyers WJ. Anesthetic efficacy of the periodontal ligament injection after an inferior alveolar nerve block. J Endod 1996;22:317–320.

25. Dumbrigue HB, Lim MV, Rudman RA, Serraon A. A comparative study of anesthetic techniques for mandibular dental extractions. Am J Dent 1997;10:275–278.

26. Meechan JG, Ledvinka JI. Pulpal anesthesia for mandibular central incisor teeth: A comparison of infiltration and intraligamentary injections. Int Endod J 2002;35:629–634.

27. Meechan JG. A comparison of ropivacaine and lidocaine with epinephrine for intraligamentary anesthesia. Oral Surg Oral Med Oral Pathol Oral Radiol Endod 2002;93:469–473.

28. Faulkner RK. The high pressure periodontal ligament injection. Br Dent J 1983;154:103–105.

29. Oztas N, Ulusu T, Bodur H, Dogan C. The Wand in pulp therapy: An alternative to inferior alveolar nerve block. Quintessence Int 2005;36:559–564.

30. Dreyer WP, van Heerden JD, de V Joubert J. The route of periodontal ligament injection of local anesthetic solution. J Endod 1983;9:471–474.

31. Fuhs QM, Walker WA, Gough RW, Schindler WG, Hartman KS. The periodontal ligament injection: Histological effects on the periodontium in dogs. J Endod 1983;9:411–415.

32. Rawson R, Orr D. Vascular penetration following intraligamental injection. J Oral Maxillofac Surg 1985;43:600–604.

33. Walton RE. Distribution of solutions with the periodontal ligament injection: Clinical, anatomical, and histological evidence. J Endod 1986;12:492–500.

34. Birchfield J, Rosenberg PA. Role of the anesthetic solution in intrapulpal anesthesia. J Endod 1975;1:26–27.

35. VanGheluwe J, Walton R. Intrapulpal injection: Factors related to effectiveness. Oral Surg Oral Med Oral Pathol 1997;19:38–40.

36. Gray R, Lomax A, Rood J. Periodontal ligament injection: With or without a vasoconstrictor? Br Dent J 1987;162:263–265.

37. Kaufman E, Solomon V, Rozen L, Peltz R. Pulpal efficacy of four lidocaine solutions injected with an intraligamentary syringe. Oral Surg Oral Med Oral Pathol Oral Radiol Endod 1994;78:17–21.

38. Kim S. Ligamental injection: A physiological explanation of its efficacy. J Endod 1986;12:486–491.

39. List G, Meister F, Nery E, Prey J. Gingival crevicular fluid response to various solutions using the intraligamentary injection. Quintessence Int 1988;19:559–563.

40. Nusstein J, Berlin J, Reader A, Beck M, Weaver J. Comparison of injection pain, heart rate increase and post-injection pain of articaine and lidocaine in a primary intraligamentary injection administered with a computer-controlled local anesthetic delivery system. Anesth Prog 2004;51:126–133.

41. Meechan JG, Thomason JM. A comparison of two topical anesthetics on the discomfort of intraligamentary injections: A double-blind split mouth volunteer clinical trial. Oral Surg Oral Med Oral Pathol Oral Radiol Endod 1999;87:362–365.

42. Nelson P. Letter to the editor. J Am Dent Assoc 1981;103:692.

43. Littner MM, Tamse A, Kaffe I. A new technique of selective anesthesia for diagnosing acute pulpitis in the mandible. J Endod 1983;9:116–119.

44. Simon D, Jacobs L, Senia E, Walker W. Intraligamentary anesthesia as an aid in endodontic diagnosis. Oral Surg Oral Med Oral Pathol 1982;54:77–82.

45. Smith G, Pashley D. Periodontal ligament injection: Evaluation of systemic effects. Oral Surg Oral Med Oral Pathol 1983;56:571–574.

46. Cannell H, Kerwala C, Webster K, Whelpton R. Are intraligamentary injections intravascular? Br Dent J 1993;175:281–284.

47. Smith G, Walton R. Periodontal ligament injections: Distribution of injected solutions. Oral Surg Oral Med Oral Pathol 1983;55:232–238.

48. Brännstrom M, Nordenvall K, Hedstrom K. Periodontal tissue changes after intraligamentary anesthesia. J Dent Child 1982;49:417–423.

49. Froum S, Tarnow D, Caiazzo A, Hochman M. Histologic response to intraligament injections using a computerized local anesthetic delivery system: A pilot study in mini-swine. J Periodontol 2000;71:1453–1459.

50. Fuhs QM, Walker WA, Gough RW, Schindler WG, Hartman KS. The periodontal ligament injection: Histological effects on the periodontium in dogs. J Endod 1983;9:411–415.

51. Galili D, Kaufman E, Garfunkel A, Michaeli Y. Intraligamental anesthesia: A histological study. Int J Oral Surg 1984;13:511–516.

52. Peterson J, Matsson L, Nation W. Cementum and epithelial attachment response to the sulcular and periodontal ligament injection techniques. Pediatr Dent 1983;5:257–260.

53. Walton RE, Garnick JJ. The periodontal ligament injection: Histologic effects on the periodontium in monkeys. J Endod 1982;8:22–26.

54. Pertot W, Dejou J. Bone and root resorption: Effects of the force developed during periodontal ligament injections in dogs. Oral Surg Oral Med Oral Pathol 1992;74:357–365.

55. Roahen JO, Marshall FJ. The effects of periodontal ligament injection on pulpal and periodontal tissues. J Endod 1990;16:28–33.

56. Cromley N, Adams D. The effect of intraligamentary injections on diseased periodontiums in dogs. Gen Dent 1991;39:33–37.

57. Lin L, Lapeyrolerie M, Skribner J, Shovlin F. Periodontal ligament injection: Effects on pulp tissue. J Endod 1985;11:529–534.

58. Peurach J. Pulpal response to intraligamentary injection in cynomologus monkey. Anesth Prog 1985;32:73–85.

59. Plamondon T, Walton R, Graham G, Houston G, Snell G. Pulp response to the combined effects of cavity preparation and periodontal ligament injection. Oper Dent 1990;15:86–93.

60. Brännstrom M, Lindskog S, Nordenvall K. Enamel hypoplasia in permanent teeth induced by periodontal ligament anesthesia of primary teeth. J Am Dent Assoc 1984;109:735–740.

61. Reader A. Taking the pain out of restorative dentistry and endodontics: Current thoughts and treatment options to help patients achieve profound anesthesia. Endod Colleagues Excell 2009;Winter:1–8.

62. Nusstein J, Wood M, Reader A, Beck M, Weaver J. Comparison of the degree of pulpal anesthesia achieved with the intraosseous injection and infiltration injection using 2% lidocaine with 1:100,000 epinephrine. Gen Dent 2005;53:50–53.

63. Beneito-Brotons R, Peñarrocha-Oltra D, Ata-Ali J, Peñarrocha M. Intraosseous anesthesia with solution injection controlled by a computerized system versus conventional oral anesthesia: A preliminary study. Med Oral Patol Oral Cir Bucal 2012;17:e426–e429.

64. Peñarrocha-Oltra D, Ata-Ali J, Oltra-Moscardó MJ, Peñarrocha-Diago MA, Peñarrocha M. Comparative study between manual injection intraosseous anesthesia and conventional oral anesthesia. Med Oral Patol Oral Cir Bucal 2012;17:e233–e235.

65. Gallatin J, Reader A, Nusstein J, Beck M, Weaver J. A comparison of two intraosseous anesthetic techniques in mandibular posterior teeth. J Am Dent Assoc 2003;134:1476–1484.

66. Replogle K, Reader A, Nist R, Beck M, Weaver J, Meyers WJ. Anesthetic efficacy of the intraosseous injection of 2% lidocaine (1:100,000 epinephrine) and 3% mepivacaine in mandibular first molars. Oral Surg Oral Med Oral Pathol Oral Radiol Endod 1997;83:30–37.

67. Coggins R, Reader A, Nist R, Beck M, Meyers WJ. Anesthetic efficacy of the intraosseous injection in maxillary and mandibular teeth. Oral Surg Oral Med Oral Pathol Oral Radiol Endod 1996;81:634–641.

68. Stabident instruction manual. Miami: Fairfax Dental, 2001.

69. X-Tip instruction manual. Tulsa, OK: Dentsply Maillefer, 2002.

70. Dunbar D, Reader A, Nist R, Beck M, Meyers WJ. Anesthetic efficacy of the intraosseous injection after an inferior alveolar nerve block. J Endod 1996;22:481–486.

71. Reitz J, Reader A, Nist R, Beck M, Meyers WJ. Anesthetic efficacy of the intraosseous injection of 0.9ml of 2% lidocaine (1:100,000 epinephrine) to augment an inferior alveolar nerve block. Oral Surg Oral Med Oral Pathol Oral Radiol Endod 1998;86:516–523.

72. Reisman D, Reader A, Nist R, Beck M, Weaver J. Anesthetic efficacy of the supplemental intraosseous injection of 3% mepivacaine in irreversible pulpitis. Oral Surg Oral Med Oral Pathol Oral Radiol Endod 1997;84:676–682.

73. Guglielmo A, Reader A, Nist R, Beck M, Weaver J. Anesthetic efficacy and heart rate effects of the supplemental intraosseous injection of 2% mepivacaine with 1:20,000 levonordefrin. Oral Surg Oral Med Oral Pathol Oral Radiol Endod 1999;87:284–293.

74. Stabile P, Reader A, Gallatin E, Beck M, Weaver J. Anesthetic efficacy and heart rate effects of the intraosseous injection of 1.5% etidocaine (1:200,000 epinephrine) after an inferior alveolar nerve block. Oral Surg Oral Med Oral Pathol Oral Radiol Endod 2000;89:407–411.

75. Gallatin E, Stabile P, Reader A, Nist R, Beck M. Anesthetic efficacy and heart rate effects of the intraosseous injection of 3% mepivacaine after an inferior alveolar nerve block. Oral Surg Oral Med Oral Pathol Oral Radiol Endod 2000;89:83–87.

76. Nusstein J, Kennedy S, Reader A, Beck M, Weaver J. Anesthetic efficacy of the supplemental X-Tip intraosseous injection in patients with irreversible pulpitis. J Endod 2003;29:724–728.

77. Chamberlain T, Davis R, Murchison D, Hansen S, Richardson B. Systemic effects of an intraosseous injection of 2% lidocaine with 1:100,000 epinephrine. Gen Dent 2000;48:299–302.

78. Sixou JL, Barbosa-Rogier ME. Efficacy of intraosseous injections of anesthetic in children and adolescents. Oral Surg Oral Med Oral Pathol Oral Radiol Endod 2008;106:173–178.

79. Hull T, Rothwell B. Intraosseous anesthesia comparing lidocaine and etidocaine [abstract]. J Dent Res 1998;77:197.

80. Bigby J, Reader A, Nusstein J, Beck M, Weaver J. Articaine for supplemental intraosseous anesthesia in patients with irreversible pulpitis. J Endod 2006;32:1044–1047.

81. Prohić S, Sulejmanagić H, Secić S. The efficacy of supplemental intraosseous anesthesia after insufficient mandibular block. Bosn J Basic Med Sci 2005;5:57–60.

82. Jensen J, Nusstein J, Drum M, Reader A, Beck M. Anesthetic efficacy of a repeated intraosseous injection following a primary intraosseous injection. J Endod 2008;34:126–130.

83. Reitz J, Reader A, Nist R, Beck M, Meyers WJ. Anesthetic efficacy of a repeated intraosseous injection given 30 min following an inferior alveolar nerve block/intraosseous injection. Anesth Prog 1998;45:143–149.

84. Replogle K, Reader A, Nist R, Beck M, Weaver J, Meyers WJ. Cardiovascular effects of intraosseous injections of 2 percent lidocaine with 1:100,000 epinephrine and 3 percent mepivacaine. J Am Dent Assoc 1999;130:649–657.

85. Wood M, Reader A, Nusstein J, Beck M, Padgett D, Weaver J. Comparison of intraosseous and infiltration injections for venous lidocaine blood concentrations and heart rate changes after injection of 2% lidocaine with 1:100,000 epinephrine. J Endod 2005;31:435–438.

86. Verma PK, Srivastava R, Ramesh KM. Anesthetic efficacy of X-Tip intraosseous injection using 2% lidocaine with 1:80,000 epinephrine in patients with irreversible pulpitis after inferior alveolar nerve block: A clinical study. J Conserv Dent 2013;16:162–166.

87. Zarei M, Ghoddusi J, Sharifi E, Forghani M, Afkhami F, Marouzi P. Comparison of the anaesthetic efficacy of and heart rate changes after periodontal ligament or intraosseous X-Tip injection in mandibular molars: A randomized controlled clinical trial. Int Endod J 2012;45:921–926.

88. Susi L, Reader A, Nusstein J, Beck M, Weaver J, Drum M. Heart rate effects of intraosseous injections using slow and fast rates of anesthetic solution deposition. Anesth Prog 2008;55:9–15.

89. Malamed S. Handbook of Local Anesthesia, ed 5. St Louis: Mosby, 2004.

90. Danielsson K, Evers H, Nordenram A. Long-acting local anesthetics in oral surgery: An experimental evaluation of bupivacaine and etidocaine for oral infiltration anesthesia. Anesth Prog 1985;32:65–68.

91. Gross R, McCartney M, Reader A, Beck M. A prospective, randomized, double-blind comparison of bupivacaine and lidocaine for maxillary infiltrations. J Endod 2007;33:1021–1024.

92. Bacsik C, Swift J, Hargreaves K. Toxic systemic reactions of bupivacaine and etidocaine. Oral Surg Oral Med Oral Pathol Oral Radiol Endod 1995;79:18–23.

93. Ingle J, Bakland L. Endodontics, ed 5. Hamilton, ON: BC Decker, 2002.

94. Gallatin J, Nusstein J, Reader A, Beck M, Weaver J. A comparison of injection pain and postoperative pain of two intraosseous anesthetic techniques. Anesth Prog 2003;50:111–120.

95. Woodmansey KF, White RK, He J. Osteonecrosis related to intraosseous anesthesia: Report of a case. J Endod 2009;35:288–291.

# Clinical Tips for Management of Routine Restorative Procedures

## 5

**After reading this chapter, the practitioner should be able to:**

- Describe how to successfully anesthetize the mandibular molars, premolars, and anterior teeth.
- Describe how to successfully anesthetize the maxillary molars, premolars, and anterior teeth.

The chapters in this book have outlined a substantial amount of information regarding pulpal anesthesia. Now that you have reviewed the information, perhaps you feel like Coach Pat Riley of the Miami Heat basketball team (February 27, 2008): "I feel like a mosquito in a nudist colony. I know what to do. I just don't know where to start."

Because we have outlined studies of pulpal anesthesia, we make our recommendations based on pulpal anesthesia requirements. Every study that has used the electric pulp tester or cold refrigerant for testing pulpal anesthesia can be repeated in a dental office. The practitioner can identify slow onset, anesthetic failures, short duration, and other problems in each individual patient by testing the teeth with a cold refrigerant.

It is important to realize that when we talk about anesthetic effects, we are talking about the majority of patients. There will always be patients outside of the norm. Some patients will be easily anesthetized for all procedures, and other patients will require supplemental techniques to achieve anesthesia. We can determine which kind of patient we are treating by simply pulp testing the teeth.

We want to ensure that the best chance of pulpal anesthesia will be obtained. Primary intraligamentary and intraosseous techniques do not provide sufficient pulpal anesthesia, or the duration is too short for most restorative procedures. Therefore, these techniques should be reserved for supplemental anesthesia. Past recommendations have been based on rather small volumes of local anesthetics. While it is important to minimize doses of local anesthesia, the scenarios list reasonable amounts of local anesthesia to accomplish profound pulpal anesthesia. The amounts are well within the limits of maximum dosages (see Table 1-1). We assume that pulpal anesthesia is required for 45 to 60 minutes because most restorative appointments are this long. We also assume that a rubber dam clamp is used so both buccal and lingual soft tissue would need to be anesthetized. Obviously, other local anesthetic regimens may also be successful. It is our intent to outline what should work the majority of the time for the majority of patients.

However, there is always the Chisholm Effect: If we propose anesthesia regimens that we're sure will meet with everybody's approval, somebody won't like it.

Practitioners should use their best professional judgment, taking into account the needs of each individual patient, when making decisions regarding local anesthesia.

# Mandibular Anesthesia

## First molar

An algorithm for anesthetizing the mandibular first molar is presented in Fig 5-1.

Administer topical anesthetic for at least 1 minute. Slowly administer an inferior alveolar nerve block (IANB) using a cartridge of 2% lidocaine with 1:100,000 epinephrine. A slow injection (at least 60 seconds) will be less painful and will increase the success rate.[1] As an alternative, a two-stage injection technique may be used.[2] The use of the CompuDent (Milestone Scientific) computer-controlled local anesthetic delivery (CCLAD) system—formerly known as the *Wand*—will also reduce the pain of injection.[3–7] Add another cartridge of 2% lidocaine with 1:100,000 epinephrine to decrease the incidence of missed block. Add a long buccal nerve block (a quarter to a half cartridge of 2% lidocaine with 1:100,000 epinephrine). Wait 10 minutes for onset of pulpal anesthesia (see Table 2-2). Check for lip numbness. If not present, wait a few more minutes. If no lip numbness occurs, perform another IANB. Once the lip is numb (soft tissue anesthesia is required in the mandible for success of the supplemental injections), test the tooth with cold refrigerant. If the patient has no response, proceed with treatment. If the patient feels the cold, add supplemental anesthesia. Anesthetic failure will occur around 23% of the time in first molars (see Table 2-1). You could wait a few additional minutes and then retest the tooth with cold refrigerant; some patients have slow onset of pulpal anesthesia (14% of the time in first molars) (see Table 2-2). Remember, if lip numbness is achieved, adding another IANB does not help pulpal anesthesia.

### *When supplemental anesthesia is needed*

Because an articaine formulation has been shown to increase efficacy in the mandibular first molar following an IANB in asymptomatic patients,[8,9] administer a cartridge of 4% articaine with 1:100,000 epinephrine as an infiltration on the buccal aspect of the first molar. Wait 5 minutes (onset of pulpal anesthesia is around 5 minutes with the buccal infiltration of articaine).[10] Retest the tooth with cold refrigerant. If there is no response, proceed with treatment. Pulpal anesthesia should be effective for approximately 60 minutes.[8] This regimen should work the majority of the time in anesthetizing the first molar. If the patient feels pain during the later stages of the appointment, repeat the buccal infiltration with 1.8 mL of 4% articaine with 1:100,000 epinephrine.[11]

It is uncommon to have a positive response to cold refrigerant after administering a cartridge of 4% articaine with 1:100,000 epinephrine. When it does occur, it is probably best to proceed to an intraosseous injection using 1.8 mL of 3% mepivacaine distal to the first molar. This recommendation is not based on the cardiovascular risks associated with a vasoconstrictor-containing anesthetic solution but rather on clinical research indicating that 3% mepivacaine is reasonably effective and does not increase the heart rate.[12,13] A few patients may overreact to the heart rate increase with epinephrine-containing solutions, which can make treatment difficult or time-consuming because the patient has to be calmed before restorative treatment can begin. However, many endodontists also use 2% lido-

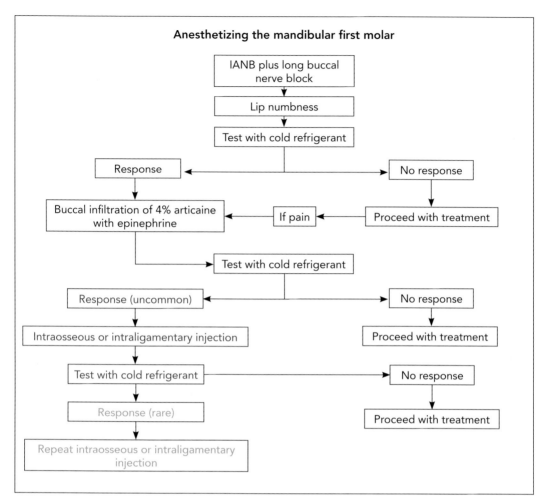

**Anesthetizing the mandibular first molar**

IANB plus long buccal nerve block

↓

Lip numbness

↓

Test with cold refrigerant

Response ← → No response

↓ ↓

Buccal infiltration of 4% articaine with epinephrine ← If pain ← Proceed with treatment

↓

Test with cold refrigerant

Response (uncommon) ← → No response

↓ ↓

Intraosseous or intraligamentary injection    Proceed with treatment

↓

Test with cold refrigerant → No response

↓ ↓

Response (rare)    Proceed with treatment

↓

Repeat intraosseous or intraligamentary injection

**Fig 5-1** Algorithm for anesthetizing the mandibular first molar. Red, uncommon; green, rare.

caine with 1:100,000 epinephrine for intraosseous anesthesia. Each clinician may want to experiment to see which anesthetic solution (3% mepivacaine or 2% lidocaine with epinephrine) works best in his or her hands. Once the intraosseous technique is learned, 1.8 mL of 2% lidocaine with 1:100,000 epinephrine could be used. Retest the tooth with cold refrigerant. If there is no response, proceed with treatment. Pulpal anesthesia should be effective for approximately 30 minutes with 3% mepivacaine[13] and 60 minutes with 2% lidocaine with 1:100,000 epinephrine.[14,15] It may be necessary to repeat the intraosseous injection at 30 minutes if 3% mepivacaine is used.

On the rare occasion that the tooth responds to cold refrigerant after the initial intraosseous injection, repeat the injection with 1.8 mL of 3% mepivacaine or 2% lidocaine with 1:100,000 epinephrine. Pulpal anesthesia should be effective for 30 to 60 minutes depending on the solution used. If the patient feels pain during the appointment, repeat the intraosseous injection.[16] Remember, it might be possible that the IANB is wearing off. Another IANB may help if the intraosseous injection does not seem to be working.

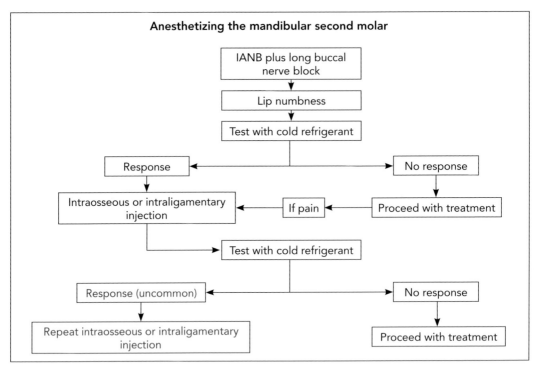

**Fig 5-2** Algorithm for anesthetizing the mandibular second molar. Red, uncommon.

### Alternative choice for supplemental anesthesia

Although not as efficacious as intraosseous anesthesia, intraligamentary anesthesia can be given on the mesial and distal aspect of the tooth using 2% lidocaine with 1:100,000 epinephrine. A plain solution of 3% mepivacaine is not effective for intraligamentary injections.[17] Retest with cold refrigerant. If there is no response, proceed with treatment. If there is a response to cold, repeat the intraligamentary injection. Remember, the intraligamentary injection may only be effective for 10 to 20 minutes. Therefore, it may need to be repeated.

If the patient desires to reduce soft tissue numbness, an injection of phentolamine mesylate (Ora-Verse, Septodont) is administered using the same location and same technique (only for the IANB and infiltration of articaine if it was used) and in the same proportion (1:1) as was used initially for the local anesthetic injection.[18]

## Second molar

An algorithm for anesthetizing the mandibular second molar is presented in Fig 5-2.

Administer topical anesthetic for at least 1 minute. Slowly administer an IANB using a cartridge of 2% lidocaine with 1:100,000 epinephrine. A slow injection (at least 60 seconds) will be less painful and will increase the success rate.[1] As an alternative, a two-stage injection technique may be used.[2] The use of the CompuDent CCLAD system will also reduce the pain of injection.[3-7] Add another cartridge of 2% lidocaine with 1:100,000 epinephrine to decrease the incidence of missed block. Add a long buccal nerve block (a quarter to a half cartridge of 2% lidocaine with 1:100,000 epinephrine). Wait 6 minutes for onset of pulpal anesthesia (see Table 2-2). Check for lip numbness; if not present, wait a few more minutes. If no lip numbness occurs, perform another IANB. Once the lip is numb (soft tissue anesthesia is required in the mandible for success of the supplemental injections), test the tooth with cold refrigerant. If the patient has no response, proceed with treatment. If the patient feels the cold, add supplemental anesthesia. Anesthetic failure will occur around 17% of the time in second molars (see Table 2-1). You could wait a few additional minutes and then test the tooth with cold refrigerant; some patients have slow onset of pulpal anesthesia (12% of the time in second molars) (see Table 2-2).

## When supplemental anesthesia is needed

A buccal infiltration of 4% articaine with epinephrine of the second molar may be used but may not be totally successful. It may be better to use intraosseous or intraligamentary anesthesia.

Intraosseous anesthesia is given mesial to the mandibular second molar using 1.8 mL of 3% mepivacaine or 2% lidocaine with 1:100,000 epinephrine. Retest the tooth with cold refrigerant. If there is no response, proceed with treatment. This regimen should work the majority of the time in anesthetizing the second molar. Although uncommon, if the patient responds to cold refrigerant testing, repeat the intraosseous injection with 1.8 mL of 3% mepivacaine or 2% lidocaine with 1:100,000 epinephrine. If the patient experiences pain in the latter stages of the appointment, readminister the intraosseous injection.[16]

Intraligamentary anesthesia is not as efficacious as intraosseous anesthesia but can be given on the mesial and distal aspect of the tooth using 2% lidocaine with 1:100,000 epinephrine. Retest with cold refrigerant. If there is no response, proceed with treatment. If there is a response to cold, repeat the intraligamentary injection. Remember, the intraligamentary injection may only be effective for 10 to 20 minutes. Therefore, it may need to be repeated.

If the patient desires to reduce soft tissue numbness, an injection of phentolamine mesylate (OraVerse) is administered at the IANB site and in the same proportion (1:1) as was used initially.[18]

# First and second premolars

An algorithm for anesthetizing the mandibular first and second premolars is presented in Fig 5-3.

Administer topical anesthetic for at least 1 minute. Slowly administer an IANB using a cartridge of 2% lidocaine with 1:100,000 epinephrine. A slow injection (at least 60 seconds) will be less painful and will increase the success rate.[1] As an alternative, a two-stage injection technique may be used.[2] The use of the CompuDent CCLAD system will also reduce the pain of injection.[3-7] Add another cartridge of 2% lidocaine with 1:100,000 epinephrine to decrease the incidence of missed block. Wait 10 minutes for onset of pulpal anesthesia (see Table 2-2). Check for lip numbness. If not present, wait a few more minutes. If no lip numbness occurs, perform another IANB. Once the lip is numb (soft tissue anesthesia is required in the mandible for success of the supplemental injections), test the tooth with cold refrigerant. If the patient has no response, proceed with treatment. If the patient feels the cold, add supplemental anesthesia. Anesthetic failure will occur from 19% to 21% of the time in premolars (see Table 2-1). You could wait a few additional minutes and then test the tooth with cold refrigerant; some patients have slow onset of pulpal anesthesia (19% to 20% of the time in premolars) (see Table 2-2).

## When supplemental anesthesia is needed

Because an articaine formulation has been shown to anesthetize premolars,[10] and because the addition of an infiltration in the premolar area after an IANB is successful,[19] administer 1.8 mL of 4% articaine with 1:100,000 epinephrine as an infiltration on the buccal aspect of the premolar under treatment. Wait 5 minutes (onset of pulpal anesthesia for a buccal infiltration of articaine is around 5 minutes),[10] and retest the tooth with cold refrigerant. If there is no response, proceed with treatment. This regimen should work the majority of the time in anesthetizing premolars. If the patient experiences pain in the latter stages of the appointment, readminister 4% articaine with 1:100,000 epinephrine.[11]

On the rare occasion that the tooth responds to cold, it is probably best to proceed to an intraosseous injection with 1.8 mL of 3% mepivacaine distal to the premolar. It is safe to administer this injec-

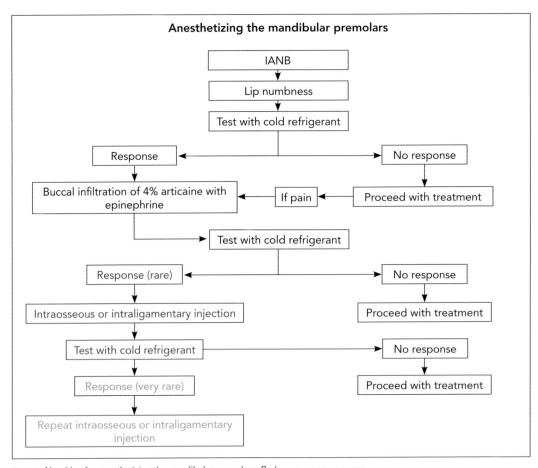

**Fig 5-3** Algorithm for anesthetizing the mandibular premolars. Red, rare; green, very rare.

tion in the premolars if the perforation site is in attached gingiva. Retest the tooth with cold refrigerant. If there is no response, proceed with treatment. If there is a response to cold, repeat the intraosseous injection with 1.8 mL of 3% mepivacaine. If the patient experiences pain in the latter stages of the appointment, readminister the intraosseous injection.[16]

### Alternative choice for supplemental anesthesia
Although not as efficacious as intraosseous anesthesia, intraligamentary anesthesia can be given on the mesial and distal aspect of the tooth using 2% lidocaine with 1:100,000 epinephrine. A plain solution of 3% mepivacaine is not effective for intraligamentary injections.[17] Retest with cold refrigerant. If there is no response, proceed with treatment. If there is a response to cold, repeat the intraligamentary injection.

 If the patient desires to reduce soft tissue numbness, an injection of phentolamine mesylate (OraVerse) is administered using the same location and same technique (for only the IANB and infiltration of articaine if it was used) and in the same proportion (1:1) as was used initially for the local anesthetic injection.[18]

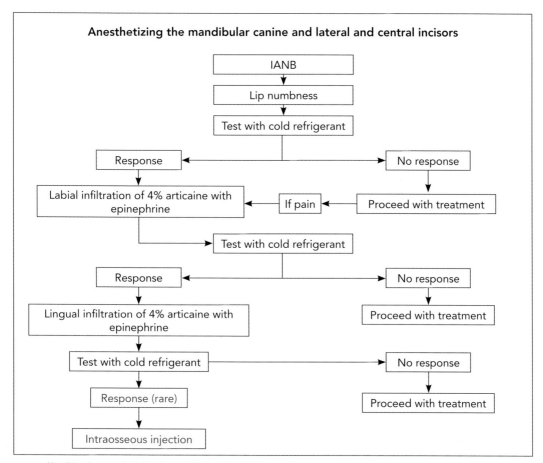

**Fig 5-4** Algorithm for anesthetizing the mandibular canine, lateral incisor, and central incisor. Red, rare.

## Canine and lateral and central incisors

An algorithm for anesthetizing the mandibular canine and lateral and central incisors is presented in Fig 5-4.

Administer topical anesthetic for at least 1 minute. Slowly administer an IANB using a cartridge of 2% lidocaine with 1:100,000 epinephrine. A slow injection (at least 60 seconds) will be less painful and will increase the success rate.[1] As an alternative, a two-stage injection technique may be used.[2] The use of the CompuDent CCLAD system will also reduce the pain of injection.[3-7] Add another cartridge of 2% lidocaine with 1:100,000 epinephrine to decrease the incidence of missed block. Wait 14 to 19 minutes because onset of pulpal anesthesia is longer for the anterior teeth than the posterior teeth (see Table 2-2). Check for lip numbness. If not present, wait a few more minutes. If no lip numbness occurs, perform another IANB. Once the lip is numb (soft tissue anesthesia is required in the mandible for success of the supplemental injections), test the tooth with cold refrigerant. If the patient has no response, proceed with treatment. If the patient feels the cold, add supplemental anesthesia. Anesthetic failure will occur 32%, 44%, and 58% of the time in canines, lateral incisors, and central incisors, respectively (see Table 2-1). You could wait a few additional minutes and then test the tooth with cold refrigerant; some patients have slow onset of pulpal anesthesia (16% to 20% of the time in anterior teeth) (see Table 2-2).

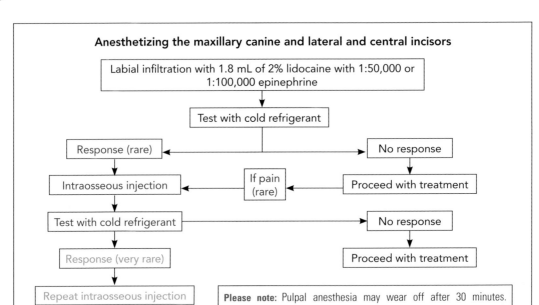

**Anesthetizing the maxillary canine and lateral and central incisors**

Labial infiltration with 1.8 mL of 2% lidocaine with 1:50,000 or 1:100,000 epinephrine

↓

Test with cold refrigerant

Response (rare) ← → No response

↓ ↓

Intraosseous injection ← If pain (rare) ← Proceed with treatment

↓

Test with cold refrigerant → No response

↓ ↓

Response (very rare) Proceed with treatment

↓

Repeat intraosseous injection

**Please note:** Pulpal anesthesia may wear off after 30 minutes. Reinjection of a cartridge of 2% lidocaine with 1:100,000 epinephrine should provide pulpal anesthesia for 60 minutes.

**Fig 5-5** Algorithm for anesthetizing the maxillary central incisor, lateral incisor, and canine. Red, rare; green, very rare.

## When supplemental anesthesia is needed

Because the addition of an infiltration in the mandibular anterior teeth after an IANB is successful,[20] add a labial infiltration of a cartridge of 4% articaine with 1:100,000 epinephrine.[20,21] Test the tooth with cold refrigerant. If there is a response to cold, add a lingual infiltration of a cartridge of 4% articaine with 1:100,000 epinephrine.[21] This regimen should work the majority of the time in anesthetizing the anterior teeth. Test the tooth with cold refrigerant. On the rare occasion that the patient responds to the cold, add an intraosseous injection of 1.8 mL of 3% mepivacaine or 2% lidocaine with 1:100,000 epinephrine distal to the anterior tooth to be anesthetized. Because intraligamentary anesthesia is not successful in anterior teeth,[22] intraosseous anesthesia is indicated. Retest the tooth with cold refrigerant. If there is no response, proceed with treatment. If there is a response to cold, repeat the intraosseous injection with 1.8 mL of 3% mepivacaine or 2% lidocaine with 1:100,000 epinephrine.

If the patient desires to reduce soft tissue numbness, an injection of phentolamine mesylate (OraVerse) is administered using the same location and same technique (only for the IANB and infiltration of articaine if it was used) and in the same proportion (1:1) as was used initially for the local anesthetic injection.[18]

# Maxillary Anesthesia

## Central and lateral incisors and canine

An algorithm for anesthetizing the maxillary central and lateral incisors and canine is presented in Fig 5-5.

Administer topical anesthetic for at least 1 minute. Slowly administer an infiltration using a cartridge of 2% lidocaine with 1:50,000 epinephrine or 1:100,000 epinephrine. The higher concentration of epinephrine (1:50,000) will provide a more effective duration.[23] A slow injection (at least 60 seconds) will be less painful. As an alternative, a two-stage injection technique may be used.[1] The use of the

CompuDent CCLAD system will also reduce the pain of injection.[3–7] If lingual soft tissue anesthesia is needed for a rubber dam clamp, administer 2% lidocaine with 1:100,000 epinephrine to the palatal tissue. The CompuDent CCLAD system will reduce the pain of a palatal injection.[24,25] Wait 4 minutes because onset of pulpal anesthesia will be around 4 minutes for the anterior teeth (see Table 3-2). Test the tooth with cold refrigerant. If there is no response, proceed with treatment. This regimen should work the majority of the time in initially anesthetizing the maxillary anterior teeth. If there is a response to cold, you could wait an additional 3 to 5 minutes and retest. Although it is uncommon, if the patient still responds to the cold refrigerant, administer supplemental anesthesia.

### Duration of pulpal anesthesia

It is important to realize that pulpal anesthesia starts to decline around 30 minutes after an initial infiltration in maxillary teeth (see Table 3-3). Therefore, at approximately 30 minutes, an additional infiltration of 1.8 mL of 2% lidocaine with 1:100,000 epinephrine can be given. The additional infiltration will prolong pulpal anesthesia until at least the 60th minute.[26]

### When supplemental anesthesia is needed

Intraosseous anesthesia is indicated as supplemental anesthesia because intraligamentary anesthesia is very painful in maxillary anterior teeth and has a success rate of 39% and a duration of only 10 minutes.[22] In some patients, infiltration anesthesia is not completely effective, and intraosseous anesthesia is very helpful. Use 1.8 mL of 3% mepivacaine or 2% lidocaine with 1:100,000 epinephrine distal to the tooth being treated. If the intraosseous injection is given, there may be a need for an additional intraosseous injection, using 1.8 mL of anesthetic solution, at approximately 30 to 45 minutes because the intraosseous injection will not provide 60 minutes of pulpal anesthesia in the maxilla.[27]

If the patient desires to reduce soft tissue numbness, an injection of phentolamine mesylate (OraVerse) is administered using the same location and same technique (only infiltration site) and in the same proportion (1:1) as was used initially for the local anesthetic injection.[18]

## Premolars and molars

An algorithm for anesthetizing the maxillary premolars and molars is presented in Fig 5-6.

Administer topical anesthetic for at least 1 minute. Slowly administer an infiltration using a cartridge of 2% lidocaine with 1:100,000 epinephrine. A slow injection (at least 60 seconds) will be less painful. As an alternative, a two-stage injection technique may be used.[2] The use of the CompuDent CCLAD system will also reduce the pain of injection.[3–7] Add another cartridge of 2% lidocaine with 1:100,000 epinephrine (total volume of 3.6 mL). The 3.6-mL volume helps to prolong the duration of anesthesia.[28] If lingual soft tissue anesthesia is needed, administer 2% lidocaine with 1:100,000 epinephrine to the palatal tissue. The CompuDent CCLAD system will reduce the pain of a palatal injection.[24,25] Wait 5 minutes; the onset of pulpal anesthesia will be 5 minutes or less (see Table 3-2). Test the tooth with cold refrigerant. If there is no response, proceed with treatment. This regimen should work the majority of the time in initially anesthetizing the maxillary premolars and molars. If there is a response to cold, you could wait an additional 3 to 5 minutes and retest. In the rare instance that the tooth still responds to cold refrigerant, administer supplemental anesthesia.

### Duration of pulpal anesthesia

In maxillary premolars and molars, pulpal anesthesia starts to decline around 45 minutes after an initial infiltration and at a slower rate than in anterior teeth (see Table 3-3). Therefore, if the patient starts to feel pain (or cold refrigerant testing reveals that the patient is no longer anesthetized) around 45 minutes, an infiltration of 1.8 mL of 2% lidocaine with 1:100,000 epinephrine can be given. The additional infiltration will prolong the duration of pulpal anesthesia.

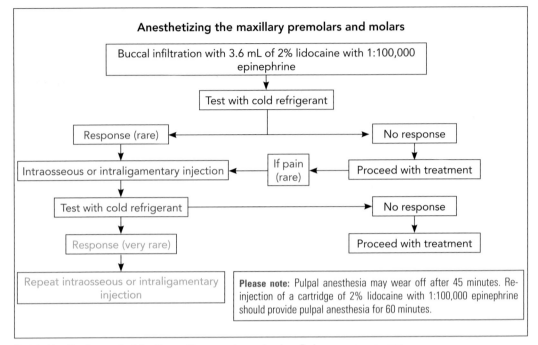

**Fig 5-6** Algorithm for anesthetizing the maxillary premolars and molars. Red, rare; green, very rare.

## *When supplemental anesthesia is needed*

In some patients, infiltration anesthesia is not completely effective; therefore, the intraosseous injection is indicated. Administer an intraosseous injection with 1.8 mL of 3% mepivacaine or 2% lidocaine with 1:100,000 epinephrine on the distal of the tooth to be anesthetized. If the tooth is a maxillary second molar, a mesial intraosseous injection site is chosen. There may be a need for an additional intraosseous injection, using 1.8 mL of anesthetic solution, at approximately 45 minutes because the intraosseous injection will not provide 60 minutes of pulpal anesthesia.

### Alternative choice for supplemental anesthesia

Although not as efficacious as intraosseous anesthesia, intraligamentary anesthesia can be given on the mesial and distal aspect of the tooth using 2% lidocaine with 1:100,000 epinephrine. Retest with cold refrigerant. If there is no response, proceed with treatment. If the tooth responds to cold, repeat the intraligamentary injection.

If the patient desires to reduce soft tissue numbness, an injection of phentolamine mesylate (Ora-Verse) is administered using the same location and same technique (only infiltration site) and in the same proportion (1:1) as was used initially for the local anesthetic injection.[18]

## Final Thoughts

The anesthesia regimens outlined should provide pulpal anesthesia in the majority of patients. The methods are fairly simple, and with a little practice the supplemental techniques can be mastered.

Remember Reader's Revision to Booker's Law: If anesthesia regimens are sufficiently difficult for the dentist to perform, most dentists will not do them.

# References

1. Kanaa M, Meechan J, Corbett I, Whitworth J. Speed of injection influences efficacy of inferior alveolar nerve blocks: A double-blind randomized controlled trial in volunteers. J Endod 2006;32:919–923.

2. Nusstein J, Steinkruger G, Reader A, Beck M, Weaver J. The effects of a 2-stage injection technique on inferior alveolar nerve block injection pain. Anesth Prog 2006;53:126–130.

3. Palm AM, Kirkegaard U, Poulsen S. The wand versus traditional injection for mandibular nerve block in children and adolescents: Perceived pain and time of onset. Pediatr Dent 2004;26:481–484.

4. Oztas N, Ulusu T, Bodur H, Dougan C. The wand in pulp therapy: An alternative to inferior alveolar nerve block. Quintessence Int 2005;36:559–564.

5. Sumer M, Misir F, Koyuturk AE. Comparison of the Wand with a conventional technique. Oral Surg Oral Med Oral Pathol Oral Radiol Endod 2006;101:106–109.

6. Yesilyurt C, Bulut G, Tasdemir T. Pain perception during inferior alveolar injection administered with the Wand or conventional syringe. Br Dent J 2008;205:258–259.

7. Yenisey M. Comparison of the pain levels of computer-controlled and conventional anesthesia techniques in prosthodontics treatment. J Appl Oral Sci 2009;17:414–420.

8. Haase A, Reader A, Nusstein J, Beck M, Drum M. Comparing anesthetic efficacy of articaine versus lidocaine as a supplemental buccal infiltration of the mandibular first molar after an inferior alveolar nerve block. J Am Dent Assoc 2008;139:1228–1235.

9. Kanaa MD, Whitworth JM, Corbett IP, Meechan JG. Articaine buccal infiltration enhances the effectiveness of lidocaine inferior alveolar nerve block. Int Endod J 2009;42:238–246.

10. Robertson D, Nusstein J, Reader A, Beck M, McCartney M. The anesthetic efficacy of articaine in buccal infiltration of mandibular posterior teeth. J Am Dent Assoc 2007;138:1104–1112.

11. Pabst L, Nusstein J, Drum M, Reader A, Beck M. The efficacy of a repeated buccal infiltration of articaine in prolonging duration of pulpal anesthesia in the mandibular first molar. Anesth Prog 2009;56:128–134.

12. Replogle K, Reader A, Nist R, Beck M, Weaver J, Meyers WJ. Cardiovascular effects of intraosseous injections of 2 percent lidocaine with 1:100,000 epinephrine and 3 percent mepivacaine. J Am Dent Assoc 1999;130:649–657.

13. Gallatin E, Stabile P, Reader A, Nist R, Beck M. Anesthetic efficacy and heart rate effects of the intraosseous injection of 3% mepivacaine after an inferior alveolar nerve block. Oral Surg Oral Med Oral Pathol Oral Radiol Endod 2000;89:83–87.

14. Dunbar D, Reader A, Nist R, Beck M, Meyers WJ. Anesthetic efficacy of the intraosseous injection after an inferior alveolar nerve block. J Endod 1996;22:481–486.

15. Guglielmo A, Reader A, Nist R, Beck M, Weaver J. Anesthetic efficacy and heart rate effects of the supplemental intraosseous injection of 2% mepivacaine with 1:20,000 levonordefrin. Oral Surg Oral Med Oral Pathol Oral Radiol Endod 1999;87:284–293.

16. Jensen J, Nusstein J, Drum M, Reader A, Beck M. Anesthetic efficacy of a repeated intraosseous injection following a primary intraosseous injection. J Endod 2008;34:126–130.

17. Schleder JR, Reader A, Beck M, Meyers WJ. The periodontal ligament injection: A comparison of 2% lidocaine, 3% mepivacaine, and 1:100,000 epinephrine to 2% lidocaine with 1:100,000 epinephrine in human mandibular premolars. J Endod 1988;14:397–404.

18. Hersh EV, Moore PA, Papas AS, et al. Reversal of soft-tissue local anesthesia with phentolamine mesylate in adolescents and adults. J Am Dent Assoc 2008;139:1080–1093.

19. Nist RA, Reader A, Beck M, Meyers WJ. An evaluation of the incisive nerve block and combination inferior alveolar and incisive nerve blocks in mandibular anesthesia. J Endod 1992;18:455–459.

20. Clark K, Reader A, Beck M, Meyers WJ. Anesthetic efficacy of an infiltration in mandibular anterior teeth following an inferior alveolar nerve block. Anesth Prog 2002;49:49–55.

21. Nuzum FM, Drum M, Nusstein J, Reader A, Beck M. Anesthetic efficacy of articaine for a combination labial plus lingual infiltration versus a labial infiltration in the mandibular lateral incisor. J Endod 2010;36:952–956.

22. White JJ, Reader A, Beck M, Meyers WJ. The periodontal ligament injection: A comparison of the efficacy in human maxillary and mandibular teeth. J Endod 1988;14:508–514.

23. Mason R, Drum M, Reader A, Nusstein, Beck M. A prospective, randomized, double-blind comparison of 2% lidocaine with 1:100,000 and 1:50,000 epinephrine and 3% mepivacaine for maxillary infiltrations. J Endod 2009;35:1173–1177.

24. Primosch RE, Brooks R. Influence of anesthetic flow rate delivered by the Wand local anesthetic system on pain response to palatal injections. Am J Dent 2002;15:15–20.

25. Nusstein J, Lee S, Reader A, Beck M, Weaver J. Injection pain and postinjection pain of the anterior middle superior alveolar injection administered with the Wand or conventional syringe. Oral Surg Oral Med Oral Pathol Endod 2004;98:124–131.

26. Scott J, Drum M, Reader A, Nusstein J, Beck M. The efficacy of a repeated infiltration in prolonging duration of pulpal anesthesia in maxillary lateral incisors. J Am Dent Assoc 2009;140:318–324.

27. Nusstein J, Wood M, Reader A, Beck M, Weaver J. Comparison of the degree of pulpal anesthesia achieved with the intraosseous injection and infiltration injection using 2% lidocaine with 1:100,000 epinephrine. Gen Dent 2005;53:50–53.

28. Mikesell A, Drum M, Reader A, Beck M. Anesthetic efficacy of 1.8 mL and 3.6 mL of 2% lidocaine with 1:100,000 epinephrine for maxillary infiltrations. J Endod 2008;34:121–125.

# 6

# Endodontic Anesthesia

**After reading this chapter, the practitioner should be able to:**

- Describe clinical factors and methods related to confirming pulpal anesthesia.
- Discuss some factors related to pain in endodontic therapy.
- Discuss success of local anesthesia in patients with irreversible pulpitis.
- Explain why patients with irreversible pulpitis do not achieve pulpal anesthesia.
- Characterize injection pain in symptomatic patients.
- Define preemptive studies trying to improve the success of the inferior alveolar nerve block in patients with irreversible pulpitis.
- Discuss supplemental and primary infiltration injections in patients presenting with irreversible pulpitis.
- Describe supplemental intraligamentary injections in patients presenting with irreversible pulpitis.
- Discuss some considerations with the use of supplemental intraligamentary injections.
- Describe supplemental and primary intraosseous injections in patients presenting with irreversible pulpitis.
- Discuss some considerations with the use of supplemental intraosseous injections.
- Explain the use of supplemental intraosseous injection in partially vital teeth.
- Explain the use of supplemental intraosseous and intraligamentary injections in teeth with necrotic pulps and periapical radiolucencies.
- Discuss the intraseptal injection.
- Discuss the intrapulpal injection.

We encourage practitioners to read the previous chapters to understand the overall clinical implications of mandibular anesthesia, maxillary anesthesia, and supplemental anesthesia in asymptomatic patients.

# Clinical Factors and Methods Related to Confirming Pulpal Anesthesia

## Lip numbness

A traditional method to confirm anesthesia usually involves questioning patients if their lip is numb. Although lip numbness can be obtained 100% of the time, successful anesthesia (ie, mild or no pain on endodontic access or initial instrumentation) using the inferior alveolar nerve block (IANB) in patients with irreversible pulpitis may only occur between 15% and 57% of the time.[1–10] However, while lip numbness does not indicate pulpal anesthesia, the lack of lip numbness following an IANB indicates that the injection was missed and that pulpal anesthesia will not be present.

   **IN CONCLUSION,** *lip numbness does not indicate pulpal anesthesia.*

## Soft tissue testing

Although soft tissue testing with a sharp explorer has a high incidence of success (90% to 100%),[11–14] pulpal anesthesia may not be present.[11–25] Therefore, soft tissue testing is a poor indicator of pulpal anesthesia.

   **IN CONCLUSION,** *soft tissue testing is a poor indicator of pulpal anesthesia.*

## Commencing with treatment

The problem with this approach is that there is no way to know if the patient is numb until we start to drill on the tooth. A typical scenario during endodontic therapy can become problematic if the patient jumps when the practitioner hits the dentin during access preparation on a mandibular molar. The endodontist may say, "Oh, did you feel that?" and try to continue with treatment. If the patient jumps again when the dentin is touched with the bur, the endodontist may say, "Hold on for a minute or two," and continue to drill to expose the pulp and then give an intrapulpal injection. This is not the best scenario for the practitioner or the patient.

   **IN CONCLUSION,** *starting treatment may increase the apprehension of the dentist and patient because neither one knows if the tooth is anesthetized.*

## Determining clinical anesthesia in patients presenting with irreversible pulpitis

After administration of local anesthesia, a cold refrigerant or electric pulp tester (EPT) can be used to test painful, vital teeth (ie, teeth with irreversible pulpitis) for pulpal anesthesia prior to beginning the endodontic procedure.[1,5,26,27] If the patient responds to the stimulus, then pulpal anesthesia has not been obtained, and supplemental anesthesia should be administered. However, in painful, vital teeth, no response to pulp testing may not guarantee pulpal anesthesia.[1,5,26,27] Therefore, if a patient experiences pain when the endodontic procedure is started after negative pulp testing, supplemental anesthesia is indicated.

Naturally, if the chamber is necrotic and the canals are vital, no objective test can predict the level of clinical anesthesia. However, as suggested by Hsiao-Wu and coauthors,[28] cold testing adjacent teeth may provide evidence of anesthesia in the working area.

**IN CONCLUSION,** *a positive response to pulp testing with a cold refrigerant or an EPT will indicate that the patient is not anesthetized.*

## Electric pulp testing

Dreven and colleagues[26] found that a negative response to pulp testing with an EPT (see Figs 1-7 and 1-8) in vital, painful teeth was only 73% successful for determining clinical anesthesia. Nusstein and coauthors[1] found a 62% success rate in a similar group of patients. Therefore, the EPT is not completely reliable in determining clinical anesthesia in vital, painful teeth. However, if the patient responds to the stimulus, the practitioner knows that pulpal anesthesia has not been obtained.

**IN CONCLUSION,** *lack of patient response to pulp testing with an EPT will not always indicate that the patient is anesthetized.*

## Cold testing

Cohen and coauthors[5] found that the cold refrigerant dichlorodifluoromethane (DDM) was 92% effective in confirming pulpal anesthesia in patients presenting with irreversible pulpitis. The cold refrigerant tetrafluoroethylene (TFE) (Hygenic Endo-Ice, Coltène/Whaledent) may not be as accurate as DDM in determining clinical anesthesia in mandibular posterior teeth with irreversible pulpitis because TFE is not as cold as DDM.[1] TFE may not be as accurate as using an EPT in mandibular posterior teeth presenting with irreversible pulpitis.[1] In maxillary teeth, TFE and an EPT may be equally effective.[1]

However, testing is much more convenient with a cold refrigerant than with an EPT. Cold testing is quick and easy, requiring seconds to complete, and does not require special equipment. If a patient does not respond to the stimulus during cold testing and still experiences pain when the endodontic procedure is started, supplemental anesthesia is indicated. However, if the patient responds to cold testing, the practitioner knows that pulpal anesthesia has not been obtained.

The technique for cold testing involves spraying the cold refrigerant on a large cotton pellet held with cotton tweezers[29] and placing the cold pellet on the tooth (see Figs 1-4 to 1-6).

**IN CONCLUSION,** *a positive response to pulp testing with a cold refrigerant will indicate if the patient is not anesthetized.*

## Pain to cold testing in patients presenting with symptomatic irreversible pulpitis

Fowler and coauthors[30] found that cold testing with Endo-Ice resulted in severe pain for patients presenting with symptomatic irreversible pulpitis. Patient reactions to cold testing demonstrated that 56% to 62% had a severe reaction.

**IN CONCLUSION,** *patients presenting with symptomatic irreversible pulpitis may experience severe pain and severe reactions to cold testing.*

## Cold testing with crowns

Pulp testing with a cold refrigerant can be performed effectively on gold crowns and porcelain-fused-to-metal crowns. In fact, pulp testing is fairly easy to use in these situations because the metal conducts the cold well. Miller and coauthors[29] also showed that pulp testing with a cold refrigerant is effective for full porcelain crowns.

**IN CONCLUSION,** *teeth with gold crowns, porcelain-fused-to-metal crowns, and full porcelain crowns can be tested with cold.*

## Effect of analgesics on pulp testing

Pulp testing is integral to the diagnosis of endodontic pulpal conditions. Some clinicians may feel that pulp testing is unreliable when patients have taken pain relievers; however, studies have generally shown otherwise. Carnes and coauthors[31] investigated the changes in pain threshold, as determined by electric pulp testing, in patients presenting with moderate to severe pain after administration of 100 mg meperidine, 220 mg naproxen sodium, 1,000 mg acetaminophen, or a placebo. The investigators concluded that clinically there was no difference in pain threshold for patients who were administered these drugs preoperatively as measured with an EPT. Kardelis and coauthors[32] studied the effects of 10 mg hydrocodone/1,000 mg acetaminophen or a placebo on pulp testing in 15 women with uninflamed teeth. They concluded that oral systemic administration of 10 mg hydrocodone/1,000 mg acetaminophen had little impact on the sensitivity of healthy pulps or mucosa in women. Jespersen and coauthors[33] found that recent analgesic use did not significantly alter the results of pulpal sensibility testing in a clinical setting. Fowler and coauthors[30] similarly found that a combination dose of 1,000 mg acetaminophen/10 mg of hydrocodone did not statistically affect cold pulpal testing in patients presenting with symptomatic irreversible pulpitis.

Read and coauthors[34] evaluated the effect of ibuprofen on masking endodontic diagnosis. They found that in a subset of teeth with inflamed vital pulps (symptomatic irreversible pulpitis/symptomatic apical periodontitis), a 25% masking of the cold response (Endo-Ice) occurred 1 hour after administration of 800 mg ibuprofen. However, there were only eight patients in this ibuprofen group, and the results were not statistically significant when compared with the placebo medication. The authors did find that bite force measurements were not masked by ibuprofen.

**IN CONCLUSION,** *generally, preoperative analgesic medication use does not affect pulp testing in patients with irreversible pulpitis.*

## Value of pulp testing in clinical practice

Almost all of the studies outlined in this chapter can be duplicated in your office. You can pulp test teeth after giving different local anesthetic formulations and techniques to evaluate pulpal anesthesia.

**IN CONCLUSION,** *pulp testing is a very valuable tool to determine if pulpal anesthesia has not been obtained.*

# Some Factors Related to Pain in Endodontic Therapy

## Anticipated pain

Rousseau and coauthors[35] found that 92% of patients undergoing endodontic therapy reported less or much less pain than anticipated. LeClaire and coauthors[36] found that approximately 96% of the patients who have had endodontic therapy would be willing to undergo endodontic therapy again if necessary. Van Wijk and Hoogstraten[37] found that patients who were given positive information about pain before endodontic treatment were less fearful of pain associated with endodontic treatment.

**IN CONCLUSION,** *patients may anticipate more pain than actually occurs during endodontic treatment. Additionally, patients should receive positive information about the pain of endodontic treatment to decrease their fears.*

## Conscious sedation and pain

Patients in pain are often anxious and fearful of dental treatment.[38] Patients reporting for emergency treatment with pain are even more fearful. The question is whether the IANB would be more successful in consciously sedated patients. Lindemann and coauthors[39] evaluated the administration of sublingual triazolam (Halcion, Pfizer) on the efficacy of the IANB in patients experiencing irreversible pulpitis. In a double-blind study, 58 emergency patients diagnosed with irreversible pulpitis of a mandibular posterior tooth randomly received either a sublingual dose of 0.25 mg of triazolam or a placebo 30 minutes before administration of a conventional IANB. Endodontic access was begun 15 minutes after completion of the IANB, and all patients were required to have profound lip numbness. Success was defined as mild or no pain upon endodontic access or initial instrumentation. The success rate for the IANB was 43% with triazolam and 57% with the placebo. There was no significant difference between the two groups. Therefore, for mandibular posterior teeth, triazolam in a sublingual dose of 0.25 mg will not result in an increase in success of the IANB in patients with irreversible pulpitis. If a painful procedure is anticipated, conscious sedation should not be used as a way to reduce pain during dental treatment. Profound local anesthesia is still required. The results of this study should not be interpreted to mean that triazolam sedation should not be used to reduce patient anxiety. Anxiety reduction may make the process of dental treatment more acceptable.

**IN CONCLUSION,** *oral conscious sedation with triazolam will not reduce pain during dental treatment.*

## Patient satisfaction with painful dental procedures

Endodontic studies evaluating patients presenting with symptomatic irreversible pulpitis have shown satisfaction ratings around 96%.[39–44] Even with some pain, most patients were highly satisfied with the overall treatment due to the level of compassion displayed by the provider during the procedure and/or the expectation that their pain would be relieved. Gale and coauthors,[45] Davidhizar and Shearer,[46] Schouten and coauthors,[47] and Fletcher and coauthors[48] found that patient satisfaction is related to four factors in the practitioner's behavior: *(1)* maintaining a positive and professional attitude, *(2)* practicing encouragement, *(3)* a caring manner, and *(4)* avoiding defensiveness. Communicative behavior of the dentist is positively related to patient satisfaction and explains why patients are satisfied with dental treatment even though pain may be involved.

**IN CONCLUSION,** *a dentist's caring manner and/or a patient's expectation that his or her pain will be relieved relates to patient satisfaction even though painful treatment may be involved. However, we should still do everything possible to minimize pain for the patient.*

## Inflammation and tissue damage to pulpal tissue

The damage to pulpal tissue from inflammation and bacterial insult causes cytokines, such as tumor necrosis factor $\alpha$ and interleukin 6, and prostaglandin $E_2$ and prostacyclin to enhance the excitability of nociceptor isoforms ($Na_v$ 1.7, $Na_v$ 1.8, and $Na_v$ 1.9) and increase the activation of transient receptor potential vanilloid-1 (TRPV-1).[49–54] Warren and coauthors[54] found a sixfold increase in $Na_v$ 1.8 in inflamed pulps. $Na_v$ 1.8 may render the tissue relatively insensitive to local anesthetics.

With prolonged peripheral pain, central sensitization occurs that may account for tactile allodynia.[49,55,56] These factors may help explain why local anesthesia is not always effective for patients in pain. For example, $Na_v$ 1.9 channels have a low sensitivity to blockade by local anesthetics.[52] Further research into specific drugs that block these cytokines or selectively block nociceptor channels will provide novel approaches to better pain control.

**IN CONCLUSION,** *various agents enhance excitability of nociceptors that makes local anesthesia less effective in patients in pain.*

# Success of Local Anesthesia in Patients with Irreversible Pulpitis

## Differences in success of the IANB in asymptomatic and symptomatic irreversible pulpitis

There is a difference between the success rates of patients with asymptomatic and symptomatic irreversible pulpitis. Patients presenting with asymptomatic irreversible pulpitis will NOT report with moderate to severe spontaneous pain at the emergency visit. They usually have an exaggerated response to cold testing.

Argueta-Figueroa and coauthors[57] found a success rate (no or mild pain on access or instrumentation) of 87% in patients presenting with asymptomatic irreversible pulpitis and a 64% success rate in patients with symptomatic irreversible pulpitis. Fragouli and coauthors[58] found that an IANB using 4% articaine with 1:100,000 epinephrine resulted in less pain when the teeth were diagnosed with reversible pulpitis than when they were diagnosed with irreversible pulpitis. Severe pain occurred in 5% of the teeth with reversible pulpitis and in 32% of the teeth diagnosed with irreversible pulpitis.

**IN CONCLUSION,** *there will be a clinical difference in success rates of the IANB between patients presenting with asymptomatic irreversible pulpitis (no spontaneous pain at the emergency appointment) and symptomatic irreversible pulpitis.*

## Differences in success of the IANB depend on preoperative pain

Additionally, there is a difference in success rates depending on the preoperative pain levels. Aggarwal and coauthors[59] found that the IANB failure rate increases with an increase in the severity of preoperative pain. For patients with mild preoperative pain, success (no or mild pain during access or instrumentation) was 33%, whereas success was only 29% for patients with moderate preoperative pain and 16% for patients with severe preoperative pain.

**IN CONCLUSION,** *there will be a clinical difference in success rates of the IANB between patients presenting with mild, moderate, and severe pain.*

## Pain scales

There are many pain scales used clinically and in experimental studies (Fig 6-1). The Heft-Parker visual analog scale (VAS) was developed to provide a more accurate scale for pain ratings.[60] The VAS includes the categorical descriptors of "faint," "weak," "mild," "moderate," "strong," and "intense" to guide participants in reporting their pain, while providing an infinite number of points along the scale that can be marked to correlate with their perceived pain (see Fig 6-1b). Heft and Parker[60] determined their VAS to be accurate by comparing the intensity of electrocutaneous shocks and reported pain ratings with two different word descriptor lists. When the descriptor words were assigned values, there was agreement between the subjects on the nonhomogenous spacing of the descriptors along the scale. Based on their findings, Heft and Parker devised the VAS that is used in many different clinical and research settings today.

**IN CONCLUSION,** *the Heft-Parker VAS is a useful clinical scale to measure pain in adult patients.*

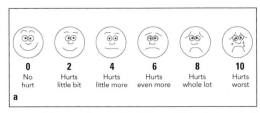

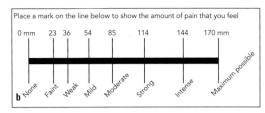

**Fig 6-1** *(a)* Faces pain scale for children. *(b)* Heft-Parker visual analog scale for adults.

## Success of maxillary infiltrations

### Lidocaine

Nusstein and coauthors[1] administered maxillary posterior buccal infiltrations of 3.6 mL of 2% lidocaine with 1:100,000 epinephrine to patients with irreversible pulpitis. Of the original 25 patients, 23 tested negative to cold, but 4% had dentinal pain, and 20% had pain upon pulpal exposure. Overall, a success rate of 88% was found (12% of the patients required intraosseous injections).

Aggarwal and coauthors[61] compared buccal infiltrations and buccal plus palatal infiltrations (2% lidocaine with 1:200,000 epinephrine) in maxillary first molars in patients presenting with symptomatic irreversible pulpitis. The authors found success rates (no or mild pain upon endodontic treatment) of 54% for buccal infiltration and 70% for buccal plus palatal infiltration.

Moradi Askari and coauthors[62] studied the effect of maxillary molar root length on the success of buccal infiltration (1.8 mL of 2% lidocaine with 1:80,000 epinephrine) in patients presenting with irreversible pulpitis. The success rate (no or mild pain on access or instrumentation) was 61%. The authors found that longer distobuccal and palatal roots had significantly higher failure.

Mehrvarzfar and coauthors[63] added fentanyl to a lidocaine formulation for infiltration anesthesia in maxillary molars in patients presenting with irreversible pulpitis. The addition of fentanyl did not increase the effectiveness of infiltration.

**IN CONCLUSION,** *maxillary posterior buccal infiltration using a one-cartridge or two-cartridge volume of 2% lidocaine with 1:100,000 epinephrine is not completely effective in patients with irreversible pulpitis.*

### Articaine

Srinivasan and coauthors[64] compared 4% articaine and 2% lidocaine, both with 1:100,000 epinephrine, for maxillary posterior buccal infiltrations in patients experiencing irreversible pulpitis in terms of success (mild or no discomfort during endodontic access). They found that the articaine formulation was more successful (100% in the first premolar and first molar) than the lidocaine formulation (80% in the first premolar and 30% in the first molar). However, the 40 patients were divided into four groups of 10 patients each. The small numbers in each group may have affected the results.

Sherman and coauthors[65] compared 4% articaine with 1:100,000 epinephrine and 2% lidocaine with 1:100,000 epinephrine using maxillary infiltrations in patients with irreversible pulpitis in posterior teeth. While they found no difference between the two anesthetic formulations, the study only used 10 subjects per group. The number of patients in each group would need to be higher to reach clinical conclusions.

Rosenberg and coauthors[66] found no significant differences between an articaine formulation and a lidocaine formulation when used as a supplemental infiltration after IANBs or maxillary infiltrations in patients with irreversible pulpitis. However, the numbers of patients were limited in the study, which could have affected the results.

Kanaa and coauthors[67] compared 4% articaine with 1:100,000 epinephrine to 2% lidocaine with 1:80,000 epinephrine in maxillary teeth in patients presenting with irreversible pulpitis. The authors found no significant difference between the two anesthetic agents. Pain-free treatment was achieved in 85% of the patients. They also found that anesthesia was easier to achieve for extraction than for pulpal removal. Hosseini and coauthors[68] compared 4% articaine with 1:100,000 epinephrine to 2% lidocaine with 1:80,000 epinephrine in maxillary first molars in patients presenting with irreversible pulpitis. Anesthetic success (no or mild pain during access or instrumentation) was 56% for lidocaine and 67% for articaine, and the difference was not statistically significant. They commented that longer palatal roots had more anesthetic failures.

Atasoy Ulusoy and coauthors[69] studied patients presenting with irreversible pulpitis and found a success rate (no or mild pain during endodontic treatment) of 62% for the maxillary first molar following a buccal infiltration of 1.5 mL of 4% articaine with 1:100,000 epinephrine (or epinephrine bitartrate). Of interest was that the buccal canals were anesthetized, but pain and an increase in heart rate were felt during instrumentation of the palatal canal.

Brandt and coauthors[70] and Kung and coauthors[71] performed a meta-analysis of articaine versus lidocaine in dentistry. The authors found that articaine was not better than lidocaine for maxillary molar infiltrations.

**IN CONCLUSION,** *maxillary posterior buccal infiltration using 4% articaine with epinephrine is not completely effective in patients with symptomatic irreversible pulpitis. There does not appear to be a difference between articaine and lidocaine formulations. Longer roots may be associated with higher rates of failure.*

## Posterior superior alveolar nerve block

Aggarwal and coauthors[61] studied the posterior superior alveolar nerve block using 2% lidocaine with 1:200,000 epinephrine in maxillary first molars in patients presenting with irreversible pulpitis. The authors found a success rate (no or mild pain upon endodontic treatment) of 64%.

**IN CONCLUSION,** *the posterior superior alveolar nerve block will not result in profound pulpal anesthesia of maxillary first molars in patients presenting with irreversible pulpitis.*

## Success of the IANB

Clinical studies in endodontics in patients with irreversible pulpitis have found that success (mild or no pain upon endodontic access or initial instrumentation) with the IANB occurred between 15% and 57% of the time.[1-10] These studies would indicate that anesthesia is often difficult to achieve in patients with irreversible pulpitis with only the IANB.

**IN CONCLUSION,** *the IANB commonly fails in patients presenting with irreversible pulpitis.*

### Clinical effectiveness of articaine for IANBs

Claffey and coauthors[4] compared the anesthetic efficacy of 4% articaine with 1:100,000 epinephrine and 2% lidocaine with 1:100,000 epinephrine for IANBs in patients experiencing symptomatic irreversible pulpitis in mandibular posterior teeth. The success rates (mild or no pain upon endodontic access or initial instrumentation) for the IANB were 24% for the articaine solution and 23% for the lidocaine solution. There was no significant difference between the articaine and lidocaine solutions. Neither solution resulted in an acceptable rate of anesthetic success in mandibular posterior teeth. Tortamano and coauthors[8] also reported that an articaine formulation was equivalent to a lidocaine formulation for IANBs in patients with irreversible pulpitis.

In a study of the IANB in patients presenting with irreversible pulpitis, Ashraf and coauthors[72] found no difference between lidocaine and articaine for nerve blocks. Sood and coauthors[73] also found no statistically significant differences between the two anesthetics. Singla and coauthors[74] found that the IANB using 1.8 mL of 4% articaine with 1:100,000 epinephrine was successful (no or mild pain upon endodontic treatment) 37% of the time. Poorni and coauthors[75] found that 4% articaine with epinephrine and 2% lidocaine with epinephrine for IANBs were equally effective for patients presenting with irreversible pulpitis. Repeated clinical trials have failed to demonstrate any statistical superiority of articaine over lidocaine for nerve blocks in terms of anesthetic efficacy.

Ahmad and coauthors[76] studied various anesthetic formulations for an IANB in patients presenting with irreversible pulpitis. The authors found an 87% success rate (no pain on endodontic treatment) for 4% articaine with 1:100,000 epinephrine versus a 40% success rate for 2% lidocaine with 1:200,000 epinephrine and a 60% success rate for 2% lidocaine with 1:80,000 epinephrine. Other studies have not shown such high success rates with an articaine formulation, which is likely the result of the small sample size of only 15 patients in each group.

In a systematic review and meta-analysis, Kung and coauthors[71] found that articaine was not superior to lidocaine for IANBs but was superior for supplemental infiltration following a failed block in patients presenting with symptomatic irreversible pulpitis. Brandt and coauthors[70] performed a meta-analysis of articaine versus lidocaine in dentistry and also found that articaine was better than lidocaine for infiltrations in the mandible.

**IN CONCLUSION,** *articaine is not better than lidocaine for IANBs in patients presenting with symptomatic irreversible pulpitis but is better for supplemental infiltrations in the mandible.*

## Success of the IANB for molars and premolars

Fowler and coauthors[77] determined the success of the IANB in first and second molars and premolars using 2% lidocaine with 1:100,000 epinephrine in 375 emergency patients presenting with symptomatic irreversible pulpitis. They found that success (no or mild pain upon endodontic access or instrumentation) of the IANB was 28% for the first molars, 25% for the second molars, and 39% for the premolars. There were no significant differences when comparing molars to premolars.

**IN CONCLUSION,** *for patients presenting with symptomatic irreversible pulpitis, the IANB will not ensure profound pulpal anesthesia in the molars or premolars.*

## Is success better with a two-cartridge volume for IANBs?

Aggarwal and coauthors,[78] using 2% lidocaine with 1:200,000 epinephrine, found that a one-cartridge volume had a lower success rate (26%) than a two-cartridge volume (54%) in patients presenting with irreversible pulpitis. Fowler and coauthors[79] determined the success of the IANB using either 3.6 mL or 1.8 mL of 2% lidocaine with 1:100,000 epinephrine in 363 emergency patients presenting with symptomatic irreversible pulpitis. They found success rates (no or mild pain upon endodontic access or instrumentation) of 27% for the 1.8-mL volume and 39% for the 3.6-mL volume. There was no statistically significant difference between the two volumes. The most likely reason for the reported differences between these two studies is the smaller number of patients sampled by Aggarwal and coauthors.

Abazarpoor and coauthors[80] compared the efficacy of 1.8 mL and 3.6 mL of articaine for an IANB when treating molars with irreversible pulpitis. No or mild pain was considered successful anesthesia. They found that the 3.6-mL volume of articaine provided a significantly higher success rate (77%) of IANBs compared with the 1.8-mL volume of the same anesthetic solution (27%). No study has shown such a high success rate with the IANB. Considering that articaine is not superior to lidocaine for IANBs and that previous studies have shown that increasing the volume to 3.6 mL does not affect success of the IANB, it is doubtful that increasing the volume of articaine would provide such high success rates.

**IN CONCLUSION,** *for patients presenting with symptomatic irreversible pulpitis, success will not be different between a 3.6-mL volume and a 1.8-mL volume of 2% lidocaine with 1:100,000 epinephrine. The success rates (27% to 39%) with either volume are not high enough to ensure complete pulpal anesthesia.*

*Is the incidence of missed blocks lower with a two-cartridge volume for IANBs?*

A *missed block* is defined as not obtaining profound lip numbness within 15 to 20 minutes following an IANB. No pulpal anesthesia will be present with a missed block. Fowler and coauthors[81] determined the incidence of missed IANBs using a one- or two-cartridge volume of 2% lidocaine with 1:100,000 epinephrine in 719 emergency patients with symptomatic irreversible pulpitis. The authors found an incidence of 8% for the one-cartridge volume and 2% for the two-cartridge volume. The two-cartridge volume was significantly better than the one-cartridge volume.

**IN CONCLUSION,** *concerning missed IANBs, the administration of a two-cartridge volume was significantly better than a one-cartridge volume in emergency patients presenting with symptomatic irreversible pulpitis.*

*Is success better if the IANB is repeated?*

Some clinicians think that repeating the IANB after achieving lip numbness will result in profound pulpal anesthesia. Kanaa and coauthors[82] studied a repeat IANB supplemental technique after a failed IANB in patients presenting with irreversible pulpitis. The success rate was 32% using 2 mL of lidocaine with epinephrine.

**IN CONCLUSION,** *in patients with symptomatic irreversible pulpitis, repeating an IANB after the first IANB fails is only 32% successful, which will not provide predictable pulpal anesthesia.*

## Success of the Gow-Gates technique

Sherman and coauthors[65] compared 4% articaine with 1:100,000 epinephrine and 2% lidocaine with 1:100,000 epinephrine using the Gow-Gates technique in patients with irreversible pulpitis in posterior teeth. While they found no difference between the two anesthetic formulations, the study only used 10 subjects per group. The number of patients in each group would have to be higher to reach clinical conclusions.

Aggarwal and coauthors[10] found that the Gow-Gates technique improved success over the conventional IANB in patients with irreversible pulpitis. The success rates were 52% and 36%, respectively. The numbers in each group of patients was small, which may have affected the results.

Click and coauthors[43] evaluated the anesthetic efficacy of the Gow-Gates technique, using 3.6 mL of 2% lidocaine with 1:100,000 epinephrine, in mandibular posterior teeth in patients presenting with symptomatic irreversible pulpitis. The authors found that subjective lip numbness was obtained 92% of the time with the Gow-Gates technique, and successful pulpal anesthesia (no or mild pain upon endodontic access or instrumentation) was obtained 35% of the time. Using a two-cartridge volume of 2% lidocaine with 1:100,000 epinephrine, the success rate with the Gow-Gates technique (35%) was similar to the 24% to 35% success rate of the IANB in previous studies in patients presenting with symptomatic irreversible pulpitis.[6,7,40,41,83] However, this is much lower than the 73% success rate found by Sherman and coauthors[65] and the 52% success rate recorded by Aggarwal and coauthors[10] for the Gow-Gates technique. Both studies used smaller volumes of anesthetic solutions (1.8 to 2.2 mL of a lidocaine formulation) for their injections.

**IN CONCLUSION,** *the Gow-Gates technique is not superior to the IANB and did not provide adequate pulpal anesthesia for mandibular posterior teeth in patients presenting with symptomatic irreversible pulpitis. The injection would require supplemental anesthesia.*

*Injection pain of the Gow-Gates technique*

Click and coauthors[43] studied injection pain with the Gow-Gates technique. They found that needle insertion resulted in 36% of the patients reporting moderate pain and 2% to 5% reporting severe pain. For needle placement, 53% of patients reported moderate pain and 5% reported severe pain. Anesthetic solution deposition resulted in a 57% incidence of moderate pain and 8% severe pain.

**IN CONCLUSION,** *the Gow-Gates technique has the potential to be painful in patients presenting with symptomatic irreversible pulpitis.*

## Success of the Vazirani-Akinosi technique

Click and coauthors[43] evaluated the anesthetic efficacy of the Vazirani-Akinosi technique, using 3.6 mL of 2% lidocaine with 1:100,000 epinephrine, in mandibular posterior teeth in patients presenting with symptomatic irreversible pulpitis. The authors found that subjective lip numbness was obtained 63% of the time with this technique. While Aggarwal and coauthors[10] found that only 1 patient in the Vazirani-Akinosi group did not have profound lip numbness, other studies[84–86] evaluating the Vazirani-Akinosi technique, using extraction models or subjects with asymptomatic vital teeth, have reported a lower incidence of lip numbness with this technique when compared to the Gow-Gates or IANB. Therefore, the Vazirani-Akinosi technique appears clinically inferior to the Gow-Gates and IANB techniques regarding lip numbness.

Click and coauthors[43] found a success rate (no or mild pain upon access or instrumentation) of 16% for the Vazirani-Akinosi technique, which is much lower than the 41% found by Aggarwal and coauthors,[10] even when using a two-cartridge volume. The Vazirani-Akinosi technique lacks bony landmarks, and the only indications of correct target placement are the initial needle orientation and the depth of insertion. It is conceivable that the placement of anesthetic solution into the pterygomandibular space may be difficult with this technique.

**IN CONCLUSION,** *the Vazirani-Akinosi technique had a 63% incidence of lip numbness and did not provide adequate pulpal anesthesia (16% success) for mandibular posterior teeth in patients presenting with symptomatic irreversible pulpitis.*

### Injection pain of the Vazirani-Akinosi technique

Click and coauthors[43] studied injection pain of the Vazirani-Akinosi technique in patients presenting with symptomatic irreversible pulpitis. They that found needle insertion resulted in 29% of the patients reporting moderate pain and 5% reporting severe pain. For needle placement, 39% reported moderate pain and 13% reported severe pain. Anesthetic solution deposition resulted in a 53% incidence of moderate pain and 11% severe pain.

**IN CONCLUSION,** *the Vazirani-Akinosi technique has the potential to be painful in patients presenting with symptomatic irreversible pulpitis.*

## Trismus

Heard and coauthors[87] found that a nerve block can reverse trismus caused by pain and muscle spasm. Kuzin and Neledva[88] felt that the Vazirani-Akinosi technique allowed increased mouth opening when trismus was present.

Although the study by Click and coauthors[43] demonstrated that the Vazirani-Akinosi technique might not be indicated for routine endodontic treatment, it certainly has a useful indication clinically for trismus. If a patient experiencing trismus is in need of endodontic treatment, the Vazirani-Akinosi injection may be a valuable primary anesthetic technique. Because the muscles of mastication protectively guard painful mouth opening in patients, the Vazirani-Akinosi technique can result in facilitated mouth opening due to anesthesia of the ipsilateral muscles of mastication or anesthesia of the inflamed/infected tissue. Once an increased opening is achieved, a conventional IANB may be administered to the trismus patient if needed.

**IN CONCLUSION,** *if a patient experiencing trismus is in need of endodontic treatment, the Vazirani-Akinosi injection may be a valuable anesthetic technique.*

# Why Patients with Irreversible Pulpitis Do Not Achieve Pulpal Anesthesia

Endodontic patients who are in pain and have pulpal pathosis have additional anesthetic problems. There are a number of explanations for failure. However, according to Fiedler: Ask five endodontists and you will get five different explanations on why anesthesia fails (six explanations if one of the endodontists went to Ohio State).

One explanation, as we discussed in previous chapters, is that conventional anesthetic techniques do not always provide profound pulpal anesthesia.

Another explanation relates to the theory that the lowered pH of inflamed tissue reduces the amount of the base form of anesthetic to penetrate the nerve membrane. Consequently, there is less of the ionized form within the nerve to achieve anesthesia. If this mechanism for failure is correct, it may be true for an infiltration injection in the maxilla. It does not explain the mandibular molar with pulpitis that is not readily anesthetized by an IANB injection. The local anesthetic is administered at some distance from the area of inflammation. Therefore, it is difficult to correlate local influences with failure of the IANB. Interestingly, a basic science investigation found that local anesthetics may be successful in inflamed tissue that is acidified.[89] More research is needed in this area.

Another explanation for failure is that nerves arising from inflamed tissue have altered resting potentials and decreased excitability thresholds.[90,91] Modaresi and coauthors[90] and Wallace and coauthors[91] demonstrated that local anesthetic agents were not sufficient to prevent impulse transmission due to these lowered excitability thresholds.

Another factor would be the tetrodotoxin-resistant (TTX-R) class of sodium channels that have been shown to be resistant to the action of local anesthetics.[92] A further factor is the increased expression of sodium channels in pulps diagnosed with irreversible pulpitis.[93]

Finally, patients in pain are often apprehensive, which lowers their pain threshold. Therefore, practitioners should consider supplemental techniques such as intraosseous[1,2,94,95] or intraligamentary injections[5] when an IANB fails to provide pulpal anesthesia for patients with irreversible pulpitis.

**IN CONCLUSION,** *many factors are involved in failure in patients presenting with irreversible pulpitis.*

## It is not your fault!

If there is one important fact that you need to remember, it is that patients do not always achieve pulpal anesthesia in endodontics, but this is not your fault.

# Injection Pain in Symptomatic Patients

## IANB injection pain

Differences in the pain response to dental injections will be found in patients presenting with painful teeth. McCartney and coauthors[96] studied the pain of the IANB in patients presenting with irreversible pulpitis. They reported that moderate-to-severe pain occurred from 57% to 89% of the time with the three phases of the IANB; 55% to 59% of the patients rated the pain of needle insertion as moderate, and 2% to 9% rated the pain as severe. The use of topical anesthesia did not eliminate the pain of needle insertion. For the placement of the needle to the target site, 35% to 70% of the patients reported moderate pain, and 10% to 35% reported severe pain. Needle placement was the most painful phase of the injection process. Interestingly, depositing 0.2 to 0.4 mL of anesthetic during needle placement did not significantly reduce pain versus just placing the needle to the target site without depositing anesthetic solution. For anesthetic solution deposition, 52% of the patients rated the pain as moderate and 14% to 21% rated the pain as severe. Therefore, there is a potential for moderate-to-severe pain in 57% to 89% of patients reporting with irreversible pulpitis when receiving the IANB. Further research is needed to decrease the pain associated with this injection.

**IN CONCLUSION,** *the IANB has the potential to be a painful injection in patients presenting with irreversible pulpitis.*

### Decreased injection pain of IANB with CCLAD

Schellenberg and coauthors[42] administered the IANB using a computer-controlled local anesthetic delivery (CCLAD) unit as follows: A 27-gauge 1½-inch needle was inserted through the mucosal tissue, the computer-assisted injection unit was activated at a slow rate, and the needle was slowly placed to the target site over a 10-second time period. The anesthetic solution was then deposited over a 1-minute time period on the slow setting, and then the CCLAD unit was activated to the faster rate as the rest of the solution was deposited for a total deposition time of 1 minute and 52 seconds. Needle placement and solution deposition resulted in a 38% to 48% incidence of moderate-to-severe pain. McCartney and coauthors[96] found a higher incidence of moderate-to-severe pain with needle placement (70% to 87%) and solution deposition (66% to 73%) in patients presenting with symptomatic irreversible pulpitis. Overall, lower values for injection pain were recorded with the CCLAD unit than with a standard syringe.[96] The majority of studies on the use of the CCLAD system have also found lower injection pain scores (see "Injection Pain" in chapter 1).

**IN CONCLUSION,** *the use of the CCLAD system will decrease the pain of needle placement and solution deposition for the IANB in patients presenting with symptomatic irreversible pulpitis.*

## Buccal nerve block injection pain

Drum and coauthors[97] used a 27-gauge 1-inch needle and a quarter cartridge of 2% lidocaine with 1:100,000 epinephrine and found that the buccal nerve block injection (injecting distal to the most distal molar as the buccal nerve passes over the anterior border of the ramus) caused a 31% incidence of moderate pain and a 10% incidence of severe pain for needle insertion. Topical anesthetic did not reduce the incidence of pain for needle insertion. Solution deposition had a 36% incidence of moderate pain and a 3% incidence of severe pain. Therefore, there is a potential for moderate-to-severe pain in approximately a third of symptomatic patients receiving the buccal nerve block.

**IN CONCLUSION,** *the buccal nerve block has the potential to be a painful injection in patients presenting with irreversible pulpitis.*

# Attempts to Improve the Success of the IANB in Patients with Irreversible Pulpitis

## Conscious sedation with oral antianxiety drugs (triazolam and alprazolam)

Patients who are anxious have reduced pain tolerances[98] and therefore may be harder to anesthetize. Because triazolam (Halcion) has been shown to reduce anxiety, it has been proposed to help the success rate of the IANB. Lindemann and coauthors[39] conducted a prospective, randomized, double-blind, placebo-controlled study to evaluate the effect of sublingual triazolam on the efficacy of the IANB in patients experiencing symptomatic irreversible pulpitis. Success (no or mild pain upon access or initial instrumentation) was 43% with triazolam and 57% with the placebo group, with no significant difference between the two. Therefore, a sublingual triazolam dose of 0.25 mg did not increase the success of the IANB in patients with irreversible pulpitis.

Khademi and coauthors[99] found that the preoperative oral administration of 0.5 mg of alprazolam (Xanax, Pfizer) did not improve the success of the IANB in patients presenting with symptomatic irreversible pulpitis. Success (no or mild pain upon access or initial instrumentation) was 53% with alprazolam and 40% with the placebo group, with no significant difference between the two.

It is important to realize that even when using conscious sedation, profound local anesthesia is still required to eliminate pain during dental treatment. Young and coauthors[100] stated that pain in sedated, unconscious patients is underreported and undertreated. Payen and coauthors[101] and Aissaoui and coauthors[102] demonstrated that sedated, unconscious patients detect, experience, and respond to pain but are unable to remember the painful event due to their unconscious state. Thus, patients who are consciously sedated will also be able to detect and experience pain unless measures are used to provide profound local anesthesia.

**IN CONCLUSION,** *antianxiety agents should not be used as a way to reduce pain during endodontic treatment.*

## How does the epinephrine concentration affect success of the IANB?

Aggarwal and coauthors[103] compared 2% lidocaine with 1:80,000 epinephrine to 2% lidocaine with 1:200,000 epinephrine for IANBs in patients with symptomatic irreversible pulpitis. The authors found success rates (no or mild pain upon endodontic treatment) of 20% and 28%, respectively, with no significant difference between the two volumes.

**IN CONCLUSION,** *epinephrine concentration does not affect success of the IANB in patients presenting with symptomatic irreversible pulpitis.*

## Does the speed of injection affect success of the IANB?

Aggarwal and coauthors[104] studied the injection speed of 3.6 mL of 2% lidocaine with 1:200,000 epinephrine in patients presenting with symptomatic irreversible pulpitis. The authors found no statistical difference in success (no or mild pain upon endodontic treatment) between a slow (120 seconds) and fast (30 seconds) injection, at 43% and 51%, respectively.

**IN CONCLUSION,** *injection speed does not affect the success of the IANB in patients presenting with symptomatic irreversible pulpitis.*

## Do buffered lidocaine formulations increase the success of the IANB?

Medical studies have suggested that buffering local anesthetic may increase the ability to achieve anesthesia. Saatchi and coauthors[105] evaluated a buffered 2% lidocaine with 1:80,000 epinephrine formulation for IANBs in patients presenting with irreversible pulpitis. They concluded that buffering did not statistically improve the success of the IANB.

What would be the results if the concentration of lidocaine was increased to a 4% formulation? Theoretically, success may increase in patients with irreversible pulpitis because more anesthetic molecules would be available to block nerve conduction than in a 2% formulation. Schellenberg and coauthors[42] determined the effect of 4% buffered lidocaine on the anesthetic success of the IANB in patients experiencing symptomatic irreversible pulpitis. In their study, 100 emergency patients diagnosed with symptomatic irreversible pulpitis of a mandibular posterior tooth randomly received a conventional IANB using either 2.8 mL of 4% lidocaine with 1:100,000 epinephrine (pH of 4.51) or 2.8 mL of 4% lidocaine with 1:100,000 epinephrine buffered with sodium bicarbonate (pH of 7.05) in a double-blind manner. For the buffered solution, each cartridge was buffered with 8.4% sodium bicarbonate, using the Onpharma system, to produce a final concentration of 0.18 mEq/mL of sodium bicarbonate. Fifteen minutes after administration of the IANB, profound lip numbness was confirmed and endodontic access was initiated. Success was defined as no or mild pain on access or instrumentation of the root canal. The authors found a success rate of 32% for the buffered group and 40% for the nonbuffered group, with no significant difference between the groups. Injection pain ratings for the IANB were not significantly different between the two formulations.

**IN CONCLUSION,** *a 2% or 4% buffered lidocaine formulation did not result in an increase in the success rate or a decrease in injection pain of the IANB in patients presenting with symptomatic irreversible pulpitis.*

## What is the effect of buccal infiltration of sodium bicarbonate on the success of the IANB?

Saatchi and coauthors[106] studied the effect of sodium bicarbonate buccal infiltration on the success of the IANB in mandibular first molars in patients presenting with symptomatic irreversible pulpitis. The authors administered a buccal infiltration of 0.7 mL 8.4% sodium bicarbonate/0.3 mL 2% lidocaine with 1:80,000 epinephrine or 0.7 mL sterile water/0.3 mL 2% lidocaine with 1:80,000 epinephrine. After 15 minutes, an IANB was given using 3.6 mL of 2% lidocaine with 1:80,000 epinephrine. Success (no or mild pain upon access or instrumentation) with the buccal infiltration of sodium bicarbonate was 78%, and the success without the bicarbonate was 44%. This difference was significant. The authors did not use a physiologic formulation as had been used in previous studies of buffered formulations (pH in these studies ranged from 7.0 to 7.5; see previous section). It seems that the authors attempted to alkalinize the surrounding area of the first molar using the sodium bicarbonate solution. The senior author of this study commented that the buccal injection of sodium bicarbonate caused severe and moderate pain. Therefore, 0.3 mL of lidocaine was added to the solution before injection. However, the United States Food and Drug Administration warns on the package insert that infiltration of sodium bicarbonate has been reported to cause chemical cellulitis, with tissue necrosis, ulceration, and sloughing. Because the pH value of sodium bicarbonate is 8.3, compared with a buffered formulation (7.0 to 7.5), it has the potential to cause tissue damage. Diluting 0.7 mL of sodium bicarbonate with 0.3 mL of lidocaine may not change the pH of the solution. Whitcomb and coauthors[107] diluted 0.6 mL of sodium bicarbonate with 3.0 mL of 2% lidocaine with 1:100,000 epinephrine because a pilot study showed that higher concentrations of sodium bicarbonate caused cellulitis and tissue injury. Because pH values were not included in the study by Saatchi and coauthors,[106] nor was there any postoperative follow-up, it is possible that tissue injury may have occurred with the buccal infiltration.

**IN CONCLUSION,** *while success was increased with the buccal infiltration of 0.7 mL sodium bicarbonate/0.3 mL lidocaine, this solution has the potential to cause tissue damage. Further studies are indicated before it can be recommended for clinical use.*

## Is acupuncture helpful in increasing success of the IANB?

Based on the premise that acupuncture inhibits pain, Jalali and coauthors[108] inserted an acupuncture needle at the L14 (Hegu) acupoint (ie, the area between the thumb and pointer finger) or used a sham acupuncture procedure prior to the IANB in patients presenting with symptomatic irreversible pulpitis. The success (no pain upon endodontic access or instrumentation) of the IANB was 60% for the acupuncture group and 20% for the sham treatment. However, there were only 20 patients per group.

Acupuncture—a jab well done.

**IN CONCLUSION,** *acupuncture may be a helpful adjunct for pulpal anesthesia in patients presenting with symptomatic irreversible pulpitis but is not enough to ensure profound pulpal anesthesia. A professional with proper training should perform acupuncture.*

## Do mannitol/lidocaine formulations affect success of the IANB?

Kreimer and coauthors[109] determined the anesthetic efficacy of lidocaine with epinephrine compared to a combination of lidocaine with epinephrine plus 0.5 M mannitol for IANBs in patients experiencing symptomatic irreversible pulpitis. Success was defined as no or mild pain upon endodontic access or instrumentation. They found that the addition of mannitol significantly increased the success rate to 39% when compared to the lidocaine formulation without mannitol (13% success rate). Talati and coauthors[110] evaluated the addition of mannitol to lidocaine in anesthetizing maxillary and mandibular teeth in patients with inflamed pulps. The authors showed that complete anesthesia in teeth with mild pain occurred 67% of the time in the lidocaine group and 83% of the time in the lidocaine/mannitol group. In teeth with moderate pain, success was 32% for the lidocaine group and 56% for the lidocaine/mannitol group. In teeth with severe pain, success was 36% for the lidocaine group and 31% for the lidocaine/mannitol group. While some of the lidocaine/mannitol groups had higher success rates, no significant differences were found between the two formulations.

IN CONCLUSION, *the combination lidocaine/mannitol formulation seems to increase success but would not result in predictable pulpal anesthesia.*

## Does magnesium sulfate affect success of the IANB?

The addition of magnesium sulfate to lidocaine has reduced the overall failure rate and extended analgesia in medicine.[111] However, Vastani and coauthors[112] found that the binding of magnesium ions depends on the conformational state of the voltage-gated sodium channel, which may explain the conflicting clinical reports on the effects of magnesium sulfate in peripheral nerve blocks. Srebro and coauthors[113] found that magnesium sulfate produced local peripheral mechanical hyperalgesia via activation of peripheral TRPA1 and N-methyl-D-aspartate receptors and peripheral production of nitric oxide.

Shetty and coauthors[111] evaluated the effect of preoperative administration of 1 mL of magnesium sulfate (60 minutes before the IANB) on the success of the IANB in patients presenting with symptomatic irreversible pulpitis. The authors found a significant increase in the success rate (no or mild pain upon access or instrumentation) of 50% when compared to the 32% success rate for the placebo. There was no discussion of the pain when administering the magnesium sulfate before the IANB.

IN CONCLUSION, *further research is needed before magnesium sulfate is used in dentistry.*

## What is the difference between mepivacaine and lidocaine for the IANB?

Visconti and coauthors[114] compared the success of 2% mepivacaine with 1:100,000 epinephrine to 2% lidocaine with 1:100,000 epinephrine in mandibular posterior teeth in patients presenting with irreversible pulpitis. Success (no or mild pain during pulpectomy) was 55% for the mepivacaine formulation and only 14% for the lidocaine formulation. However, only 21 patients were used in each group.

IN CONCLUSION, *further studies are needed to confirm the differences between mepivacaine and lidocaine for the IANB in patients with irreversible pulpitis.*

## What is the effect of a combination of mepivacaine and tramadol on IANB success?

Based on the premise that tramadol has some ability to block nerve conduction, Rodriguez-Wong and coauthors[115] used a combination of mepivacaine and tramadol (1.3 mL of 2% mepivacaine with 1:100,000 epinephrine plus 0.5 mL of tramadol [50 mg/mL]) to determine if an increase in success of the IANB in patients with symptomatic irreversible pulpitis could be achieved versus 1.8 mL of 2% mepivacaine with 1:100,000 epinephrine. The authors found no significant difference between the combination formulation (57% success) and the 2% mepivacaine formulation (46%).

**IN CONCLUSION,** *the combination of mepivacaine and tramadol does not appear to increase the success of the IANB in patients presenting with symptomatic irreversible pulpitis.*

## How does tramadol affect IANB success?

Isiordia-Espinoza and coauthors[116] found that submucosal tramadol, which has a brief local anesthetic–like action, increased the anesthetic efficacy of the IANB. However, Beyazova and coauthors[117] found that the dose of tramadol needed to be increased to provide a clinically useful nerve block, which may limit clinical applicability due to systemic side effects.

**IN CONCLUSION,** *further research is needed before tramadol is used clinically.*

## What is the effect of lidocaine/clonidine on the success of the IANB?

Shadmehr and coauthors[118] compared 2% lidocaine with clonidine (15 µg/mL) to 2% lidocaine with epinephrine (12.5 µg/mL) in patients with irreversible pulpitis. Clonidine produces vasoconstriction (selective $\alpha 2$ adrenoceptor agonist). It has also been reported to directly inhibit C-fiber activation and enhance clinical anesthesia. Success (no or mild pain on access or instrumentation) was 59% for the lidocaine/clonidine formulation and 29% for the lidocaine/epinephrine formulation; this difference was significant.

**IN CONCLUSION,** *further research is needed to confirm the results of using lidocaine/clonidine in patients with irreversible pulpitis.*

## Does hyaluronidase affect IANB success?

Satish and coauthors[119] studied 40 patients diagnosed with irreversible pulpitis. The IANB was administered using 2% lidocaine with epinephrine. Hyaluronidase (75 IU) or a placebo was injected 30 minutes after the beginning of pulpal anesthesia. The duration of the effect in the pulpal and gingival tissues was evaluated by the response to painful electrical stimuli applied to the adjacent premolar and by mechanical stimuli (pinprick) to the buccal gingiva, respectively. The authors found that pulpal and gingival anesthesia was longer when hyaluronidase was given 30 minutes after the IANB. However, only 20 patients were used in each group.

**IN CONCLUSION,** *further research is needed before hyaluronidase is used clinically.*

## Bupivacaine versus lidocaine

Sampaio and coauthors[120] compared the administration of 3.6 mL of either bupivacaine with 1:200,000 epinephrine or 2% lidocaine with 1:100,000 epinephrine in patients presenting with symptomatic irreversible pulpitis. The success rates (no or mild pain upon endodontic treatment) were 63% for the lidocaine formulation and 80% for the bupivacaine formulation, with no statistically significant difference between the formulations. Both success rates were higher than reported in previous studies.

Parirokh and coauthors[121] compared the administration of 1.8 mL of either 0.5% bupivacaine with 1:200,000 epinephrine or 2% lidocaine with 1:80,000 epinephrine in patients presenting with asymptomatic irreversible pulpitis. The success rates (no or mild pain upon access or instrumentation) were 25% for the lidocaine formulation and 20% for the bupivacaine formulation, with no statistically significant difference between the formulations.

Fernandez and coauthors[122] found that lidocaine had a significantly faster onset of pulpal anesthesia than bupivacaine.

**IN CONCLUSION,** *lidocaine and bupivacaine seem to have similar efficacy for IANBs in patients presenting with irreversible pulpitis. However, bupivacaine may have a slower onset of anesthesia.*

## What is the effect of a combination mental/incisive nerve block and IANB in symptomatic irreversible pulpitis?

Aggarwal and coauthors[123] studied the combination of the mental/incisive nerve block plus IANB in mandibular premolars in patients presenting with symptomatic irreversible pulpitis. Success (no or mild pain during access and instrumentation) of the combination technique was 82%. The mental/incisive nerve block and IANB were successful 53% and 47% of the time, respectively.

**IN CONCLUSION,** *the combination of the mental/incisive nerve block plus IANB was more successful (82%) in symptomatic mandibular premolars than either nerve block alone.*

## Effect of preemptive ibuprofen and acetaminophen

One preemptive approach to improve anesthesia in patients with irreversible pulpitis is to give ibuprofen or acetaminophen 1 hour before anesthetic administration. The rationale is that prostaglandin induces sensitization of peripheral nociceptors.[124,125] Interventions that decrease the overall concentration of prostaglandins, such as ibuprofen, lead to reduced activation of these receptors.[125] Therefore, there may be a potential for preoperative medications to increase the effectiveness of the IANB.

Modaresi and coauthors[126] recommended the use of ibuprofen for this purpose. However, they evaluated success (the assumption of profound anesthesia) using tooth sensitivity level evaluated by an EPT, and a lowered stimulus reading or lack of response from an EPT in patients with irreversible pulpitis will *not* ensure profound anesthesia.[127,128] Ianiro and coauthors[129] used either acetaminophen or a combination of acetaminophen and ibuprofen preoperatively and found a trend toward higher success rates (no pain on access) of 71% and 76%, respectively, when compared with the placebo group (46%). However, the differences were not significant.

Oleson and coauthors[7] evaluated the effect of administration of 800 mg of preoperative ibuprofen on the success of the IANB in patients presenting with irreversible pulpitis. The success rate (mild or no pain on access or initial instrumentation) of the IANB was 41% with ibuprofen and 35% with the placebo, with no significant difference between the two groups. Therefore, a preoperative dose of 800 mg of ibuprofen did not result in an increase in success in patients presenting with symptomatic irreversible pulpitis. Aggarwal and coauthors[130] evaluated the effect of preoperative ibuprofen (600 mg) on the success (no or mild pain on access or initial instrumentation) of the IANB in patients presenting with symptomatic irreversible pulpitis and found no significant difference between a placebo (29% success) and ibuprofen (27% success).

Simpson and coauthors[83] determined the effect of preoperative administration of a combination of 800 mg of ibuprofen and 1,000 mg of acetaminophen on the success of the IANB in patients presenting with symptomatic irreversible pulpitis. The success rate (no or mild pain on access or initial instrumentation) of the IANB was 32% with the ibuprofen/acetaminophen combination and 24% with the placebo, with no significant difference between the two groups. Therefore, a preoperative dose of 800 mg ibuprofen/1,000 mg acetaminophen did not result in an increase in success in patients presenting with symptomatic irreversible pulpitis.

Parirokh and coauthors[131] investigated the effect of preoperative administration of 600 mg of ibuprofen on the success of the IANB in patients presenting with asymptomatic irreversible pulpitis. The success rate (no or mild pain on access or initial instrumentation) of the IANB was significantly higher with ibuprofen (78%) than with the placebo (32%). However, none of the patients had spontaneous pain at the time of the appointment; therefore, these results would only apply to patients presenting with no spontaneous pain at the endodontic appointment.

Noguera-Gonzalez and coauthors[132] found that preoperative oral administration of 600 mg of ibuprofen 1 hour before the administration of an IANB using 2% mepivacaine with 1:100,000 epinephrine statistically increased success to 72% when compared with a placebo (36% success) in patients presenting with irreversible pulpitis. However, only 25 patients were studied in each group. Jena and Shashirekha[133] studied preoperative oral administration of various medications 30 minutes before the administration of an IANB using 2% lignocaine with 1:100,000 epinephrine in patients presenting with irreversible pulpitis. They reported a success rate of 55% for ibuprofen (600 mg), which was not statistically significant when compared to a placebo (40% success rate). However, there were only 20 patients per group. Shahi and coauthors[134] compared the effects of preoperative dexamethasone and ibuprofen on the success rates of an IANB in patients with irreversible pulpitis. They found that success (no or mild pain during treatment) was higher with the dexamethasone than with the placebo. There was no significant difference between the ibuprofen and placebo groups.

Ramachandran and coauthors[135] compared the effect of preoperative ibuprofen (800 mg) and a placebo given 1 hour before the endodontic procedure in patients presenting with irreversible pulpitis in maxillary first molars. Following infiltration with 1.8 mL of 2% lidocaine with 1:200,000 epinephrine, the authors found success rates (no or mild pain upon treatment) of 93% with ibuprofen and 26% with the placebo. Ibuprofen was significantly more effective than the placebo. Nusstein and coauthors[1] administered maxillary posterior buccal infiltrations of 3.6 mL of 2% lidocaine with 1:100,000 epinephrine to patients with symptomatic irreversible pulpitis and found an 88% success rate. Aggarwal and coauthors[61] found that a buccal infiltration of 2% lidocaine with 1:200,000 epinephrine in maxillary first molars in patients presenting with irreversible pulpitis was 54% successful (no or mild pain upon endodontic treatment). In light of these findings, it is difficult to explain why Ramachandran and coauthors[135] had such a low success rate of 26% with the infiltration of 2% lidocaine with epinephrine.

**IN CONCLUSION,** *preemptive ibuprofen and/or acetaminophen will not clinically improve the success of the IANB in patients with symptomatic irreversible pulpitis.*

## Effect of preemptive acetaminophen/hydrocodone

Acetaminophen has analgesic and antipyretic activity comparable to that of aspirin. The mechanism of action seems to be the inhibition of prostaglandin synthesis and interaction with both cannabinoid and serotoninergic pathways. Hydrocodone is an opioid that can modulate pain by acting at opioid receptors in the brain that are not associated with the descending pain inhibitory system.[136] The peripheral analgesic effect of opioids is associated with opioid receptors located on the terminals of nociceptors. With tissue insult, opioid receptors are upregulated. By introducing exogenous opioid agonists that can then bind to these receptors, analgesia is produced at the site of tissue insult.[136]

Fullmer and coauthors[41] evaluated the effect of administration of the combination 1,000 mg acetaminophen/10 mg hydrocodone, given 60 minutes before the IANB, on the anesthetic success of the IANB in patients experiencing symptomatic irreversible pulpitis. Success was defined as no or mild pain on access or instrumentation. The authors found a 32% success rate for the IANB with the combination dose of acetaminophen/hydrocodone and a 28% success rate with the placebo, with no statistically significant difference between the two groups.

**IN CONCLUSION,** *for mandibular posterior teeth, a combination dose of 1,000 mg of acetaminophen and 10 mg of hydrocodone given 60 minutes before administration of the IANB did not result in a statistically significant increase in IANB success in patients diagnosed with symptomatic irreversible pulpitis.*

## Effect of preemptive ketorolac

In another attempt to improve anesthesia, Mellor and coauthors[137] injected ketorolac (30 mg/mL) adjacent to the tooth under treatment 15 minutes before a maxillary infiltration or IANB in patients with symptomatic irreversible pulpitis. They found that ketorolac did not improve the pain of pulp extirpation and caused significant pain during injection. However, as pointed out by Hargreaves,[138] it is possible that the lack of detected effect is because of the limited sample size (five subjects in the experimental group and five subjects in the placebo group), the pain course employed, and the time course evaluated. Aggarwal and coauthors[130] also investigated preoperative ketorolac in patients with symptomatic irreversible pulpitis and found no significant effect on the success rate of the IANB. However, their study used fewer than 24 patients per medication group.

Jena and Shashirekha[133] studied the effects of preoperative oral administration of various medications 30 minutes before the administration of an IANB using 2% lignocaine with 1:100,000 epinephrine in patients presenting with irreversible pulpitis. The reported success rate was 70% for ketorolac (10 mg). This increase was not statistically significant when compared to a placebo (40% success rate). However, there were only 20 patients per group. Yadav and coauthors[139] evaluated the success of IANBs with buccal and lingual infiltrations of articaine and lidocaine with or without preoperative oral ketorolac (10 mg) for supplemental anesthesia in patients with irreversible pulpitis. The authors found that the IANB using 4% articaine with 1:100,000 epinephrine with buccal and lingual infiltrations plus oral ketorolac was 76% successful (no or mild pain upon access or instrumentation), whereas without the ketorolac the IANB was only 64% successful. The IANB using 2% lidocaine with 1:80,000 epinephrine with buccal and lingual infiltrations was only 32% successful. However, each group was divided into 25 patients per group. This may have affected the success rate when compared with other studies that have used a larger number of patients. There was no power analysis to determine the number of patients required per group.

Saha and coauthors[140] studied the effect of preoperative oral administration of ketorolac (10 mg), diclofenac potassium (50 mg), and a placebo on the efficacy of the IANB in patients with symptomatic irreversible pulpitis. They found success rates (no or mild pain) of 76% for ketorolac, 55% for diclofenac, and 29% for the placebo.

**IN CONCLUSION,** *further research is indicated regarding preemptive ketorolac for patients with irreversible pulpitis.*

## Various preemptive analgesics

Parirokh and coauthors[131] determined the effect of preoperative administration of 75 mg of indomethacin on the success of the IANB in patients presenting with asymptomatic irreversible pulpitis. The success rate (no or mild pain on access or initial instrumentation) of the IANB was significantly higher with indomethacin (62%) than with the placebo (32%). However, none of the patients had spontaneous pain at the time of the appointment. Therefore, these results would only apply to patients presenting with no spontaneous pain at the endodontic appointment.

Prasanna and coauthors[141] determined the effect of administration of preoperative lornoxicam or diclofenac on the success of the IANB in patients with irreversible pulpitis. They found success rates (no pain on access or instrumentation) of 71% for lornoxicam, 53% for diclofenac, and 28% for the placebo. There was a significant difference between lornoxicam and the placebo. Jena and Shashirekha[133] studied preoperative oral administration of various medications 30 minutes before the administration of an IANB using 2% lignocaine with 1:100,000 epinephrine in patients presenting with irreversible pulpitis. The reported success rates were 55% for the combination of etodolac (400 mg) plus paracetamol (500 mg) and 50% for the combination of aceclofenac (100 mg) plus paracetamol (500 mg). These success rates were not statistically significant when compared with the placebo (40% success rate). However, there were only 20 patients per group. Shahi and coauthors[134] studied the effect of preemptive dexamethasone on the success rates of an IANB in patients with irreversible pulpitis. They found that success (no or mild pain during treatment) was higher with the dexamethasone than with the placebo.

Ramachandran and coauthors[135] compared the effects of preoperative administration of paracetamol (1,000 mg), aceclofenac (100 mg), and a placebo, given 1 hour before the endodontic procedure in maxillary first molars, on the success of IANBs in patients presenting with irreversible pulpitis. Following infiltration with 1.8 mL of 2% lidocaine with 1:200,000 epinephrine, the authors found success rates (no or mild pain upon treatment) of 90% with aceclofenac, 73% with paracetamol, and 26% with the placebo. All active medications were significantly better than the placebo.

**IN CONCLUSION,** *further research is indicated regarding various preemptive analgesics for patients with irreversible pulpitis.*

## Meta-analysis of the effect of preemptive medications

Li and coauthors[142] performed a meta-analysis on the use of preoperative medications to increase the success of the IANB in patients presenting with irreversible pulpitis. The authors suggested a relationship but felt that more studies were necessary to confirm an outcome. Lapidus and coauthors[143] analyzed nine clinical trials evaluating preemptive medications versus a placebo as a supplement to the IANB in patients with irreversible pulpitis. They felt there was some evidence to support the use of nonsteroidal anti-inflammatory drugs (NSAIDs) preoperatively, particularly ibuprofen, to provide additional analgesia.

**IN CONCLUSION,** *further analysis of the use of preemptive medications should be performed in patients presenting with symptomatic irreversible pulpitis.*

### Asymptomatic versus symptomatic irreversible pulpitis

While some studies of preemptive medications have used patients presenting with symptomatic irreversible pulpitis, other studies have used patients presenting with asymptomatic irreversible pulpitis, or the studies made no clear distinction between the diagnoses. As shown by Argueta-Figueroa and coauthors[57] and Fragouli and coauthors,[58] success rates are higher in patients presenting with asymptomatic irreversible pulpitis than in patients presenting with symptomatic irreversible pulpitis.

Additionally, there is a difference in success depending on the level of preoperative pain. Aggarwal and coauthors[59] found that the IANB failure rate increases with an increase in the severity of preoperative pain.

**IN CONCLUSION,** *there will be a clinical difference in success rates of preemptive medications between patients presenting with asymptomatic irreversible pulpitis (no spontaneous pain at the emergency appointment) and symptomatic irreversible pulpitis. That is, asymptomatic patients will have higher success rates.*

## Effect of preemptive nitrous oxide

Nitrous oxide is the most commonly used inhalation anesthetic in dentistry.[144] It has an impressive safety record and is excellent for providing conscious sedation for apprehensive dental patients. Moreover, nitrous oxide provides a mild analgesic effect.[144] The most common estimate of analgesic efficacy suggests that 30% nitrous oxide is equivalent to 10 to 15 mg of morphine.[145] Nitrous oxide may have potential benefits in endodontic treatment because of its sedation and analgesic effects.

Stanley and coauthors[40] investigated the effect of nitrous oxide on the anesthetic success of the IANB in patients experiencing symptomatic irreversible pulpitis. Each patient was randomly assigned to receive an inhalation regimen of nitrous oxide/oxygen mix or room air/oxygen mix (placebo). Success was defined as no or mild pain on access or instrumentation. The authors found a success rate of 50% for the nitrous oxide group and 28% for the placebo group; this difference was statistically significant.

**IN CONCLUSION,** *the administration of 30% to 50% nitrous oxide resulted in a statistically significant increase in success of the IANB.*

# Postoperative Pain Reduction in Irreversible Pulpitis

## Use of anesthetics and analgesic medications

Attar and coauthors[146] used single-dose ibuprofen for postoperative endodontic pain. They found that a single-dose pretreatment analgesic alone did not significantly reduce postoperative pain beyond the reduction in pain from endodontic treatment. Al-Kahtani[147] evaluated postoperative pain following endodontic treatment in patients with irreversible pulpitis receiving either lidocaine or bupivacaine. The authors found significantly less pain at 6 and 12 hours in the bupivacaine group. Pain significantly decreased overall by 24 hours. However, only 20 patients were evaluated in each group.

Ramazani and coauthors[148] compared the effects of ibuprofen and Zintoma (Goldaru) on postoperative pain of molars with irreversible pulpitis. The authors concluded Zintoma (a ginger extract) was not an effective pain-relieving agent. Sethi and coauthors[149] evaluated postoperative pain following endodontic treatment in patients with irreversible pulpitis receiving 10 mg of ketorolac, 400 mg of etodolac, or 100 mg of tapentadol. The authors found that a single dose of ketorolac and tapentadol significantly reduced postoperative endodontic pain when compared with etodolac. However, only 20 patients were evaluated in each group.

Parirokh and coauthors[150] evaluated the effects of taking ibuprofen on a regular bases versus on demand after endodontic treatment on postoperative pain in patients presenting with asymptomatic irreversible pulpitis (no spontaneous pain). They found that prescribing ibuprofen on a regular basis had no effect on postoperative pain relief compared with an on-demand regimen up to 48 hours after endodontic treatment.

Mokhtari and coauthors[151] evaluated the effect of premedication with indomethacin (25 mg) and ibuprofen (400 mg) compared with a placebo on postoperative endodontic pain in patients with irreversible pulpitis. Both medications reduced postoperative pain at 8 hours, but there was no significant difference between them at 12 and 24 hours after treatment. However, there were only 22 patients in each of the three groups.

Elzaki and coauthors[152] evaluated four NSAIDs for their ability to control postoperative endodontic pain in patients with irreversible pulpitis: paracetamol (1,000 mg), paracetamol (1,000 mg) plus ibuprofen (600 mg), paracetamol (1,000 mg) plus mefenamic acid (500 mg), and paracetamol (1,000 mg) plus diclofenac (50 mg). Each medication was administered to 33 to 35 patients, and there was also a group that received only a placebo. The authors found that the paracetamol plus ibuprofen performed the best during the 8-hour postobservation time.

Remember the adage for postoperative pain: "The pain will go away when it stops hurting."

**IN CONCLUSION,** *the use of postoperative pain medications following endodontic treatment in patients presenting with symptomatic irreversible pulpitis needs further study.*

## Does liposomal bupivacaine (Exparel) significantly reduce postoperative pain/numbness when endodontic treatment is not possible?

Liposomal bupivacaine (Exparel, Pacira Pharmaceuticals) was cleared for use by the US Food and Drug Administration in 2011. Exparel combines bupivacaine with DepoFoam, which is a delivery system of microscopic spherical lipid-based chambers (Fig 6-2), each containing a small amount of bupivacaine at a concentration of 13.3 mg/mL (expressed as anhydrous bupivacaine hydrochloride equivalent).[153,154] Due to erosion and lipid membrane reorganization, chambers release the bupivacaine, allowing for continued drug release for up to 72 hours. A small amount (approximately 3%) is free bupivacaine and supposedly allows immediate numbness, while the rest of the drug is released from the liposome over time. The lipids (phospholipids, cholesterol, and triglycerides) are naturally occurring or close analogs of endogenous lipids, so they are well tolerated and cleared by normal pathways.[154]

Several medical trials have been performed evaluating the efficacy and safety of liposomal bupivacaine. Various surgical settings have been used in studies, including bunionectomy,[155] total knee arthroplasty,[156–159] total hip arthroplasty,[160] implant-based breast reconstruction,[161] colectomy,[162,163] ileostomy reversal,[164,165] hemorrhoidectomy,[166–167] mammoplasty,[169,170] abdominoplasty,[171] and rhytidectomy.[172] Because liposomal bupivacaine is *not cleared for use* for nerve blocks, all of these studies restricted its use to infiltration anesthesia. Postoperative pain was reduced in some studies, and some studies showed a reduction in the use of postoperative narcotics. However, other studies showed no difference in pain/and or opioid use postoperatively.

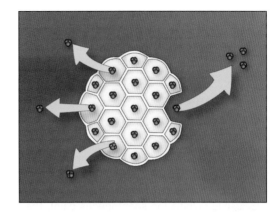

**Fig 6-2** The DepoFoam carrier matrix is made up of microscopic polyhedral particles composed of numerous nonconcentric internal aqueous chambers that encapsulate drugs without altering their molecular structure and then release them over a desired period of time. Each chamber is separated from adjacent chambers by lipid membranes. Following injection, the DepoFoam particles release medication over time due to erosion and/or reorganization of the lipid membranes. (Courtesy of Pacira Pharmaceuticals.)

Bultema and coauthors[173] evaluated pain reduction and numbness in untreated symptomatic irreversible pulpitis by comparing bupivacaine to liposomal bupivacaine (Exparel). In their study, 100 patients randomly received a 4-mL buccal infiltration of either bupivacaine or liposomal bupivacaine. No endodontic treatment was performed. For postoperative pain, patients were given ibuprofen/acetaminophen, and they could receive narcotic pain medication as an escape. Patients recorded their level of numbness, pain, and medication use the night of the appointment and over the next 5 days. No significant differences were found between treatment groups for tooth numbness, pain, and use of non-narcotic and narcotic pain medications. A statistically significant difference in lip numbness was found for days 1 to 3 for the liposomal bupivacaine group.

**IN CONCLUSION,** *for untreated irreversible pulpitis, a 4-mL infiltration of liposomal bupivacaine will not provide prolonged pain control, nor will it reduce analgesic consumption when compared to bupivacaine.*

## Postoperative pain reduction in patients with irreversible pulpitis when endodontic treatment is not possible

Endodontic debridement (pulpectomy or pulpotomy) is the most predictable method to relieve the pain of irreversible pulpitis.[174] When debridement is not possible, clinicians may prescribe strong analgesics and penicillin to try and relieve the pain. Unfortunately, the pain persists, and the use of penicillin has no effect on the pain of untreated irreversible pulpitis.[175–177] While there is an indication for pain medications, antibiotics should not be given for irreversible pulpitis.

Gallatin and coauthors[178] evaluated pain reduction in untreated irreversible pulpitis using an intraosseous injection of long-acting methylprednisolone acetate (Depo-Medrol, Pfizer). The authors found that methylprednisolone acetate clinically reduced the patient's pain to manageable levels for up to 7 days before receiving endodontic treatment, which supports this as a method to control patient pain until definitive endodontic treatment can be performed. Bane and coauthors[179] compared local intraosseous injection of Depo-Medrol to pulpotomy in patients presenting with irreversible pulpitis. They found that the Depo-Medrol group had less intense spontaneous and percussion pain in days 0 to 7 than the patients in the pulpotomy group.

Because pulpal inflammation is initially reduced by the methylprednisolone acetate dosage,[180] this regimen potentially could result in more successful anesthesia when the patient returns for endodontic treatment. Unfortunately, Agarwala and coauthors[181] and Stein and coauthors[182] found that the success rate of the IANB was not improved following the methylprednisolone acetate regimen. Therefore, the preemptive use of methylprednisolone acetate did not result in an acceptable success rate in patients returning with untreated irreversible pulpitis.

**IN CONCLUSION,** *methylprednisolone acetate reduces patient pain to manageable levels for up to 7 days before receiving endodontic treatment, which supports this as a method to control patient pain until definitive endodontic treatment can be performed. Methylprednisolone acetate did not improve the success rate of the IANB when the patient returned for endodontic treatment.*

## Pulpotomy as an interim treatment

Patients often have to decide between extraction and endodontic treatment for irreversible pulpitis. Because of financial circumstances, patients may choose extraction. McDougal and coauthors[183] performed pulpotomies in patients with irreversible pulpitis and restored the teeth with intermediate restorative material (IRM) or an IRM base and glass-ionomer core. They found that pain was present in 10% of patients at 6 months and in 22% of patients at 12 months. While not ideal, the option of pulpotomy and provisional restoration may allow the patient time to find the means to finance complete endodontic treatment.[183,184] Teixeria[185] found that an intrapulpal injection of local anesthesia to a 2-mm depth during a pulpotomy did not interfere with the healing process of pulpotomized teeth.

**IN CONCLUSION,** *pulpotomy may be a potential interim treatment for patients who need more time to finance complete endodontic treatment.*

# Supplemental and Primary Infiltration Injections in Patients with Irreversible Pulpitis

## Supplemental buccal infiltration of articaine following an IANB

Matthews and coauthors[6] determined the anesthetic efficacy of the supplemental buccal infiltration injection of a cartridge of 4% articaine with 1:100,000 epinephrine in mandibular posterior teeth diagnosed with symptomatic irreversible pulpitis when the conventional IANB failed. They found that success (mild or no pain upon endodontic access or instrumentation) of the supplemental buccal infiltration occurred 58% of the time.

In similar studies, Oleson and coauthors[7] and Simpson and coauthors[83] used an identical methodology to Matthews and coauthors[6] and reported success rates of 38% and 52%, respectively. Aggarwal and coauthors[186] found a 54% success rate for the supplemental buccal infiltration of articaine and a 62% success rate for infiltration of articaine plus ketorolac. They also found a 45% success rate for a supplemental dexamethasone infiltration.[186]

Fan and coauthors[187] evaluated the anesthetic efficacy of the IANB plus a buccal infiltration of articaine in patients with irreversible pulpitis. They found an anesthetic success rate (mild or no pain upon endodontic access) of 82%. However, it was not known how many of the patients would have been successfully anesthetized with the IANB alone before the buccal infiltration was given. In the studies of Matthew and coauthors,[6] Oleson and coauthors,[7] and Simpson and coauthors,[83] only patients who had failure with the IANB received the buccal infiltration of articaine. This omission in study design could have affected the results of the study by Fan and coauthors.[187]

Poorni and coauthors[75] found that 4% articaine with epinephrine and 2% lidocaine with epinephrine for IANB were equally effective (75% versus 69%) for patients presenting with symptomatic irreversible pulpitis. The buccal infiltration of 4% articaine with epinephrine alone was also successful 69% of the time. These success rates are high when compared with other studies.

Kanaa and coauthors[82] studied supplemental techniques after a failed IANB in patients presenting with irreversible pulpitis. The success rate (no or mild pain upon access or instrumentation) for the supplemental buccal infiltration of articaine (2 mL) was 84%, which is much higher than that found in previous studies. Dou and coauthors[188] investigated the effect of supplemental lingual infiltration (0.9 mL of articaine) in mandibular molars following an IANB (4 mL of lidocaine) plus buccal infiltration (0.9 mL of articaine) in patients presenting with irreversible pulpitis. The authors found success rates (no or mild pain upon access or initial instrumentation) of 70% for the buccal plus lingual supplemental injections versus 62% for the supplemental buccal infiltration. There was no significant difference between the two regimens. Supplemental lingual infiltrations of articaine do not improve the success rate in mandibular molars with irreversible pulpitis over the IANB plus buccal infiltration. In a study of the IANB and supplemental buccal infiltration in patients presenting with irreversible pulpitis, Ashraf and coauthors[72] found no difference between lidocaine and articaine for the nerve blocks. The supplemental buccal infiltration was 57% successful (58 of 102 patients). In these 58 patients, articaine was 71% successful (41 of 58 patients) and lidocaine was 29% successful (17 of 58 patients). While we know articaine is more successful for buccal infiltration than lidocaine following a failed IANB, a 71% success rate achieved with articaine is far above the success rates reported in other studies (38% to 54%). Rogers and coauthors[189] evaluated articaine versus lidocaine for buccal infiltration after a failed IANB in patients with irreversible pulpitis. They found a success rate (no or mild pain upon access or instrumentation) of 26% with the IANB using articaine. The buccal infiltration was 62% successful with articaine and 37% successful for lidocaine. Monteiro and coauthors[190] found that a 4% articaine buccal infiltration was 40% successful after a failed IANB in patients with irreversible pulpitis. Schellenberg and coauthors[42] similarly found a 37% success rate (no or mild pain upon access or instrumentation) for a buccal infiltration of articaine after a failed IANB in patients presenting with symptomatic irreversible pulpitis.

Fowler and coauthors[77] determined the anesthetic success of a supplemental articaine buccal infiltration following a failed IANB in first and second molars and premolars in 204 emergency patients presenting with symptomatic irreversible pulpitis. Success was defined as the ability to access and instrument the tooth with no pain or only mild pain. They reported success rates of 42% for the first molars, 48% for the second molars, and 73% for the premolars. There were no significant differences when comparing the molars, but there was a significant difference when comparing the premolars with the molars. However, the success rates of supplemental buccal infiltration of articaine of the molars and premolars would not be high enough to ensure profound pulpal anesthesia.

In a systematic review and meta-analysis, Kung and coauthors[71] found that articaine was not superior to lidocaine for IANBs but was superior for supplemental infiltration following a failed block in patients presenting with symptomatic irreversible pulpitis. Brandt and coauthors[70] performed a meta-analysis of articaine versus lidocaine in dentistry and also found articaine to be better than lidocaine for infiltrations in the mandible.

Unfortunately, the modest success rates of the supplemental buccal infiltration would not provide predictable pulpal anesthesia for all patients requiring profound anesthesia. This is in contradiction to the finding in asymptomatic teeth, where the buccal infiltration of a cartridge of 4% articaine with 1:100,000 epinephrine following an IANB was successful 88% of the time.[191]

**IN CONCLUSION,** *a buccal infiltration of articaine following a failed IANB is not reliable for pulpal anesthesia in patients presenting with symptomatic irreversible pulpitis.*

## *Increasing the volume of articaine for a supplemental buccal infiltration of articaine*

Singla and coauthors[74] compared different volumes of supplemental 4% articaine (1.8 mL and 3.6 mL) after failed IANBs in patients presenting with irreversible pulpitis. The authors found that the IANB using 1.8 mL of 4% articaine with 1:100,000 epinephrine was successful (no or mild pain upon endodontic treatment) 37% of the time. The supplemental buccal infiltrations were 62% (1.8-mL volume) and 64% (3.6-mL volume) successful, with no significant difference between the two volumes.

**IN CONCLUSION,** *increasing the volume of articaine to a two-cartridge volume did not increase the success rate of a supplemental buccal infiltration after a failed IANB in patients with irreversible pulpitis.*

## Supplemental buccal infiltrations of lidocaine following an IANB

Parirokh and coauthors[27] found a 65% success rate when an infiltration of 1.8 mL of 2% lidocaine with 1:80,000 epinephrine was administered buccal to the mandibular first molar after an IANB in patients with irreversible pulpitis. However, it was not known how many of the patients would have been successfully anesthetized with the IANB alone before the buccal infiltration was given. That is, the authors did not test for failure before administering the buccal infiltration. This omission in study design could have affected the results.

In general, a supplemental buccal infiltration of a cartridge of 2% lidocaine with 1:80,000 epinephrine will not be as effective as an intraosseous injection for posterior mandibular teeth.

**IN CONCLUSION,** *a buccal infiltration of 2% lidocaine with 1:80,000 epinephrine following a failed IANB is not reliable for pulpal anesthesia in patients presenting with irreversible pulpitis.*

## Supplemental buccal plus lingual infiltrations of articaine following an IANB

Aggarwal and coauthors[9] found articaine to be more successful (67%) than lidocaine (47%) for buccal and lingual infiltrations following an IANB in patients with irreversible pulpitis. However, it was not known how many of the patients would have been successfully anesthetized with the IANB alone before the buccal and lingual infiltrations were given. That is, the authors did not test for failure before administering the infiltrations. This omission in study design could have affected the results.

**IN CONCLUSION,** *buccal and lingual infiltrations of articaine following an IANB are not reliable for pulpal anesthesia in patients presenting with irreversible pulpitis.*

## Primary buccal plus lingual infiltrations of articaine

Aggarwal and coauthors[10] found that primary buccal (1.1 mL) plus lingual infiltrations (1.1 mL) of 4% articaine with 1:100,000 epinephrine had only a 27% success rate in mandibular first and second molars for patients presenting with irreversible pulpitis.

**IN CONCLUSION,** *primary buccal plus lingual infiltrations (1.1 mL) of articaine are not reliable for pulpal anesthesia in patients presenting with irreversible pulpitis.*

## Primary buccal infiltration of 4% articaine

Zain and coauthors[192] evaluated the success of a primary buccal infiltration of 4% articaine in mandibular first molars in patients presenting with irreversible pulpitis. The success rate was 77%. This success rate is very high considering that Aggarwal and coauthors[10] found a success rate of 27% using a primary buccal and lingual infiltration of 4% articaine for patients presenting with irreversible pulpitis.

**IN CONCLUSION,** *further research is needed to confirm the high success rate of a primary buccal infiltration of 4% articaine.*

## Supplemental buccal infiltration of ketorolac to improve the success of the IANB

Akhlaghi and coauthors[193] determined whether ketorolac buccal infiltrations (30 mg/mL) improved the success of the IANB in patients with acute irreversible pulpitis. Successful anesthesia (no or mild pain) was 40% for the ketorolac group and 15% for the control group (saline injection). However, there were only 20 patients in each group.

**IN CONCLUSION,** *further research is needed to confirm the results of using a buccal infiltration of ketorolac to improve the success of the IANB.*

# Supplemental Intraligamentary Injection in Patients with Irreversible Pulpitis

## Success rates using lidocaine

The success of supplemental intraligamentary injections in achieving pulpal anesthesia for endodontic procedures has been reported to be 50% to 96%.[5,194–196] Walton and Abbott[196] reported a 63% success rate of the supplemental intraligamentary injection during endodontic and restorative procedures. If the first intraligamentary injection failed, reinjection was shown to be successful in 71% of the patients for an overall success rate of 92%. Smith and coauthors[195] reported similar results. Cohen and coauthors[5] studied endodontic patients with irreversible pulpitis and found that a supplemental intraligamentary injection was 74% successful. Reinjection increased success to 96%. The intraligamentary injection will not be successful in mandibular anterior teeth.[197,198]

Kanaa and coauthors[82] studied supplemental techniques after a failed IANB in patients presenting with irreversible pulpitis. The success rate (no or mild pain upon access or instrumentation) was 48% using an intraligamentary injection (0.36 mL of lidocaine with epinephrine). Zarei and coauthors[199] evaluated supplemental intraligamentary anesthesia following a failed IANB in patients presenting with irreversible pulpitis. Success (no or mild pain upon access or instrumentation) was 70% with the intraligamentary technique. There was no increase in heart rate with the intraligamentary injection.

Parirokh and coauthors[200] studied a combination of the IANB plus buccal infiltration plus intraligamentary injection versus a traditional IANB. Success (no or mild pain during endodontic treatment) was 22% for the IANB and 58% for the combination technique.

Mohajeri and coauthors[201] evaluated supplemental intraligamentary injection of meperidine/lidocaine in patients presenting with symptomatic irreversible pulpitis. The authors found that the addition of 0.4 mL of 5% meperidine to lidocaine did not improve anesthetic efficacy.

In a survey of endodontists (response rate of 33%), Bangerter and coauthors[202] found that the intraligamentary injection was used more often than intraosseous techniques, with older endodontists using the intraligamentary injection more often than their younger colleagues. The reported finding may be because many endodontists have not been taught the newer intraosseous systems.

Comment: The senior author of this book used the supplemental intraligamentary technique for many years until the intraosseous systems were introduced. It seemed the technique required reinjection to obtain a successful result about 25% to 37% of the time. It also required strong back pressure, which I found disconcerting due to the sustained force required during delivery. In addition, if I had a long tooth (25 to 28 mm), it did not seem to work very well. The duration was short because of the small amount of anesthetic delivered with this technique, which meant that if I left the patient unattended very long, he or she might not be numb when I returned. Then I would have to repeat the injection. So I always felt rushed. Supplemental intraosseous anesthesia is more efficient because you do not need to reinject to increase initial success (unless 3% mepivacaine plain is used), and it provides a longer duration of pulpal anesthesia than intraligamentary supplemental anesthesia.

**IN CONCLUSION,** *supplemental intraligamentary anesthesia is less successful than intraosseous anesthesia. Additionally, the intraligamentary technique requires reinjection for higher success rates.*

## Success rates using articaine

Fan and coauthors[187] evaluated the anesthetic efficacy of the IANB plus the intraligamentary injection using articaine in patients with irreversible pulpitis. They found an anesthetic success rate (mild or no pain upon endodontic access) of 83%. It was not known how many of the patients would have been successfully anesthetized with the IANB alone before the intraligamentary injection was given. This omission in study design may have affected the results.

**IN CONCLUSION,** *further research of a supplemental intraligamentary injection using articaine when the IANB fails needs to be performed on patients presenting with irreversible pulpitis.*

## Success rates using CCLAD

Nusstein and coauthors[203] investigated the anesthetic effectiveness of the supplemental intraligamentary injection of 2% lidocaine with 1:100,000 epinephrine administered with the CompuDent (Milestone Scientific) CCLAD system—formerly known as the *Wand*—in mandibular posterior teeth diagnosed with irreversible pulpitis when the conventional IANB failed. Success of the intraligamentary injection (mild or no pain upon endodontic access or initial instrumentation) was obtained in 56% of the patients. The results were disappointing because the CCLAD system should have been capable of delivering approximately 1.4 mL of anesthetic solution via the intraligamentary injection by consistently maintaining a precise flow rate. Because the study used a prototype pressure-sensing unit, it may be helpful if a further study could use a currently marketed pressure sensing unit (eg, STA Single Tooth Anesthesia unit [Milestone Scientific] with dynamic pressure-sensing technology).

**IN CONCLUSION,** *a supplemental intraligamentary injection using the CompuDent CCLAD prototype pressure-sensing unit following a failed IANB was successful 56% of the time in patients presenting with irreversible pulpitis.*

# Considerations with the Use of Supplemental Intraligamentary Injections

## Injection discomfort

Cohen and coauthors[5] used a high-pressure syringe to administer supplemental intraligamentary anesthesia after the IANB had failed in patients with symptomatic vital teeth (irreversible pulpitis). They felt that the intraligamentary injection did not produce discomfort. However, Dreven and coauthors[26] reported moderate pain with the intraligamentary injection in patients with irreversible pulpitis. Nusstein and coauthors[203] used an intraligamentary injection with the CompuDent CCLAD unit and reported pain for needle insertion and placement as 18% moderate pain and 4% severe pain. Deposition of the anesthetic solution resulted in 10% of the patients reporting moderate pain and 1% reporting severe pain. The clinician should be aware that moderate-to-severe pain may be experienced when using a supplemental intraligamentary injection in patients with irreversible pulpitis.

**IN CONCLUSION,** *the incidence is less than 20% for moderate-to-severe pain when using a supplemental intraligamentary injection in patients presenting with irreversible pulpitis.*

## Onset and duration of anesthesia

Onset is basically immediate. When used as a supplemental technique with the CompuDent CCLAD system in endodontic therapy, 56% of patients who had success maintained anesthesia for the debridement appointment (approximately 35 minutes).[203] The duration with the CompuDent CCLAD unit is longer than with intraligamentary syringes.[203,204]

**IN CONCLUSION,** *onset is immediate, and when successful, duration of a supplemental intraligamentary injection will last for approximately 35 minutes when the CompuDent CCLAD unit is used.*

## Postoperative pain and precautions

The postoperative discomfort of the supplemental intraligamentary injection will be additive to the normal postoperative pain of the endodontic treatment.

Do not use intraligamentary injections in painful teeth with necrotic pulps and periapical radiolucencies or in teeth exhibiting cellulitis or abscess formation. This would be very painful and would likely not provide profound anesthesia.

In addition, patients with clinical manifestations of bisphosphonate-related osteonecrosis of the jaw should not receive intraligamentary injections. Although not studied, patients taking oral bisphosphonates may be able to receive intraligamentary injections. Further information is needed.

# Supplemental and Primary Intraosseous Injections in Patients with Irreversible Pulpitis

The intraosseous injection is not a new technique and was included in a textbook from 1935, *Anesthesia in Dental Surgery* by Sterling V. Mead. The last line of his short description of intraosseous anesthesia gives the impression that anesthesia was predictable in the 1930s: "It seems to me this method has no real advantages and is not necessary."[205] Interesting.

## Success of a supplemental intraosseous injection following an IANB

### Stabident system using lidocaine

Nusstein and coauthors[1] found that a supplemental mandibular intraosseous injection of 1.8 mL of 2% lidocaine with 1:100,000 epinephrine with the Stabident system (Fairfax Dental, see Fig 4-11), was 90% successful (mild or no pain upon endodontic access or initial instrumentation) in gaining pulpal anesthesia for posterior teeth diagnosed with irreversible pulpitis. Likewise, in similar studies, Oleson and coauthors[7] and Simpson and coauthors[83] found a 94% and 86% success rate, respectively. Parente and coauthors[95] used the Stabident intraosseous injection in patients with irreversible pulpitis when conventional local anesthetic techniques failed. They found an initial supplemental intraosseous injection using 0.45 to 0.9 mL of 2% lidocaine with 1:100,000 epinephrine to be successful in 79% of posterior mandibular teeth. A second intraosseous injection increased success to 91%. Therefore, a quarter to a half cartridge of a lidocaine formulation seems to be less effective than a full cartridge.[1,95]

Kanaa and coauthors[82] studied supplemental techniques after a failed IANB in patients presenting with irreversible pulpitis. The success rate (no or mild pain upon access or instrumentation) was only 68% with the intraosseous technique using 1 mL of lidocaine with epinephrine. The lower success rate with the intraosseous injection was the result of using only 1 mL instead of the 1.8-mL volume used in previous studies.

**IN CONCLUSION,** *the supplemental intraosseous injection of a cartridge of 2% lidocaine with 1:100,000 epinephrine will be successful approximately 90% of the time in mandibular posterior teeth.*

### Stabident system using mepivacaine

Reisman and coauthors[2] reported that the supplemental intraosseous injection of 1.8 mL of 3% mepivacaine increased success (mild or no pain upon endodontic access or initial instrumentation) in mandibular teeth diagnosed with irreversible pulpitis to 80% when compared with the IANB alone (25% success). A repeated intraosseous injection of a cartridge of 3% mepivacaine increased success to 98%. Therefore, one cartridge of 3% mepivacaine plain is not as efficacious as one cartridge of 2% lidocaine with 1:100,000 epinephrine, but 3% mepivacaine does not have the heart rate increase seen with epinephrine-containing solutions.

**IN CONCLUSION,** *the supplemental intraosseous injection of a cartridge of 3% mepivacaine will be successful 80% of the time in mandibular posterior teeth. Repeating the intraosseous injection with another cartridge of 3% mepivacaine will increase success to 98%.*

## Stabident system using articaine

Bigby and coauthors[206] found that for posterior teeth diagnosed with irreversible pulpitis, the supplemental intraosseous injection of 1.8 mL of 4% articaine with 1:100,000 epinephrine was 86% successful (mild or no pain upon endodontic access or initial instrumentation) when the IANB failed. Therefore, the success rate of the articaine formulation was similar to that for a formulation of lidocaine.

**IN CONCLUSION,** *articaine is similar to lidocaine for a supplemental intraosseous injection when the IANB fails.*

## X-Tip system

Nusstein and coauthors[94] used an X-Tip system (Dentsply Maillefer, see Fig 4-12) to provide supplemental intraosseous injections in patients with symptomatic irreversible pulpitis when a conventional IANB failed. The X-Tip injection site was 3 to 7 mm apical to the mucogingival junction of the mandibular molar or premolar, and 1.8 mL of 2% lidocaine with 1:100,000 epinephrine was administered. They found that 6 of the 33 (18%) X-Tip injections resulted in backflow of the anesthetic solution into the oral cavity. None of the backflow injections were successful in obtaining anesthesia. The 27 remaining X-Tip injections (82%) were successful (mild or no pain upon endodontic access or initial instrumentation). They concluded that when the IANB fails to provide profound pulpal anesthesia, and when used in an apical location, the X-Tip system was successful in achieving pulpal anesthesia in mandibular posterior teeth of patients presenting with irreversible pulpitis. Zarei and coauthors[199] evaluated supplemental X-Tip intraosseous anesthesia following a failed IANB in patients presenting with irreversible pulpitis. Success was 100% with the intraosseous technique. Verma and coauthors[207] found a 93% success rate using the supplemental X-Tip intraosseous technique in patients with irreversible pulpitis. Idris and coauthors[208] evaluated the effectiveness of the X-Tip using 4% articaine with 1:100,000 epinephrine when the IANB failed. The X-Tip was successful (no or mild pain upon endodontic treatment) 87% of the time.

**IN CONCLUSION,** *the supplemental intraosseous injection using the X-Tip and a cartridge of 2% lidocaine with 1:100,000 epinephrine will result in high success rates and will be similar to a Stabident intraosseous injection.*

## Success of primary intraligamentary and intraosseous injections

Jing and coauthors[209] used primary intraligamentary injections (CCLAD) of 4% articaine with 1:100,000 epinephrine in posterior teeth in patients with asymptomatic irreversible pulpitis. Success rates were 92% for the premolars, 53% for the first molar, and 93% for the second molar. Even with patients presenting with asymptomatic irreversible pulpitis, it is difficult to explain such high success rates. Pereira and coauthors[210] used a primary X-Tip intraosseous injection of 0.9 mL (injection rate of 0.45 mL/min) of 2% lidocaine with either 1:100,000 or 1:200,000 epinephrine in mandibular molars in patients presenting with irreversible pulpitis. While they reported success rates (no pain during the endodontic procedure) of 97% and 93%, respectively, for an average 90-minute appointment and no increase in heart rate, perhaps the use of 31 and 29 patients in each group affected the results. No other study has reported such high success rates, and none has reported no increase in heart rate using intraosseous injection. More research is needed to confirm the results of this study. Razavian and coauthors[211] used the X-Tip as a primary technique in patients with irreversible pulpitis and found an 85% success rate; however, only 20 patients were included in the study.

The IntraFlow system (Pro-Dex, see Fig 4-15) combines a slow-speed handpiece with an anesthetic cartridge dispenser system and a rotating needle/drill. The anesthetic solution is delivered after the cortical bone is perforated. Reemers and coauthors[212] studied the IntraFlow system as a primary injection technique in 15 patients with irreversible pulpitis and found an 87% success rate (two consecutive 80 readings with an EPT). However, the authors did not test the assumption of pulpal anesthesia by performing access openings and measuring pain. Additionally, some lingual anesthesia would be required for the rubber dam clamp and placement of the radiographic digital sensor or film. A separate injection of anesthetic solution would be required. The authors showed that the needle/drill became clogged and resulted in leakage around the transfuser assembly and subsequent failure. When the needle/drill is clogged, the anesthetic solution slowly leaks almost imperceptibly from the transfuser assembly. Therefore, there is no feedback when this occurs other than the lack of pulpal anesthesia. The IntraFlow system is no longer marketed.

Comment: Our impression from clinical experience is that when the IANB *does not* result in lip numbness, the intraosseous or intraligamentary injection used as supplemental anesthesia will usually not provide pulpal anesthesia. Therefore, we would not expect a primary intraosseous or intraligamentary injection to be successful.

**IN CONCLUSION,** *further research on primary intraosseous and intraligamentary injections needs to be performed on patients presenting with irreversible pulpitis before either can be recommended.*

## The key to success

The key to success with the supplemental intraosseous injection is flow of the anesthetic into the cancellous space. If anesthetic solution flows out of the perforation site into the oral cavity, no anesthetic effect will be realized. Reperforation or choosing another perforation site would be a good choice to gain access to the cancellous bone.

In less than 10% of intraosseous injections, constricted cancellous spaces may limit the distribution of the anesthetic solution around the apices of the teeth.[1,2,16,20,21,23,94,203,204,206,213–215] Therefore, failure may result even when the anesthetic solution is delivered intraosseously.

**IN CONCLUSION,** *the anesthetic solution must be delivered into the cancellous space.*

# Considerations with the Use of Supplemental Intraosseous Injections

## What to tell patients when administering intraosseous anesthesia

An example of an explanation of intraosseous anesthesia would be, "Your tooth isn't as numb as we would like. Therefore, we are going to give additional numbing solution next to your tooth. You will feel some vibrations and possibly your heart may beat a little faster," if using a solution with a vasoconstrictor. We should not say, "We are going to drill through your gum and bone and then give you a shot of the anesthetic." For the IANB we do not give detailed description such as, "We are going to go through the mucosal surface, then some connective tissue and possibly muscle, then hit the bone, and try to hit the nerve." We simply say, "We are going to get you comfortable by numbing your tooth." The explanation for an intraosseous injection should be no different than what we say when administering other local anesthetic injections.

**IN CONCLUSION,** *the explanation should be simple and similar to the details given for any other intraoral injection.*

## Pain of perforation and solution deposition

In mandibular posterior teeth with irreversible pulpitis, Nusstein and coauthors,[1] Reisman and coauthors,[2] and Bigby and coauthors[206] found that 0%, 9%, and 16% of patients, respectively, reported moderate-to-severe pain with the Stabident perforation. In addition, 5%, 31%, and 22%, respectively, reported moderate-to-severe pain during anesthetic solution deposition. For use of the X-Tip system in patients with irreversible pulpitis, Nusstein and coauthors[94] reported a 48% incidence of moderate-to-severe pain with perforation. Solution deposition resulted in a 27% incidence of moderate pain. Verma and coauthors[207] evaluated supplemental intraosseous (X-Tip) anesthesia following a failed IANB in patients presenting with irreversible pulpitis. They found that, during perforation, 97% of patients reported no or mild pain, while 3% reported moderate-to-severe pain. During solution deposition, 25% of patients reported moderate-to-severe pain. For both intraosseous systems, pain upon perforation only lasted a few seconds and occurred during the actual rotating of the drill. Solution deposition pain usually occurred when initial pressure was applied to deposit the solution. Generally, the clinician should be aware that a transient but moderate-to-severe pain may be experienced when using the Stabident or X-Tip systems for perforation and solution deposition in patients with irreversible pulpitis. The higher pain ratings, compared with asymptomatic teeth, are related to the patients being in pain and possibly being anxious.

IN CONCLUSION, *the supplemental intraosseous injection has the potential to be painful in patients with irreversible pulpitis.*

### Onset and duration
The onset is immediate. There is no waiting period.

In patients with irreversible pulpitis, the supplemental intraosseous injection provided anesthesia for the entire debridement appointment (at least 35 minutes) using the Stabident or X-Tip systems.[1,2,94,206]

IN CONCLUSION, *onset is immediate, and the supplemental intraosseous injection will last at least 35 minutes.*

### Repeating the intraosseous injection
Jensen and coauthors[215] found that repeating the intraosseous injection using 1.4 mL of 2% lidocaine with 1:100,000 epinephrine 30 minutes after the initial intraosseous injection provided an additional 15 to 20 minutes of pulpal anesthesia. Therefore, if the patient starts to feel discomfort during the later stages of the endodontic appointment, repeating the intraosseous injection may be helpful. However, in some cases, the IANB may be wearing off in the later stages of the appointment. Therefore, repeating the IANB may also be helpful.

IN CONCLUSION, *repeating the intraosseous injection will provide an additional 15 to 20 minutes of pulpal anesthesia.*

### When does pain occur during endodontic treatment after a failed IANB?
After a failed IANB, endodontic access into dentin will result in a 38% incidence of moderate pain and a 14% incidence of severe pain.[1,3,4,39] If the access is successful through dentin, exposing the pulp will result in an 18% incidence of moderate pain and an 11% incidence of severe pain.[1,3,4,39] If access in dentin and pulp exposure is successful, initial instrumentation will result in a 6% incidence of moderate pain and a 7% incidence of severe pain.[1,3,4,39] Therefore, the biggest problem is gaining access in dentin before the pulp is exposed. It would seem logical to administer supplemental anesthesia during this stage of access rather than causing pain trying to gain further access to expose the pulp.

IN CONCLUSION, *52% of patients will experience moderate-to-severe pain upon access in dentin after a failed IANB before the pulp is exposed.*

## *When should the intraosseous injection be given?*

Considering the high failure rate of the initial IANB, it would be prudent to give many patients with irreversible pulpitis a supplemental intraosseous injection following an IANB. That is, administer an IANB and then test the tooth with a cold refrigerant. If negative, proceed with treatment. If positive, administer an intraosseous injection. An infiltration of 1.8 mL of 4% articaine with 1:100,000 epinephrine is first given over the site of the proposed intraosseous injection to help decrease the pain of the perforation and supplemental anesthesia. The intraosseous injection will significantly decrease patients' pain and allow a quicker onset of treatment.

More endodontists do not yet use this regimen because many clinicians do what they were taught in their initial clinical training, and sometimes it is hard to change. For example, a 1998 study in the *Journal of the American Medical Association* urged the use of anesthesia during circumcision.[216] At the time of the study, up to 96% of babies did not receive anesthesia. Physicians were taught in their residencies not to administer anesthesia, and consequently it will be a slow process to change them over. This is a common problem in many health care disciplines and emphasizes the need to stay current with new advances.

This book has presented good information regarding intraosseous anesthesia, and we feel that the reader should adopt some of the strategies presented. This follows Torquemada's Law: When you are sure you are right, you have the moral duty to impose your will upon anyone who disagrees with you.

**IN CONCLUSION,** *administering a supplemental intraosseous injection after an IANB will significantly decrease patient pain and allow a quicker onset of treatment in patients with irreversible pulpitis.*

## Postoperative pain and problems

In patients with irreversible pulpitis, the postoperative pain of the intraosseous injection would likely be additive to any postoperative pain of the endodontic procedure. In addition, the incidence of patients developing swelling and/or exudate at the site of perforation should be similar to the incidence in asymptomatic patients (around 5%). See chapter 4 for further discussion.

# Supplemental Intraosseous Injection in Partially Vital Teeth

The supplemental intraosseous injection should work in teeth where the chamber is necrotic, the canals are vital or partially vital, and there is a widening of the periodontal ligament radiographically (Fig 6-3). A recent history of hot and cold sensitivity should differentiate this condition from one of a patient with a symptomatic tooth with a necrotic pulp and associated periapical radiolucencies experiencing an acute exacerbation (Phoenix abscess).

**IN CONCLUSION,** *supplemental intraosseous injections should be successful in teeth with partially vital pulps.*

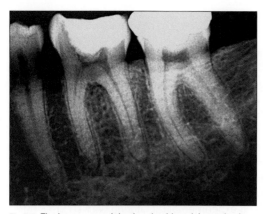

Fig 6-3 The intraosseous injection should work in teeth where the chamber is necrotic, the canals are vital or partially vital, and there is a widening of the periodontal ligament radiographically.

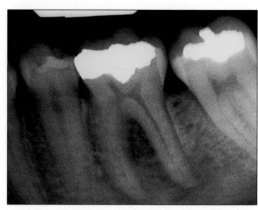

Fig 6-4 The intraosseous injection is painful in necrotic teeth with periapical radiolucencies.

# Supplemental Intraosseous and Intraligamentary Injections in Teeth with Necrotic Pulps and Periapical Radiolucencies

## Symptomatic teeth

No study has investigated the success rate in these teeth. More than likely, anesthetic solution deposition would be very painful, and profound anesthesia may not be provided, or if obtained, it may be of short duration.

In a preliminary study we performed at The Ohio State University, anesthetic solution deposition with the supplemental intraosseous and intraligamentary injections was very painful in symptomatic teeth with necrotic pulps and periapical radiolucencies (Fig 6-4), and the study had to be terminated. Therefore, until future studies can address this issue, intraosseous and intraligamentary injections should not be used in painful teeth with necrotic pulps and radiolucent areas.

**IN CONCLUSION,** *supplemental intraosseous and intraligamentary injections should not be used in painful teeth with necrotic pulps and radiolucent areas.*

## Asymptomatic teeth

Although rarely needed, supplemental intraosseous and intraligamentary injections should be successful in asymptomatic teeth with necrotic pulps and radiolucent areas.

## Precautions

Do not use intraosseous injections in painful teeth with necrotic pulps and periapical radiolucencies or teeth exhibiting cellulitis or abscess formation. This would be very painful and would likely not provide profound anesthesia. Patients with clinical manifestations of bisphosphonate-related osteonecrosis of the jaw should not receive intraosseous injections. Although not studied, patients taking oral bisphosphonates may be able to receive intraosseous injections. Further information is needed.

# Intraseptal Anesthesia

Intraseptal anesthesia is the deposition of the anesthetic solution directly into the interdental septum, thereby allowing solution to flow through the porous crestal alveolar bone and into the cancellous bone surrounding the tooth.[217–223] The injection is further described by Saadoun and Malamed[222] as being given in buccal keratinized tissue at a point "located at the center of the papillary triangle…equal distance from the adjacent teeth." In a 2005 review of the injection technique, Woodmansey[223] suggests advancing the needle "until it contacts the underlying bone," impaling the osseous crest, and then firmly advancing into the interdental septum where the anesthetic should be delivered. Woodmansey also recommended repeating the intraseptal injection at mesial and distal aspects of the tooth.[223] Success rates of intraseptal anesthesia have ranged from 76% to 90%, depending on how success was measured (extractions, restorative procedures, and experimental monitoring with an EPT.[217–223]

Webster and coauthors[44] determined the anesthetic efficacy of the supplemental intraseptal technique in mandibular posterior teeth diagnosed with symptomatic irreversible pulpitis when the conventional IANB failed. Patients were administered mesial and distal supplemental intraseptal injections using 0.7 mL of 4% articaine with 1:100,000 epinephrine administered with a CCLAD unit. Success was defined as the ability to perform endodontic access and instrumentation with mild or no pain. The supplemental intraseptal injection provided success in 29% of patients.

**IN CONCLUSION,** *the supplemental intraseptal injection's low level of success (29%) would not provide predictable levels of anesthesia for patients requiring emergency endodontic treatment for symptomatic irreversible pulpitis in mandibular posterior teeth.*

# Intrapulpal Injection

In about 5% to 10% of mandibular posterior teeth with irreversible pulpitis, supplemental injections, even when repeated, do not produce profound anesthesia. Pain persists when the pulp is entered. This is an indication for an intrapulpal injection.

## Technique

Before starting, the patient must be informed that a little extra anesthetic will ensure their comfort and to expect a sharp sensation.

One technique creates back pressure by stoppering the access with a cotton pellet to prevent backflow of anesthetic. Other stoppers such as gutta-percha, waxes, or pieces of rubber have been used. If possible, the roof of the pulp chamber should be penetrated by a half-round bur; the needle will then fit snugly in the bur hole.

Another approach is an injection into each canal after the chamber is partially unroofed. A standard syringe is usually equipped with a 27-gauge short needle. With fingers or a hemostat supporting the needle shaft to prevent buckling, the needle is positioned in the access opening and then moved down the canal, while slowly expressing the anesthetic, to the point of wedging. Maximum pressure is then applied slowly on the syringe handle for 5 to 10 seconds. If there is no back pressure, anesthetic solution will flow out of the access opening. The needle should then be wedged deeper or withdrawn and replaced with a larger-gauge needle (25-gauge), and the injection should be repeated. This may be necessary in each canal of a molar.

Grubbs and coauthors[224] studied patients with irreversible pulpitis and found that a needle-mounted obturator (Fig 6-5) resulted in increased pressure and may result in increased anesthesia when intrapulpal anesthesia is given. A clinical study is indicated.

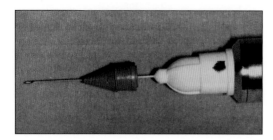

**Fig 6-5** Needle-mounted obturator for intrapulpal injection. (Reprinted from Grubbs et al[224] with permission.)

## Considerations

The major drawback of the technique is that needle placement and injection are directly into a vital and very sensitive pulp. The injection may be moderately to severely painful.[1] In the *Journal of Endodontics*, Miles[225] (a dentally trained neurophysiologist needing endodontic treatment) reported intense pain when the intrapulpal injection was administered. While he reported it as successful, success was achieved at a price. Miles stated that there was decreased confidence in the endodontist and increased apprehension. Because we currently have more successful methods of supplemental anesthesia, the intrapulpal injection should only be given after all other supplemental techniques have failed.

Another disadvantage of the technique is that the duration of pulpal anesthesia may be short (10 minutes or less). Therefore, the bulk of the pulpal tissue must be removed quickly, at the correct working length, to prevent recurrence of pain during instrumentation. Another disadvantage is that the pulp must be exposed to permit direct injection. Frequently anesthetic problems occur prior to exposure while still in dentin.[1,3,4,39]

The advantage of the intrapulpal injection is that it works well for profound anesthesia if given under back pressure.[226,227] Onset will be immediate, and no special syringes or needles are required. Strong back pressure has been shown to be a major factor in producing anesthesia.[226,227] Depositing anesthetic passively into the chamber is not adequate; the solution will not diffuse throughout the pulp.

**IN CONCLUSION,** *the intrapulpal injection will work if back pressure is achieved, but the intrapulpal injection should only be given after all other supplemental techniques have failed.*

## Topical anesthetic

DeNunzio[228] reported on a technique of using a topical anesthetic during pulpectomies. Topical anesthetic is placed on the files and pushed down the canal supposedly to anesthetize the remaining pulpal tissue. The author stated that there might be minor discomfort for approximately 10 seconds. Although the author reported that the technique worked well, no objective study of this method has been performed. Sooraparaju and coauthors[229] found that combining 20% benzocaine gel mixed with hyaluronidase reduced the pain of the intrapulpal injection.

Moghadamnia and coauthors[230] studied the use of 2% amitriptyline gel as an adjunct to local anesthetics in patients with irreversible pulpitis. Amitriptyline (a tricyclic antidepressant) has been shown to block sodium channels but has not been used systemically because of adverse side effects. The authors found that when applied to exposed pulps, the amitriptyline decreased VAS pain scores 9 minutes after administration. The clinical problem is that pain may be experienced in dentin before the pulp is exposed.

**IN CONCLUSION,** *further research is indicated regarding topical anesthetics for intrapulpal anesthesia.*

**Fig 6-6** Postoperative pain for debridement versus no debridement by day. Debridement resulted in decreased postoperative pain. (Reprinted from Sebastian et al[232] with permission.)

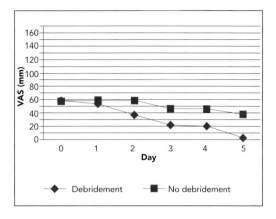

## Symptomatic teeth with pulpal necrosis and associated periapical radiolucencies

### Ibuprofen versus ibuprofen/acetaminophen for postoperative endodontic pain

Wells and coauthors[231] compared ibuprofen versus ibuprofen/acetaminophen usage for postoperative endodontic pain in symptomatic emergency patients with a pulpal diagnosis of necrosis experiencing moderate-to-severe preoperative pain. An emergency debridement of the tooth was completed with hand and rotary instrumentation. At the end of the appointment, the patients randomly received either 600 mg of ibuprofen or 600 mg of ibuprofen combined with 1,000 mg of acetaminophen (blinded to both operator and patient). Patients also received a 6-day diary to be completed after anesthesia wore off and every morning for 5 days. Patients were asked to record pain and symptoms and the number of medications taken. Patients received escape medication (Vicodin, AbbVie) if the study medication was not controlling their pain. The combination ibuprofen/acetaminophen was not more effective for postoperative pain control than the ibuprofen alone. Because approximately 20% of patients in both groups required escape medication to control pain, the combination ibuprofen/acetaminophen or ibuprofen was not completely effective at controlling postoperative pain in symptomatic patients with necrotic pulps and associated periapical radiolucencies.

**IN CONCLUSION,** *the combination ibuprofen/acetaminophen was not more effective for postoperative pain control than the ibuprofen alone. Neither the combination ibuprofen/acetaminophen nor ibuprofen was completely effective at controlling postoperative pain in symptomatic patients with necrotic pulps and associated periapical radiolucencies.*

### What is the effect of no endodontic debridement on postoperative pain for symptomatic teeth with pulpal necrosis?

Patients without a dentist or access to care often present to hospital emergency departments with painful teeth. These patients are typically prescribed pain medication and an antibiotic. If they do not seek immediate dental treatment, what postoperative pain do they experience?

Sebastian and coauthors[232] compared the effect of complete endodontic debridement versus no endodontic debridement on postoperative pain in emergency patients with symptomatic teeth, a pulpal diagnosis of necrosis, and a periapical radiolucency. Success was defined as no or mild postoperative pain and no use of narcotic medication. All patients had a decrease in postoperative pain over the 5 days (Fig 6-6). Debridement resulted in a statistically higher success rate, but there was no significant difference in the need for escape narcotic medication.

**IN CONCLUSION,** *complete endodontic debridement at the emergency visit resulted in a statistically higher success rate than no debridement. All patients had a decrease in postoperative pain over the 5 days.*

## Does liposomal bupivacaine (Exparel) significantly reduce postoperative pain/numbness in symptomatic teeth with a diagnosis of necrosis?

Moderate-to-severe postoperative pain may persist for days following endodontic treatment of symptomatic teeth with a pulpal diagnosis of necrosis, and a narcotic medication may be required to manage this postoperative pain.[231,232] While the analgesic period may be prolonged when bupivacaine is administered postoperatively, it does not usually extend long enough to cover the whole time of postoperative discomfort. Therefore, prescribing strong analgesic medications may be the only option to control postoperative pain in these patients. Perhaps the use of a longer-acting anesthetic bupivacaine formulation would extend the postoperative analgesic period.

Glenn and coauthors[233] compared bupivacaine to liposomal bupivacaine (Exparel) for postoperative numbness and pain in symptomatic patients diagnosed with pulpal necrosis experiencing moderate-to-severe preoperative pain and a periapical radiolucency. In their study, 100 patients randomly received a 4-mL buccal infiltration of either bupivacaine or liposomal bupivacaine following endodontic debridement. The study used an infiltration because Exparel is currently *not cleared* for use in nerve block injections. For postoperative pain, patients were given ibuprofen/acetaminophen, and they could receive narcotic pain medication as an escape. Patients recorded their level of numbness, pain, and medication use the night of the appointment and over the next 5 days. Success was defined as no or mild postoperative pain and no narcotic use. The authors found success rates of 29% for the liposomal group and 22% for the bupivacaine group, with no significant difference between the groups. Liposomal bupivacaine had some effect on soft tissue numbness, pain, and use of non-narcotic medications, but it would not be clinically significant. There was no significant difference in the need for escape medication.

**IN CONCLUSION,** *for symptomatic patients diagnosed with pulpal necrosis experiencing moderate-to-severe preoperative pain, a 4-mL infiltration of liposomal bupivacaine will not result in significant pain control, nor will it reduce analgesic consumption when compared to bupivacaine.*

## Incision and drainage—Buffered anesthetics

In dentistry, incision and drainage of a symptomatic patient with odontogenic facial swelling is a common emergency procedure. Singer and coauthors[234] found that incision and drainage of abscesses in a medical emergency department was the second most painful procedure performed after nasogastric intubation. In dentistry, adequate pain control during the incision and drainage procedure is difficult. One explanation for the failure of local anesthetics is the low pH associated with inflamed/infected tissues, particularly in acute apical abscesses. The pH of pus collected from apical abscesses had a mean pH of 6.68.[235] The presence of acute inflammation/infection may limit the formation of the non-ionized base form of the local anesthetic. Buffered local anesthetics may be more efficient in achieving pain control, particularly during painful procedures such as incision and drainage. The reasoning behind buffering of local anesthetics is logical according to the Henderson-Hasselbalch equation: If a local anesthetic solution is buffered to a pH that is closer to its pKa, more of the free base form will be available upon injection to enter the nerve sheath. The most common method for buffering local anesthetics is by the addition of sodium bicarbonate, which will increase the pH of the solution.

Balasco and coauthors[236] studied the pain of infiltration and the pain of an incision and drainage procedure of a buffered versus a nonbuffered 2% lidocaine formulation in symptomatic emergency patients presenting with a diagnosis of pulpal necrosis, associated periapical area, and an acute clinical swelling. The patients received two infiltrations (of the same formulation, mesial and distal to the swelling) using either 2% lidocaine with 1:100,000 epinephrine buffered with 0.18 mL of 8.4% sodium bicarbonate (pH of 7.0) or 2% lidocaine with 1:100,000 epinephrine (pH of 4.6). Patients rated pain of needle insertion, placement, and solution deposition for each infiltration on a 170-mm VAS. An incision and drainage procedure was performed, and the pain of incision, drainage, and dissection was recorded. The mesial and distal needle insertion and needle placement phases of the injection for both formulations resulted in a 30% to 43% incidence of moderate-to-severe pain, with no significant difference between the two anesthetic formulations. The mesial and distal solution deposition phase of the injection for both formulations resulted in a 34% to 51% incidence of moderate-to-severe pain, with no significant difference between the two anesthetic formulations. The authors found moderate-to-severe pain ratings in 56% to 74% of patients for the incision phase, 64% to 72% for the drainage phase, and 68% to 87% for the dissection phase, with no significant difference between the two anesthetic formulations.

In a similar study, Harreld and coauthors[237] studied the pain of infiltration and the pain of an incision and drainage procedure of a buffered (pH of 7.0) versus a nonbuffered 4% lidocaine with epinephrine formulation (pH of 4.5) in symptomatic emergency patients presenting with a diagnosis of pulpal necrosis, associated periapical area, and an acute clinical swelling. The authors used a 4% formulation because a higher concentration of lidocaine may be more effective due to more anesthetic molecules being delivered to the site for the incision and drainage procedure. The mesial and distal needle insertion and needle placement phases of the injection for both formulations resulted in a 33% to 60% incidence of moderate-to-severe pain, with no significant difference between the two anesthetic formulations. The mesial and distal solution deposition phase of the injection for both formulations resulted in a 46% to 63% incidence of moderate-to-severe pain, with no significant difference between the two anesthetic formulations. The authors found moderate-to-severe pain ratings in 38% to 51% of patients for the incision and drainage procedure, with no significant difference between the two anesthetic formulations. The 4% lidocaine formulation appeared to be more effective in reducing pain than the 2% lidocaine formulation used by Balasco and coauthors.[236] However, the incidence of moderate-to-severe pain was still 38% to 51%.

While the theory of buffering local anesthetics is logical, in reality the presence of a buffer in the local anesthetic may not be enough to overcome the lowered excitability thresholds and peripheral sensitization associated with such significant inflammatory and infectious conditions of a patient with pulpal necrosis and associated acute swelling.

Punnia-Moorthy[238] found no support for the hypothesis that tissue acidity in inflammation is an important factor in the failure of local anesthetics to act in inflamed tissue. Likewise, Tsuchiya[239] stated that "The drug and membrane interaction causable in inflamed tissue acidification does not support the conventional theory on local anaesthetic failure associated with inflammation."

**IN CONCLUSION,** *moderate-to-severe pain was experienced in a large number of patients with anesthetic solution deposition and the incision and drainage procedure. Buffering did not significantly decrease the pain of infiltrations or the pain of the incision and drainage procedure, when compared with a nonbuffered 2% or 4% lidocaine formulation, in symptomatic patients with a diagnosis of pulpal necrosis and an associated acute swelling.*

## Patient satisfaction with the incision and drainage procedure

Despite the findings that most patients experienced moderate-to-severe pain during the incision and drainage procedure,[236,237] 93% to 95% of patients were moderately to completely satisfied with their experience. Patient satisfaction may be related to the chairside manner of the dentist or satisfaction with completion of the emergency procedure in the hope that their discomfort will be abated. Other studies have shown that patients were moderately or completely satisfied with endodontic treatment for symptomatic irreversible pulpitis even though moderate-to-severe pain was experienced during treatment.[39–44] This is an important clinical finding because it helps explain why patients accept painful dental and medical procedures.

**IN CONCLUSION,** *patient satisfaction ratings for incision and drainage procedures (93% to 95%) are similar to those found in endodontic studies evaluating patients presenting with symptomatic irreversible pulpitis (96% satisfaction rating). However, we should do everything possible to prevent pain during endodontic treatment.*

# Final Thoughts

Supplemental injections are critical to the practice of endodontics. These techniques are simple enough to learn, so they can be easily adopted into clinical practice.

Remember that everything looks more complicated to most people than it actually is.

# References

1. Nusstein J, Reader A, Nist R, Beck M, Meyers WJ. Anesthetic efficacy of the supplemental intraosseous injection of 2% lidocaine with 1:100,000 epinephrine in irreversible pulpitis. J Endod 1998;24:487–491.
2. Reisman D, Reader A, Nist R, Beck M, Weaver J. Anesthetic efficacy of the supplemental intraosseous injection of 3% mepivacaine in irreversible pulpitis. Oral Surg Oral Med Oral Pathol Oral Radiol Endod 1997;84:676–682.
3. Kennedy S, Reader A, Nusstein J, Beck M, Weaver J. The significance of needle deflection in success of the inferior alveolar nerve block in patients with irreversible pulpitis. J Endod 2003;29:630–633.
4. Claffey E, Reader A, Nusstein J, Beck M, Weaver J. Anesthetic efficacy of articaine for inferior alveolar nerve blocks in patients with irreversible pulpitis. J Endod 2004;30:568–571.
5. Cohen H, Cha B, Spangberg L. Endodontic anesthesia in mandibular molars: A clinical study. J Endod 1993;19: 370–373.
6. Matthews R, Drum M, Reader A, Nusstein J, Beck M. Articaine for supplemental, buccal mandibular infiltration anesthesia in patients with irreversible pulpitis when the inferior alveolar nerve block fails. J Endod 2009;35:343–346.
7. Oleson M, Drum M, Reader A, Nusstein J, Beck M. Effect of preoperative ibuprofen on the success of the inferior alveolar nerve block in patients with irreversible pulpitis. J Endod 2010;36:379–382.
8. Tortamano IP, Siviero M, Costa CG, Buscariolo IA, Armonia PL. A comparison of the anesthetic efficacy of articaine and lidocaine in patients with irreversible pulpitis. J Endod 2009;35:165–168.
9. Aggarwal V, Jain A, Debipada K. Anesthetic efficacy of supplemental buccal and lingual infiltrations of articaine and lidocaine following an inferior alveolar nerve block in patients with irreversible pulpitis. J Endod 2009;35:925–929.
10. Aggarwal V, Singla M, Kabi D. Comparative evaluation of anesthetic efficacy of Gow-Gates mandibular conduction anesthesia, Vazirani-Akinosi technique, buccal-plus-lingual infiltrations, and conventional inferior alveolar nerve anesthesia in patients with irreversible pulpitis. Oral Surg Oral Med Oral Pathol Oral Radiol Endod 2010;109:303–308.
11. Vreeland DL, Reader A, Beck M, Meyers W, Weaver J. An evaluation of volumes and concentrations of lidocaine in human inferior alveolar nerve block. J Endod 1989;15:6–12.
12. Hinkley SA, Reader A, Beck M, Meyers WJ. An evaluation of 4% prilocaine with 1:200,000 epinephrine and 2% mepivacaine with 1:20,000 levonordefrin compared with 2% lidocaine with 1:100,000 epinephrine for inferior alveolar nerve block. Anesth Prog 1991;38:84–89.
13. McLean C, Reader A, Beck M, Meyers WJ. An evaluation of 4% prilocaine and 3% mepivacaine compared with 2% lidocaine (1:100,000 epinephrine) for inferior alveolar nerve block. J Endod 1993;19:146–150.
14. Chaney MA, Kerby R, Reader A, Beck FM, Meyers WJ, Weaver J. An evaluation of lidocaine hydrocarbonate compared with lidocaine hydrocloride for inferior alveolar nerve block. Anesth Prog 1991;38:212–216.
15. Ågren E, Danielsson K. Conduction block analgesia in the mandible. A comparative investigation of the techniques of Fischer and Gow-Gates. Swed Dent J 1981;5:81–89.
16. Dunbar D, Reader A, Nist R, Beck M, Meyers WJ. Anesthetic efficacy of the intraosseous injection after an inferior alveolar nerve block. J Endod 1996;22:481–486.
17. Nist RA, Reader A, Beck M, Meyers WJ. An evaluation of the incisive nerve block and combination inferior alveolar and incisive nerve blocks in mandibular anesthesia. J Endod 1992;18:455–459.
18. Childers M, Reader A, Nist R, Beck M, Meyers WJ. Anesthetic efficacy of the periodontal ligament injection after an inferior alveolar nerve block. J Endod 1996;22:317–320.
19. Clark S, Reader A, Beck M, Meyers WJ. Anesthetic efficacy of the mylohyoid nerve block and combination inferior alveolar nerve block/mylohyoid nerve block. Oral Surg Oral Med Oral Pathol Oral Radiol Endod 1999;87:557–563.
20. Reitz J, Reader A, Nist R, Beck M, Meyers WJ. Anesthetic efficacy of the intraosseous injection of 0.9ml of 2% lidocaine (1:100,000 epinephrine) to augment an inferior alveolar nerve block. Oral Surg Oral Med Oral Pathol Oral Radiol Endod 1998;86:516–523.
21. Stabile P, Reader A, Gallatin E, Beck M, Weaver J. Anesthetic efficacy and heart rate effects of the intraosseous injection of 1.5% etidocaine (1:200,000 epinephrine) after an inferior alveolar nerve block. Oral Surg Oral Med Oral Pathol Oral Radiol Endod 2000;89:407–411.

22. Gallatin E, Stabile P, Reader A, Nist R, Beck M. Anesthetic efficacy and heart rate effects of the intraosseous injection of 3% mepivacaine after an inferior alveolar nerve block. Oral Surg Oral Med Oral Pathol Oral Radiol Endod 2000;89:83–87.

23. Guglielmo A, Reader A, Nist R, Beck M, Weaver J. Anesthetic efficacy and heart rate effects of the supplemental intraosseous injection of 2% mepivacaine with 1:20,000 levonordefrin. Oral Surg Oral Med Oral Pathol Oral Radiol Endod 1999;87:284–293.

24. Hannan L, Reader A, Nist R, Beck M, Meyers WJ. The use of ultrasound for guiding needle placement for inferior alveolar nerve blocks. Oral Surg Oral Med Oral Pathol Oral Radiol Endod 1999;87:658–665.

25. Ridenour S, Reader A, Beck M, Weaver J. Anesthetic efficacy of a combination of hyaluronidase and lidocaine with epinephrine in inferior alveolar nerve blocks. Anesth Prog 2001;48:9–15.

26. Dreven LJ, Reader A, Beck M, Meyers WJ, Weaver J. An evaluation of an electric pulp tester as a measure of analgesia in human vital teeth. J Endod 1987;13:233–238.

27. Parirokh M, Satvati SA, Sharifi R, et al. Efficacy of combining a buccal infiltration with an inferior alveolar nerve block for mandibular molars with irreversible pulpitis. Oral Surg Oral Med Oral Pathol Oral Radiol Endod 2010;109:468–473.

28. Hsiao-Wu GW, Susarla SM, White RR. Use of cold test as a measure of pulpal anesthesia during endodontic therapy: A randomized, blinded, placebo-controlled clinical trial. J Endod 2007;33:406–410.

29. Miller SO, Johnson JD, Allemang JD, Strother JM. Cold testing through full-coverage restorations. J Endod 2004;30:695–700.

30. Fowler S, Fullmer S, Drum M, Reader A. Does acetaminophen/hydrocodone affect cold pulpal testing in patients with symptomatic irreversible pulpitis? A prospective, randomized, double-blind, placebo-controlled study. J Endod 2014;40:1958–1960.

31. Carnes PL, Cook B, Eleazer PD, Scheetz JP. Change in pain threshold by meperidine, naproxen sodium, and acetaminophen as determined by electric pulp testing. Anesth Prog 1999;45:139–142.

32. Kardelis AC, Meinberg TA, Sulte HR, Gound TG, Marx DB, Reinhardt RA. Effect of narcotic pain reliever on pulp tests in women. J Endod 2002;28:537–539.

33. Jespersen JJ, Hellstein J, Williamson A, Johnson WT, Qian F. Evaluation of dental sensibility tests in a clinical setting. J Endod 2014;40:351–354.

34. Read JK, McClanahan SB, Khan AA, Lunos S, Bowles WR. Effect of ibuprofen on masking endodontic diagnosis. J Endod 2014;40:1058–1062.

35. Rousseau WH, Clark SJ, Newcomb BE, Walker ED, Eleazer PD, Scheetz JP. A comparison of pain levels during pulpectomy, extractions, and restorative procedures. J Endod 2002;28:108–110.

36. LeClaire AJ, Skidmore AE, Griffin JA Jr, Balaban FS. Endodontic fear survey. J Endod 1998;14:459–476.

37. Van Wijk AJ, Hoogstraten J. Reducing fear of pain associated with endodontic therapy. Int Endod J 2006;39:384–388.

38. Jackson DL, Johnson BS. Conscious sedation for dentistry: Risk management and patient selection. Dent Clin N Am 2000;46:767–780.

39. Lindemann M, Reader A, Nusstein J, Drum M, Beck M. Effect of sublingual triazolam on the success of inferior alveolar nerve block in patients with irreversible pulpitis. J Endod 2008;34:1167–1170.

40. Stanley W, Drum M, Nusstein J, Reader A, Beck M. Effect of nitrous oxide on the efficacy of the inferior alveolar nerve block in patients with symptomatic irreversible pulpitis. J Endod 2012;38:565–569.

41. Fullmer S, Drum M, Reader A, Nusstein J, Beck M. Effect of preoperative acetaminophen/hydrocodone on the efficacy of the inferior alveolar nerve block in patients with symptomatic irreversible pulpitis: A prospective, randomized, double-blind, placebo-controlled study. J Endod 2014;40:1–5.

42. Schellenberg J, Drum M, Reader A, Nusstein J, Fowler S, Beck M. Effect of buffered 4% lidocaine on the success of the inferior alveolar nerve block in patients with symptomatic irreversible pulpitis: A prospective, randomized, double-blind study. J Endod 2015;41:791–796.

43. Click V, Drum M, Reader A, Nusstein J, Beck M. Evaluation of the Gow-Gates and Vazirani-Akinosi techniques in patients with symptomatic irreversible pulpitis: A prospective randomized study. J Endod 2015;41:16–21.

44. Webster S Jr, Drum M, Reader A, Fowler S, Nusstein J, Beck M. How effective is supplemental intraseptal anesthesia in patients with symptomatic irreversible pulpitis? J Endod 2016;42:1453–1457.

45. Gale EN, Carlsson SG, Eriksson A, Jontell M. Effects of dentists' behavior on patients' attitudes. J Am Dent Assoc 1984;109:444–446.

46. Davidhizar R, Shearer R. Improving your bedside manner. J Pract Nurs 1998;48:10–14.

47. Schouten BC, Eijkman MA, Hoogstraten J. Dentists' and patients' communicative behavior and their satisfaction with the dental encounter. Community Dent Health 2003;20:11–15.

48. Fletcher KE, Furney SL, Stern DT. Patients speak: What's really important about bedside interactions with physician teams. Teach Learn Med 2007;19:120–127.

49. Strichartz GR. Novel ideas of local anaesthetic actions on various ion channels to ameliorate postoperative pain. Br J Anaesth 2008;101:45–47.

50. Cohen JS, Reader A, Fertel R, Beck M, Meyers WJ. A radioimmunoassay determination of the concentrations of prostaglandins E2 and F2alpha in painful and asymptomatic human dental pulps. J Endod 1985;11:330–335.

51. Isett J, Reader A, Gallatin E, Beck M, Padgett D. Effect of an intraosseous injection of depomedrol on pulpal concentrations of PGE2 and IL8 in untreated irreversible pulpitis. J Endod 2003;29:268–271.

52. Wells JE, Bingham V, Rowland KC, Hatton J. Expression of Nav1.9 channels in human dental pulp and trigeminal ganglion. J Endod 2007;33:1172–1176.

53. Luo S, Perry GM, Levinson SR, Henry MA. $Na_v1.7$ expression is increased in painful human dental pulp [abstract]. Mol Pain 2008;21:16.

54. Warren CA, Mok L, Gordon S, Fouad AF, Gold MS. Quantification of neural proteins in extirpated tooth pulps. J Endod 2008;34:7–10.

55. Hargreaves K, Keiser K. Local anesthetic failure in endodontics: Mechanisms and management. Endod Topics 2003;1:26–39.

56. Owatz CB, Khan AA, Schindler WG, Schwartz SA, Keiser K, Hargreaves KM. The incidence of mechanical allodynia in patients with irreversible pulpitis. J Endod 2007;33:552–556.

57. Argueta-Figueroa L, Arzate-Sosa G, Mendieta-Zeron H. Anesthetic efficacy of articaine for inferior alveolar nerve blocks in patients with symptomatic versus asymptomatic irreversible pulpitis. Gen Dent 2012;60:39E–43E.

58. Fragouli E, Panopoulos P, Georgopoulou M. Efficacy of inferior alveolar nerve block using 1.7 mL of 4% articaine with 1:100,00 epinephrine in reversible and irreversible pulpitis. ENDO (Lond Engl) 2011;5:285–291.

59. Aggarwal V, Singla M, Subbiya A, et al. Effect of preoperative pain on inferior alveolar nerve block. Anesth Prog 2015;62:135–139.

60. Heft M, Parker SR. An experimental basis for revising the graphic rating scale for pain. Pain 1984;19:153–161.

61. Aggarwal V, Singla M, Miglani S, Ansari I, Kohli S. A prospective, randomized, single-blind comparative evaluation of anesthetic efficacy of posterior superior alveolar nerve blocks, buccal infiltrations, and buccal plus palatal infiltrations in patients with irreversible pulpitis. J Endod 2011;37:1491–1494.

62. Moradi Askari E, Parirokh M, Nakhaee N, Hosseini HR, Abbott PV. The effect of maxillary first molar root length on the success rate of buccal infiltration anesthesia. J Endod 2016;42:1462–1466.

63. Mehrvarzfar P, Pourhashemi A, Khodaei F, et al. The effect of adding fentanyl to epinephrine-containing lidocaine on the anesthesia of maxillary teeth with irreversible pulpitis: A randomized clinical trial. Iran Endod J 2014;9:290–294.

64. Srinivasan N, Kavitha M, Loganathan CS, Padmini G. Comparison of anesthetic efficacy of 4% articaine and 2% lidocaine for maxillary buccal infiltration in patients with irreversible pulpitis. Oral Surg Oral Med Oral Pathol Oral Radiol Endod 2009;107:133–136.

65. Sherman MG, Flax M, Namerow K, Murray PE. Anesthetic efficacy of the Gow-Gates injection and maxillary infiltration with articaine and lidocaine for irreversible pulpitis. J Endod 2008;34:656–659.

66. Rosenberg PA, Amin KG, Zibari Y, Lin LM. Comparison of 4% articaine with 1:100,000 epinephrine and 2% lidocaine with 1:100,000 epinephrine when used as a supplemental anesthetic. J Endod 2007;33:403–405.

67. Kanaa MD, Whitworth JM, Meechan JG. A comparison of the efficacy of 4% articaine with 1:100,000 epinephrine and 2% lidocaine with 1:80,000 epinephrine in achieving pulpal anesthesia in maxillary teeth with irreversible pulpitis. J Endod 2012;38:279–282.

68. Hosseini HR, Parirokh M, Nakhaee N, V Abbott P, Samani S. Efficacy of articaine and lidocaine for buccal infiltration of first maxillary molars with symptomatic irreversible pulpitis: A randomized double-blinded clinical trial. Iran Endod J 2016;11:79–84.

69. Atasoy Ulusoy ÖI, Alaçam T. Efficacy of single buccal infiltrations for maxillary first molars in patients with irreversible pulpitis: A randomized controlled clinical trial. Int Endod J 2014;47:222–227.

70. Brandt RG, Anderson PF, McDonald NJ, Sohn W, Peters MC. The pulpal anesthetic efficacy of articaine versus lidocaine in dentistry: A meta-analysis. J Am Dent Assoc 2011;142:493–504.

71. Kung J, McDonagh M, Sedgley CM. Does articaine provide an advantage over lidocaine in patients with symptomatic irreversible pulpitis? A systematic review and meta-analysis. J Endod 2015;41:1784–1794.

72. Ashraf H, Kazem M, Dianat O, Noghrehkar F. Efficacy of articaine versus lidocaine in block and infiltration anesthesia administered in teeth with irreversible pulpitis: A prospective, randomized, double-blind study. J Endod 2013;39:6–10.

73. Sood R, Hans MK, Shetty S. Comparison of anesthetic efficacy of 4% articaine with 1:100,000 epinephrine and 2% lidocaine with 1:80,000 epinephrine for inferior alveolar nerve block in patients with irreversible pulpitis. J Clin Exp Dent 2014;6:520E–523E.

74. Singla M, Subbiya A, Aggarwal V, et al. Comparison of the anaesthetic efficacy of different volumes of 4% articaine (1.8 and 3.6 mL) as supplemental buccal infiltration after failed inferior alveolar nerve block. Int Endod J 2015;48:103–108.

75. Poorni S, Veniashok B, Senthilkumar AD, Indira R, Ramachandran S. Anesthetic efficacy of four percent articaine for pulpal anesthesia by using inferior alveolar nerve block and buccal infiltration techniques in patients with irreversible pulpitis: A prospective randomized double-blind clinical trial. J Endod 2011;37:1603–1607.

76. Ahmad ZH, Ravikumar H, Karale R, Preethanath RS, Sukumaran A. Study of the anesthetic efficacy of inferior alveolar nerve block using articaine in irreversible pulpitis. J Contemp Dent Pract 2014;15:71–74.

77. Fowler S, Drum M, Reader A, Beck M. Anesthetic success of an inferior alveolar nerve block and supplemental articaine buccal infiltration for molars and premolars in patients with symptomatic irreversible pulpitis. J Endod 2016;42:390–392.

78. Aggarwal V, Singla M, Miglani S, Kohli S, Singh S. Comparative evaluation of 1.8 mL and 3.6 mL of 2% lidocaine with 1:200,000 epinephrine for inferior alveolar nerve block in patients with irreversible pulpitis: A prospective, randomized single-blind study. J Endod 2012;38:753–756.

79. Fowler S, Reader A. Is a volume of 3.6 mL better than 1.8 mL for inferior alveolar nerve blocks in patients with symptomatic irreversible pulpitis? J Endod 2013;39:970–972.

80. Abazarpoor R, Parirokh M, Nakhaee N, Abbott PV. A comparison of different volumes of articaine for inferior alveolar nerve block for molar teeth with symptomatic irreversible pulpitis. J Endod 2015;41:1408–1411.

81. Fowler S, Reader A, Beck M. Incidence of missed inferior alveolar nerve blocks in vital asymptomatic subjects and in patients with symptomatic irreversible pulpitis. J Endod 2015;41:637–639.

82. Kanaa MD, Whitworth JM, Meechan JG. A prospective randomized trial of different supplementary local anesthetic techniques after failure of inferior alveolar nerve block in patients with irreversible pulpitis in mandibular teeth. J Endod 2012;38:421–425.

83. Simpson M, Drum M, Reader A, Nusstein J, Beck M. Effect of preoperative ibuprofen/acetaminophen on the success of the inferior alveolar nerve block in patients with symptomatic irreversible pulpitis. J Endod 2011;37:593–597.

84. Goldberg S, Reader A, Drum M, Nusstein J, Beck M. Comparison of the anesthetic efficacy of the conventional inferior alveolar, Gow-Gates, and Vazirani-Akinosi techniques. J Endod 2008;34:1306–1311.

85. Donkor P, Wong J, Punnia-Moorthy A. An evaluation of the closed mouth mandibular block technique. Int J Oral Maxillofac Surg 1990;19:216–219.

86. Yücel E, Hutchison IL. A comparative evaluation of the conventional and closed-mouth technique for inferior alveolar nerve block. Aust Dent J 1995;40:15–16.

87. Heard AM, Green RJ, Lacquiere DA, Sillifant P. The use of mandibular nerve block to predict safe anaesthetic induction in patients with acute trismus. Anaesthesia 2009;64:1196–1198.

88. Kuzin AV, Neledva VV. Indications, feasibility and clinical experience with Vazirani-Akinosi mandibular block in limiting mouth opening and difficult anatomical conditions [in Russian]. Stomatologiia (Mosk) 2015;94(2):27–29.

89. Tsuschiya H, Mizogami M, Ueno T, Takakura K. Interaction of local anaesthetics with lipid membranes under inflammatory conditions. Inflammopharmacology 2007;15:164–170.

90. Modaresi J, Dianat O, Soluti A. Effect of pulp inflammation on nerve impulse quality with or without anesthesia. J Endod 2008;34:438–441.

91. Wallace JA, Michanowicz AE, Mundell RD, Wilson EG. A pilot study of the clinical problem of regionally anesthetizing the pulp of an acutely inflamed mandibular molar. Oral Sur Oral Med Oral Pathol 1985;59:517–521.

92. Roy M, Narahashi T. Differential properties of tetrodotoxin-sensitive and tetrodotoxin-resistant sodium channels in rat dorsal root ganglion neurons. J Neurosci 1992;12:2104–2111.

93. Sorensen H, Skidmore L, Rzasa R, Kleier S, Levinson S, Henry M. Comparison of pulpal sodium channel density in normal teeth to diseased teeth with severe spontaneous pain [abstract]. J Endod 2004;30:287.

94. Nusstein J, Kennedy S, Reader A, Beck M, Weaver J. Anesthetic efficacy of the supplemental X-Tip intraosseous injection in patients with irreversible pulpitis. J Endod 2003;29:724–728.

95. Parente SA, Anderson RW, Herman WW, Kimbrough WF, Weller RN. Anesthetic efficacy of the supplemental intraosseous injection for teeth with irreversible pulpitis. J Endod 1998;24:826–828.

96. McCartney M, Reader A, Beck M. Injection pain of the inferior alveolar nerve block in patients with irreversible pulpitis. Oral Surg Oral Med Oral Pathol Oral Radiol Endod 2007;104:571–575.

97. Drum M, Reader A, Beck M. Long buccal nerve block injection pain in patients with irreversible pulpitis. Oral Surg Oral Med Oral Pathol Oral Radiol Endod 2011;112(1):e51–54.

98. Carter LE, McNeil DW, Vowles KE, et al. Effects of emotion on pain reports, tolerance and physiology. Pain Res Manag 2002;7:21–30.

99. Khademi AA, Saatchi M, Minaiyan M, Rostamizadeh N, Sharafi F. Effect of preoperative alprazolam on the success of inferior alveolar nerve block for teeth with irreversible pulpitis. J Endod 2012;38:1337–1339.

100. Young J, Siffleet J, Nikoletti S, Shaw T. Use of Behavioral Pain Scale to assess pain in ventilated, unconscious and/or sedated patients. Intensive Crit Care Nurs 2006;22:32–39.

101. Payen JF, Bru O, Bosson JL, et al. Assessing pain in critically ill sedated patients by using a behavioral pain scale. Crit Care Med 2001;29:2258–2263.

102. Aissaoui Y, Zeggwagh AA, Zekraoui A, Abidi K, Abouqal R. Validation of a behavioral pain scale in critically ill, sedated, and mechanically ventilated patients. Anesth Analg 2005;101:1470–1476.

103. Aggarwal V, Singla M, Miglani S, Kohli S. Comparison of the anesthetic efficacy of epinephrine concentrations (1 : 80 000 and 1 : 200 000) in 2% lidocaine for inferior alveolar nerve block in patients with symptomatic irreversible pulpitis: A randomized, double-blind clinical trial. Int Endod J 2014;47:373–379.

104. Aggarwal V, Singla M, Miglani S, Kohli S, Irfan M. A prospective, randomized single-blind evaluation of effect of injection speed on anesthetic efficacy of inferior alveolar nerve block in patients with symptomatic irreversible pulpitis. J Endod 2012;38:1578–1580.

105. Saatchi M, Khademi A, Baghaei B, Noormohammadi H. Effect of sodium bicarbonate-buffered lidocaine on the success of inferior alveolar nerve block for teeth with symptomatic irreversible pulpitis: A prospective, randomized double-blind study. J Endod 2015;41: 33–35.

106. Saatchi M, Farhad AR, Shenasa N, Haghighi SK. Effect of sodium bicarbonate buccal infiltration on the success of inferior alveolar nerve block in mandibular first molars with symptomatic irreversible pulpitis: A prospective, randomized double-blind study. J Endod 2016;42:1458–1461.

107. Whitcomb M, Drum M, Reader A, Nusstein J, Beck M. A prospective, randomized double-blind study of the anesthetic efficacy of sodium bicarbonate buffered 2% lidocaine with 1:100,000 epinephrine in inferior alveolar nerve blocks. Anesth Prog 2010;57:59–66.

108. Jalali S, Moradi Majd N, Torabi S, Habibi M, Homayouni H, Mohammadi N. The effect of acupuncture on the success of inferior alveolar nerve block for teeth with symptomatic irreversible pulpitis: A triple-blind randomized clinical trial. J Endod 2015;41:1397–1402.

109. Kreimer T, Kiser R 2nd, Reader A, Nusstein J, Drum M, Beck M. Anesthetic efficacy of combinations of 0.5 mol/L mannitol and lidocaine with epinephrine for inferior alveolar nerve blocks in patients with symptomatic irreversible pulpitis. J Endod 2012;38:598–603.

110. Talati A, Bidar M, Sadeghi G, Nezami H. A comparative study of lidocaine and lidocaine- mannitol in anesthetizing human teeth with inflamed pulps. Iran Endod J 2006;1:19–23.

111. Shetty KP, Satish SV, Kilaru KR, Sardar P, Luke AM. Comparison of anesthetic efficacy between lidocaine with and without magnesium sulfate USP 50% for inferior alveolar nerve blocks in patients with symptomatic irreversible pulpitis. J Endod 2015;41:431–433.

112. Vastani N, Seifert B, Spahn DR, Maurer K. Sensitivities of rat primary sensory afferent nerves to magnesium: Implications for differential nerve blocks. Eur J Anaesthesiol 2013;30:21–28.

113. Srebro DP, Vučković SM, Savić Vujović KR, Prostran MŠ. TRPA1, NMDA receptors and nitric oxide mediate mechanical hyperalgesia induced by local injection of magnesium sulfate into the rat hind paw. Physiol Behav 2015;139:267–273.

114. Visconti RP, Tortamano IP, Buscariolo IA. Comparison of the anesthetic efficacy of mepivacaine and lidocaine in patients with irreversible pulpitis: A double-blind randomized clinical trial. J Endod 2016;42:1314–1319.

115. Rodríguez-Wong L, Pozos-Guillen A, Silva-Herzog D, Chavarría-Bolaños D. Efficacy of mepivacaine-tramadol combination on the success of inferior alveolar nerve blocks in patients with symptomatic irreversible pulpitis: A randomized clinical trial. Int Endod J 2016;49:325–333.

116. Isiordia-Espinoza MA, Orozco-Solis M, Tobías-Azúa FJ, Méndez-Gutiérrez EP. Submucous tramadol increases the anesthetic efficacy of mepivacaine with epinephrine in inferior alveolar nerve block. Br J Oral Maxillofac Surg 2012;50:157–160.

117. Beyazova M, Öztürk E, Zinnuroğlu M, Gökyar I, Babacan A, Kaya K. Effects of perineural tramadol on nerve conduction of sural nerve. Agri 2011;23(2):51–56.

118. Shadmehr E, Aminozarbian MG, Akhavan A, Mahdavian P, Davoudi A. Anaesthetic efficacy of lidocaine/clonidine for inferior alveolar nerve block in patients with irreversible pulpitis [epub ahead of print 13 May 2016]. Int Endod J doi:10.1111/iej.12659.

119. Satish SV, Shetty KP, Kilaru K, Bhargavi P, Reddy ES, Bellutgi A. Comparative evaluation of the efficacy of 2% lidocaine containing 1:200,000 epinephrine with and without hyaluronidase (75 IU) in patients with irreversible pulpitis. J Endod 2013;39:1116–1118.

120. Sampaio RM, Carnaval TG, Lanfredi CB, Horliana AC, Rocha RG, Tortamano IP. Comparison of the anesthetic efficacy between bupivacaine and lidocaine in patients with irreversible pulpitis of mandibular molar. J Endod 2012;38:594–597.

121. Parirokh M, Yosefi MH, Nakhaee N, Abbott PV, Manochehrifar H. The success rate of bupivacaine and lidocaine as anesthetic agents in inferior alveolar nerve block in teeth with irreversible pulpitis without spontaneous pain. Restor Dent Endod 2015;40:155–160.

122. Fernandez C, Reader A, Beck M, Nusstein J. A prospective, randomized, double-blind comparison of bupivacaine and lidocaine for inferior alveolar nerve blocks. J Endod 2005;31:499–503.

123. Aggarwal V, Singla M, Miglani S, Kohli S. Comparative evaluation of mental incisal nerve block, inferior alveolar nerve block, and their combination on the anesthetic success rate in symptomatic mandibular premolars: A randomized double-blind clinical trial. J Endod 2016;42:843–845.

124. Henry MA, Hargreaves KM. Peripheral mechanisms of odontogenic pain. Dent Clin North Am 2007;51:19–44.

125. Obrien TP, Roszkowski MT, Wolff LF, Hinrichs JE, Hargreaves KM. Effect of a non-steroidal anti-inflammatory drug on tissue levels of immunoreactive prostaglandin E2, immunoreactive leukotriene, and pain after periodontal surgery. J Periodontol 1996;67:1307–1316.

126. Modaresi J, Dianat O, Mozayeni MA. The efficacy comparison of ibuprofen, acetaminophen-codeine, and placebo premedication therapy on the depth of anesthesia during treatment of inflamed teeth. Oral Surg Oral Med Oral Pathol Oral Radiol Endod 2006;102:399–403.

127. Nusstein J, Reader A, Nist R, Beck M, Meyers WJ. Anesthetic efficacy of the supplemental intraosseous injection of 2% lidocaine with 1:100,000 epinephrine in irreversible pulpitis. J Endod 1998;24:487–491.

128. Dreven LJ, Reader A, Beck M, Meyers WJ, Weaver J. An evaluation of an electric pulp tester as a measure of analgesia in human vital teeth. J Endod 1987;13:233–238.

129. Ianiro SR, Jeansonne BJ, McNeal SF, Eleazer PD. The effect of preoperative acetaminophen or a combination of acetaminophen and ibuprofen on the success of the inferior alveolar nerve block for teeth with irreversible pulpitis. J Endod 2007;33:11–14.

130. Aggarwal V, Singla M, Kabi D. Comparative evaluation of effect of preoperative oral medication of ibuprofen and ketorolac on anesthetic efficacy of inferior alveolar nerve block with lidocaine in patients with irreversible pulpitis: A prospective, double-blind, randomized clinical trial. J Endod 2010;36:375–378.

131. Parirokh M, Ashouri R, Rekabi AR, et al. The effect of premedication with ibuprofen and indomethacin on the success of inferior alveolar nerve block for teeth with irreversible pulpitis. J Endod 2010;36:1450–1454.

132. Noguera-Gonzalez D, Cerda-Cristerna B, Chavarria-Bolaños D, Flores-Reyes H, Pozos-Guillen A. Efficacy of preoperative ibuprofen on the success of inferior alveolar nerve block in patients with symptomatic irreversible pulpitis: A randomized clinical trial. Int Endod J 2013;46:1056–1062.

133. Jena A, Shashirekha G. Effect of preoperative medications on the efficacy of inferior alveolar nerve block in patients with irreversible pulpitis: A placebo-controlled clinical study. J Conserv Dent 2013;16:171–174.

134. Shahi S, Mokhtari H, Rahimi S, et al. Effect of premedication with ibuprofen and dexamethasone on success rate of inferior alveolar nerve block for teeth with asymptomatic irreversible pulpitis: A randomized clinical trial. J Endod 2013;39:160–162.

135. Ramachandran A, Khan SI, Mohanavelu D, Kumar KS. The efficacy of pre-operative oral medication of paracetamol, ibuprofen, and aceclofenac on the success of maxillary infiltration anesthesia in patients with irreversible pulpitis: A double-blind, randomized controlled clinical trial. J Conserv Dent 2012;15:310–314.

136. Yagiela JA, Dowd FJ, Johnson BS, Mariotti AJ, Neidle EA. Pharmacology and Therapeutics for Dentistry, ed 6. St Louis: Mosby, 2011.

137. Mellor AC, Dorman ML, Girdler NM. The use of an intra-oral injection of ketorolac in the treatment of irreversible pulpitis. Int Endod J 2005;38:789–792.

138. Hargreaves KM. Letter to the editor. Int Endod J 2006;39:334–335.

139. Yadav M, Grewal MS, Grewal S, Deshwal P. Comparison of preoperative oral ketorolac on anesthetic efficacy of inferior alveolar nerve block and buccal and lingual infiltration with articaine and lidocaine in patients with irreversible pulpitis: A prospective, randomized, controlled, double-blind study. J Endod 2015;41:1773–1777.

140. Saha SG, Jain S, Dubey S, Kala S, Misuriya A, Kataria D. Effect of oral premedication on the efficacy of inferior alveolar nerve block in patients with symptomatic irreversible pulpitis: A prospective, double-blind, randomized controlled clinical trial. J Clin Diagn Res 2016;10(2):ZC25–ZC29.

141. Prasanna N, Subbarao CV, Gutmann JL. The efficacy of pre-operative oral medication of lornoxicam and diclofenac potassium on the success of inferior alveolar nerve block in patients with irreversible pulpitis: A double-blind, randomised controlled clinical trial. Int Endod J 2011;44:330–336.

142. Li C, Yang X, Ma X, Li L, Shi Z. Preoperative oral nonsteroidal anti-inflammatory drugs for the success of the inferior alveolar nerve block in irreversible pulpitis treatment: A systematic review and meta-analysis based on randomized controlled trials. Quintessence Int 2012;43:209–219.

143. Lapidus D, Goldberg J, Hobbs EH, Ram S, Clark GT, Enciso R. Effect of premedication to provide analgesia as a supplement to inferior alveolar nerve block in patients with irreversible pulpitis. J Am Dent Assoc 2016;147:427–437.

144. Becker DE, Rosenberg M. Nitrous oxide and the inhalation anesthetics. Anesth Prog 2008;55:124–130.

145. Jastak JT, Donaldson D. Nitrous oxide. Anesth Prog 1991;38:142–153.

146. Attar S, Bowles WR, Baisden MK, Hodges JS, McClanahan SB. Evaluation of pretreatment analgesia and endodontic treatment for postoperative endodontic pain. J Endod 2008;34:652–655.

147. Al-Kahtani A. Effect of long acting local anesthetic on postoperative pain in teeth with irreversible pulpitis: Randomized clinical trial. Saudi Pharm J 2014;22:39–42.

148. Ramazani M, Hamidi MR, Moghaddamnia AA, Ramazani N, Zarenejad N. The prophylactic effects of zintoma and ibuprofen on post-endodontic pain of molars with irreversible pulpitis: A randomized clinical trial. Iran Endod J 2013;8:129–134.

149. Sethi P, Agarwal M, Chourasia HR, Singh MP. Effect of single dose pretreatment analgesia with three different analgesics on postoperative endodontic pain: A randomized clinical trial. J Conserv Dent 2014;17:517–521.

150. Parirokh M, Sadr S, Nakhaee N, Abbott PV, Manochehrifar H. Comparison between prescription of regular or on-demand ibuprofen on postoperative pain after single-visit root canal treatment of teeth with irreversible pulpitis. J Endod 2014;40:151–154.

151. Mokhtari F, Yazdi K, Mahabadi AM, Modaresi SJ, Hamzeheil Z. Effect of premedication with indomethacin and ibuprofen on postoperative endodontic pain: A clinical trial. Iran Endod J 2016;11:57–62.

152. Elzaki WM, Abubakr NH, Ziada HM, Ibrahim YE. Double-blind randomized placebo-controlled clinical trial of efficiency of nonsteroidal anti-inflammatory drugs in the control of post-endodontic pain. J Endod 2016;42:835–842.

153. Pacira Pharmaceuticals, Inc. How DepoFoam Works. http://www.pacira.com/depofoam-platform/how-it-works. Accessed 23 June 2015.

154. Massaro F. Liposomal bupivacaine: A long-acting local anesthetic for postsurgical analgesia. Formulary 2012;47:212–226.

155. Golf M, Daniels SE, Onel E. A phase 3, randomized, placebo-controlled trial of DepoFoam bupivacaine (extended-release bupivacaine local analgesia) in bunionectomy. Adv Ther 2011;28:776–788.

156. Bagsby DT, Ireland PH, Meneghini RM. Liposomal bupivacaine versus traditional periarticular injection for pain control after total knee arthroplasty. J Arthroplasty 2014;29:1687–1690.

157. Bramlett K, Onel E, Viscusi ER, Jones K. A randomized, double-blind, dose-ranging study comparing wound infiltration of DepoFoam bupivacaine, an extended-release liposomal bupivacaine, to bupivacaine HCl for postsurgical analgesia in total knee arthroplasty. Knee 2012;19:530–536.

158. Skolnik A, Gan TJ. New formulations of bupivacaine for the treatment of postoperative pain: Liposomal bupivacaine and SABER-Bupivacaine. Expert Opin Pharmacother 2014;15:1535–1542.

159. Surdam JW, Licini DJ, Baynes NT, Arce BR. The use of exparel (liposomal bupivacaine) to manage postoperative pain in unilateral total knee arthroplasty patients. J Arthroplasty 2015;30:325–329.

160. Domb BG, Gupta A, Hammarstedt JE, Stake CE, Sharp K, Redmond JM. The effect of liposomal bupivacaine injection during total hip arthroplasty: A controlled cohort study. BMC Musculoskelet Disord 2014;15:310.

161. Butz DR, Shenaq DS, Rundell VL, et al. Postoperative pain and length of stay lowered by use of Exparel in immediate, implant-based breast reconstruction. Plast Reconstr Surg Glob Open 2015;3:391E.

162. Candiotti KA, Sands LR, Lee E, et al. Liposome bupivacaine for postsurgical analgesia in adult patients undergoing laparoscopic colectomy: Results from prospective phase IV sequential cohort studies assessing health economic outcomes. Curr Ther Res Clin Exp 2013;76:1–6.

163. Cohen SM, Vogel JD, Marcet JE, Candiotti KA. Liposome bupivacaine for improvement in economic outcomes and opioid burden in GI surgery: IMPROVE Study pooled analysis. J Pain Res 2014;7:359–366.

164. Marcet JE, Nfonsam VN, Larach S. An extended pain relief trial utilizing the infiltration of a long-acting multivesicular liposome formulation of bupivacaine, Exparel (IMPROVE): A phase IV health economic trial in adult patients undergoing ileostomy reversal. J Pain Res 2013;6:549–555.

165. Vogel JD. Liposome bupivacaine (EXPAREL) for extended pain relief in patients undergoing ileostomy reversal at a single institution with a fast-track discharge protocol: An IMPROVE phase IV health economics trial. J Pain Res 2013;6:605–610.

166. Gorfine SR, Onel E, Patou G, Krivokapic ZV. Bupivacaine extended-release liposome injection for prolonged postsurgical analgesia in patients undergoing hemorrhoidectomy: A multicenter, randomized, double-blind placebo-controlled trial. Dis Colon Rectum 2011;54:1552–1559.

167. Haas E, Onel E, Miller H, Ragupathi M, White PF. A double-blind, randomized, active-controlled study for post-hemorrhoidectomy pain management with liposome bupivacaine, a novel local analgesic formulation. Am Surg 2012;78:574–581.

168. Onel E, Miller H, Patou G, White PF. Exparel, a liposomal bupivacaine local analgesic, extends pain relief and decreases opioid use [Proceedings of the American Society of Anesthesiologists 2010 Annual Meeting, 16–20 Oct 2010, San Diego, CA]. Schaumburg, IL: American Society of Anesthesiologists, 2010.

169. Smoot JD, Bergese SD, Onel E, Williams HT, Hedden W. The efficacy and safety of DepoFoam bupivacaine in patients undergoing bilateral, cosmetic, submuscular augmentation mammaplasty: A randomized, double-blind, active control study. Aesthetic Surg J 2012;32:69–76.

170. Minkowitz H, Onel E, Patronella CK, Smoot JD. A two-year observational study assessing the safety of DepoFoam bupivacaine after augmentation mammoplasty. Aesthetic Surg J 2012;32:186–193.

171. Morales R Jr, Mentz H 3rd, Newall G, Patronella C, Masters O 3rd. Use of abdominal field block injections with liposomal bupivicaine to control postoperative pain after abdominoplasty. Aesthet Surg J 2013;33:1148–1153.

172. Man D. The incorporation of liposome bupivacaine into an opioid-sparing strategy for patients undergoing rhytidectomy. Plast Reconstr Surg 2014;134(4S-1):124.

173. Bultema K, Fowler S, Drum M, Reader A, Nusstein J, Beck M. Pain reduction in untreated symptomatic irreversible pulpitis using liposomal bupivacaine (Exparel): A prospective, randomized, double-blind trial. J Endod (in press).

174. Oguntebi B, DeSchepper E, Taylor T, White C, Pink F. Postoperative pain incidence related to the type of emergency treatment of symptomatic pulpitis. Oral Surg Oral Med Oral Pathol Oral Radiol Endod 1992;73:479–483.

175. Nagle D, Reader A, Beck M, Weaver J. Effect of systemic penicillin on pain in untreated irreversible pulpitis. Oral Surg Oral Med Oral Pathol Oral Radiol Endod 2000;90:636–640.

176. Keenan JV, Farman AG, Fedorowicz Z, Newton JT. A Cochrane systematic review finds no evidence to support the use of antibiotics for pain relief in irreversible pulpitis. J Endod 2006;32:87–92.

177. Sutherland S. Antibiotics do not reduce toothache caused by irreversible pulpitis. Are systematic antibiotics effective in providing pain relief in people who have irreversible pulpitis? Evid Based Dent 2005;6:67.

178. Gallatin E, Reader A, Nist R, Beck M. Pain reduction in untreated irreversible pulpitis using an intraosseous injection of Depo-Medrol. J Endod 2000;26:633–638.

179. Bane K, Charpentier E, Bronnec F, et al. Randomized clinical trial of intraosseous methylprednisolone injection for acute pulpitis pain. J Endod 2016;42:2–7.

180. Isett J, Reader A, Gallatin E, Beck M, Padgett D. Effect of an intraosseous injection of depo-medrol on pulpal concentrations of PGE2 and IL8 in untreated irreversible pulpitis. J Endod 2003;29:268–271.

181. Agarwala V, Reader A, Nusstein JM, Beck M. Anesthetic effect of a preemptive intraosseous injection of Depo-Medrol in untreated irreversible pulpitis [abstract]. J Endod 2006;32:238.

182. Stein K, Reader A, Agarwala V, Nusstein J, Beck M. Anesthetic effectiveness of a preemptive injection of Depo-Medrol in untreated irreversible pulpitis [abstract]. J Endod 2007;33:332.

183. McDougal RA, Delano EO, Caplan D, Sigurdsson A, Trope M. Success of an alternative for interim management of irreversible pulpitis. J Am Dent Assoc 2004;135:1707–1712.

184. DeRosa T. A retrospective evaluation of pulpotomy as an alternative to extraction. Gen Dent 2006;54:37–40.

185. Teixeira LS, Demarco FF, Coppola MC, Bonow ML. Clinical and radiographic evaluation of pulpotomies performed under intrapulpal injection of anaesthetic solution. Int Endod J 2001;34:440–446.

186. Aggarwal V, Singla M, Rizvi A, Miglani S. Comparative evaluation of local infiltration of articaine, articaine plus ketorolac, and dexamethasone on anesthetic success of inferior alveolar nerve block with lidocaine in patients with irreversible pulpitis. J Endod 2011;37:445–449.

187. Fan S, Chen WL, Pan CB, et al. Anesthetic efficacy of inferior alveolar nerve block plus buccal infiltration or periodontal ligament injections with articaine in patients with irreversible pulpitis in the mandibular first molar. Oral Surg Oral Med Oral Pathol Oral Radiol Endod 2009;108:89–93.

188. Dou L, Luo J, Yang D. Anaesthetic efficacy of supplemental lingual infiltration of mandibular molars after inferior alveolar nerve block plus buccal infiltration in patients with irreversible pulpitis. Int Endod J 2013;46:660–665.

189. Rogers BS, Botero TM, McDonald NJ, Gardner RJ, Peters MC. Efficacy of articaine versus lidocaine as a supplemental buccal infiltration in mandibular molars with irreversible pulpitis: A prospective, randomized, double-blind study. J Endod 2014;40:753–758.

190. Monteiro MR, Groppo FC, Haiter-Neto F, Volpato MC, Almeida JF. 4% articaine buccal infiltration versus 2% lidocaine inferior alveolar nerve block for emergency root canal treatment in mandibular molars with irreversible pulpits: A randomized clinical study. Int Endod J 2015;48:145–152.

191. Haase A, Reader A, Nusstein J, Beck M, Drum M. Comparing anesthetic efficacy of articaine versus lidocaine as a supplemental buccal infiltration of the mandibular first molar after an inferior alveolar nerve block. J Am Dent Assoc 2008;139:1128–1135.

192. Zain M, Rehman Khattak SU, Sikandar H, Shah SA, Fayyaz. Comparison of anaesthetic efficacy of 4% articaine primary buccal infiltration versus 2% lidocaine inferior alveolar nerve block in symptomatic mandibular first molar teeth. J Coll Physicians Surg Pak 2016;26:4–8.

193. Akhlaghi NM, Hormozi B, Abbott PV, Khalilak Z. Efficacy of ketorolac buccal infiltrations and inferior alveolar nerve blocks in patients with irreversible pulpitis: A prospective, double-blind, randomized clinical trial. J Endod 2016;42:691–695.

194. Malamed S. The periodontal ligament (PDL) injection: An alternative to inferior alveolar nerve block. Oral Surg Oral Med Oral Pathol 1982;53:117–121.

195. Smith GN, Walton RE, Abbott BJ. Clinical evaluation of periodontal ligament anesthesia using a pressure syringe. J Am Dent Assoc 1983;107:953–956.

196. Walton RE, Abbott BJ. Periodontal ligament injection: A clinical evaluation. J Am Dent Assoc 1981;103:571–575.

197. Meechan JG, Ledvinka JI. Pulpal anesthesia for mandibular central incisor teeth: A comparison of infiltration and intraligamentary injections. Int Endod J 2002;35:629–634.

198. White JJ, Reader A, Beck M, Meyers WJ. The periodontal ligament injection: A comparison of the efficacy in human maxillary and mandibular teeth. J Endod 1988;14:508–514.

199. Zarei M, Ghoddusi J, Sharifi E, Forghani M, Afkhami F, Marouzi P. Comparison of the anaesthetic efficacy of and heart rate changes after periodontal ligament or intraosseous X-Tip injection in mandibular molars: A randomized controlled clinical trial. Int Endod J 2012;45:921–926.

200. Parirokh M, Sadr S, Nakhaee N, Abbott PV, Askarifard S. Efficacy of supplementary buccal infiltrations and intraligamentary injections to inferior alveolar nerve blocks in mandibular first molars with asymptomatic irreversible pulpitis: A randomized controlled trial. Int Endod J 2014;47:926–933.

201. Mohajeri L, Salehi F, Mehrvarzfar P, Arfaee H, Bohluli B, Hamedy R. Anesthetic efficacy of meperidine in teeth with symptomatic irreversible pulpitis. Anesth Prog 2015;62:14–19.

202. Bangerter C, Mines P, Sweet M. The use of intraosseous anesthesia among endodontists: Results of a questionnaire. J Endod 2009;35:15–18.

203. Nusstein J, Claffey E, Reader A, Beck M, Weaver J. Anesthetic effectiveness of the supplemental intraligamentary injection, administered with a computer-controlled local anesthetic delivery system, in patients with irreversible pulpitis. J Endod 2005;31:354–358.

204. Berlin J, Nusstein J, Reader A, Beck M, Weaver J. Efficacy of articaine and lidocaine in a primary intraligamentary injection administered with a computer-controlled local anesthetic delivery system. Oral Surg Oral Med Oral Pathol Oral Radiol Endod 2005;99:361–366.

205. Mead S. Anesthesia in Dental Surgery. St Louis: Mosby, 1935.

206. Bigby J, Reader A, Nusstein J, Beck M, Weaver J. Articaine for supplemental intraosseous anesthesia in patients with irreversible pulpitis. J Endod 2006;32:1044–1047.

207. Verma PK, Srivastava R, Ramesh KM. Anesthetic efficacy of X-Tip intraosseous injection using 2% lidocaine with 1:80,000 epinephrine in patients with irreversible pulpitis after inferior alveolar nerve block: A clinical study. J Conserv Dent 2013;16:162–166.

208. Idris M, Sakkir N, Naik KG, Jayaram NK. Intraosseous injection as an adjunct to conventional local anesthetic techniques: A clinical study. J Conserv Dent 2014;17:432–435.

209. Jing Q, Wan K, Wang XJ, Ma L. Effectiveness and safety of computer-controlled periodontal ligament injection system in endodontic access to the mandibular posterior teeth. Chin Med Sci J 2014;29:23–27.

210. Pereira LA, Groppo FC, Bergamaschi Cde C, et al. Articaine (4%) with epinephrine (1:100,000 or 1:200,000) in intraosseous injections in symptomatic irreversible pulpitis of mandibular molars: Anesthetic efficacy and cardiovascular effects. Oral Surg Oral Med Oral Pathol Oral Radiol 2013;116:85E–91E.

211. Razavian H, Kazemi S, Khazaei S, Jahromi MZ. X-Tip intraosseous injection system as a primary anesthesia for irreversible pulpitis of posterior mandibular teeth: A randomized clinical trail. Dent Res J (Isfahan) 2013;10:210–213.

212. Reemers T, Glickman G, Spears R, He J. The efficacy of the IntraFlow intraosseous injection as a primary anesthesia technique. J Endod 2008;34:280–283.

213. Coggins R, Reader A, Nist R, Beck M, Meyers WJ. Anesthetic efficacy of the intraosseous injection in maxillary and mandibular teeth. Oral Surg Oral Med Oral Pathol Oral Radiol Endod 1996;81:634–641.

214. Gallatin J, Reader A, Nusstein J, Beck M, Weaver J. A comparison of two intraosseous anesthetic techniques in mandibular posterior teeth. J Am Dent Assoc 2003;134:1476–1484.

215. Jensen J, Nusstein J, Drum M, Reader A, Beck M. Anesthetic efficacy of a repeated intraosseous injection following a primary intraosseous injection. J Endod 2008;34:126–130.

216. Andersson C. Local anesthesia for infants undergoing circumcision. J Am Med Assoc 1998;279:1169–1170.

217. Brkovic BM, Savic BM, Andric M, Jurisic M, Todorovic L. Intraseptal vs. periodontal ligament anaesthesia for maxillary tooth extraction: Quality of local anaesthesia and haemodynamic response. Clin Oral Investig 2010;14:675–681.

218. Biocanin V, Brkovic B, Milicic B, Stojic D. Efficacy and safety of intraseptal and periodontal ligament anesthesia achieved by computer-controlled articaine + epinephrine delivery: A dose-finding study. Clin Oral Investig 2013;17:525–533.

219. Borodina OE, Petrkas AZh. Intraceptal anesthesia of lower and upper teeth [in Russian]. Stomatologiia (Mosk) 2009;88(5):19–20.

220. Doman SM. An audit of the use of intra-septal local anaesthesia in a dental practice in the South of England. Prim Dent Care 2011;18:67–71.

221. Marin MK. Intraseptal anesthesia in the general dental practice. Compendium 1987;8:204–209.

222. Saadoun AP, Malamed S. Intraseptal anesthesia in periodontal surgery. J Am Dent Assoc 1985;111:249–256.

223. Woodmansey K. Intraseptal anesthesia: A review of a relevant injection technique. Gen Dent 2005;53:418–420.

224. Grubbs SL, Alley LW, Eleazer PD. An ex vivo comparison of pressures within dental pulp space using conventional anesthetic technique versus needle-mounted obturator. J Endod 2014;40:907–909.

225. Miles T. Dental pain: Self-observations by a neurophysiologist. J Endod 1993;19:613–615.

226. Birchfield J, Rosenberg PA. Role of the anesthetic solution in intrapulpal anesthesia. J Endod 1975;1:26–27.

227. VanGheluwe J, Walton R. Intrapulpal injection: Factors related to effectiveness. Oral Surg Oral Med Oral Pathol 1997;19:38–40.

228. DeNunzio M. Topical anesthetic as an adjunct to local anesthesia during pulpectomies. J Endod 1998;24:202–203.

229. Sooraparaju SG, Abarajithan M, Sathish ES, Suryakumari NB, Ealla KK, Gade W. Anaesthetic efficacy of topical benzocaine gel combined with hyaluronidase for supplemental intrapulpal injection in teeth with irreversible pulpitis—A double blinded clinical trial. J Clin Diagn Res 2015;9(8):ZC95–ZC97.

230. Moghadamnia AA, Partovi M, Mohammadianfar I, et al. Evaluation of the effect of locally administered amitriptyline gel as adjunct to local anesthetics in irreversible pulpitis pain. Indian J Dent Res 2009;20:3–6.

231. Wells LK, Drum M, Nusstein J, Reader A, Beck M. Efficacy of ibuprofen and ibuprofen/acetaminophen on postoperative pain in symptomatic patients with a pulpal diagnosis of necrosis. J Endod 2011;37:1608–1612.

232. Sebastian R, Drum M, Reader A, Nusstein J, Fowler S, Beck M. What is the effect of no endodontic debridement on postoperative pain for symptomatic teeth with pulpal necrosis? J Endod 2016;42:378–382.

233. Glenn B, Drum M, Reader A, Fowler S, Nusstein J, Beck M. Does liposomal bupivacaine (Exparel) significantly reduce postoperative pain/numbness in symptomatic teeth with a diagnosis of necrosis? A prospective, randomized, double-blind trial. J Endod 2016;42:1301–1306.

234. Singer AJ, Richman PB, Kowalska A, Thode HC Jr. Comparison of patient and practitioner assessments of pain from commonly performed emergency department procedures. Ann Emerg Med 1999;33:652–658.

235. Nekoofar MH, Namazikhah MS, Sheykhrezae MS, et al. pH of pus collected from periapical abscesses. Int Endod J 2009;42:534–538.

236. Balasco M, Drum M, Reader A, Nusstein J, Beck M. Buffered lidocaine for incision and drainage: A prospective, randomized double-blind study. J Endod 2013;39:1329–1334.

237. Harreld TK, Fowler S, Drum M, Reader A, Nusstein J, Beck M. Efficacy of a buffered 4% lidocaine formulation for incision and drainage: A prospective, randomized, double-blind study. J Endod 2015;41:1583–1588.

238. Punnia-Moorthy A. Buffering capacity of normal and inflamed tissues following the injection of local anaesthetic solutions. Br J Anaesth 1988;61:154–159.

239. Tsuchiya H, Mizogami M, Ueno T, Takakura K. Interaction of local anaesthetics with lipid membranes under inflammatory acidic conditions. Inflammopharmacology 2007;15:164–170.

# Clinical Tips for Management of Specific Endodontic Situations

**After reading this chapter, the practitioner should be able to:**

- Describe how to successfully anesthetize the mandibular molars, premolars, and anterior teeth.
- Describe how to successfully anesthetize the maxillary molars, premolars, and anterior teeth.
- Define other considerations for endodontic anesthesia.
- Evaluate future directions.

The chapters in this book have outlined a substantial amount of information regarding pulpal anesthesia. Therefore, we make our recommendations based on pulpal anesthesia requirements. It is important to realize that when we talk about anesthetic effects, we are talking about the majority of patients. There will always be patients outside of the norm. Some patients will be easily anesthetized for all procedures, and some patients will only achieve anesthesia with multiple supplemental injections.

In order to ensure that the best chance for pulpal anesthesia will be obtained, we have made recommendations based on the results of studies outlined in this book. Practitioners should use their best professional judgment, taking into account the needs of each individual patient, when making decisions regarding local anesthesia.

Remember the Optimum Optimorum Principle: There comes a time when one must use the existing information and implement one pretty good solution.

## Considerations for Irreversible Pulpitis

For endodontists, the teeth with irreversible pulpitis that are the most difficult to anesthetize are the mandibular molars followed by mandibular premolars, maxillary molars, and maxillary premolars. The least problems are associated with maxillary anterior teeth.

In some teeth, vital, inflamed tissue is present in the apical portion of the canals, but the tissue in the chamber is necrotic and does not respond to pulp testing. In such cases, the pulp chamber can be entered with no problem, but severe pain will result when attempting

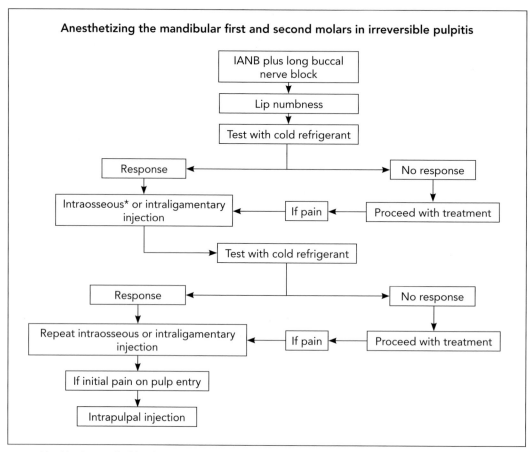

**Fig 7-1** Algorithm for anesthetizing the mandibular first and second molars in irreversible pulpitis. *Before an intraosseous injection, provide a buccal infiltration of 4% articaine with epinephrine. IANB, inferior alveolar nerve block.

to place a file to length. Intraosseous injections will be helpful, and an intrapulpal injection could be used. However, this condition of irreversible pulpitis must be differentiated from a symptomatic tooth with a necrotic pulp and periapical areas (not just a thickened periodontal ligament space). In this condition, intraosseous and intrapulpal injections are painful and may not be effective. There also exists the possibility of forcing bacteria into the periapical tissues with the intrapulpal injection.

In the 1970s, before supplemental techniques of intraligamentary and intraosseous injections were used, we would administer conventional anesthesia. After signs of soft tissue anesthesia were evident, the pain abated and the patient relaxed. Local anesthesia produced the classic soft tissue signs and relieved the painful symptoms. However, when the access opening was begun or the pulp was entered, pain frequently resulted. Currently, the use of supplemental injections can significantly reduce pain during endodontic treatment.

# Mandibular Anesthesia

## First and second molars

An algorithm for anesthetizing the first and second molars in irreversible pulpitis is presented in Fig 7-1.

Administer topical anesthetic for at least 1 minute. Slowly administer an inferior alveolar nerve block (IANB) using a two-cartridge volume of 2% lidocaine with 1:100,000 epinephrine. A slow injection (at least 60 seconds) will be less painful.[1] As an alternative, a two-stage injection technique may be used.[2] The use of the CompuDent (Miles Scientific) computer-controlled local anesthetic delivery (CCLAD) system—formerly known as the *Wand*—will also reduce the pain of injection.[3–7] Add a long buccal nerve block (a quarter to a half cartridge of 2% lidocaine with 1:100,000 epinephrine). Wait 10 minutes. Check for lip numbness. If it is not present, wait a few more minutes. If no lip numbness occurs, perform another IANB or Gow-Gates injection. Once the lip is numb (soft tissue anesthesia is required in the mandible for success of the supplemental injections), test the tooth with cold refrigerant. If the patient feels the cold, add supplemental anesthesia. You could wait a few additional minutes and then retest the tooth with cold refrigerant because some patients have slow onset of pulpal anesthesia. If the patient has no response to cold, proceed with treatment. If the patient responds to the cold, add supplemental anesthesia. Remember, if lip numbness is achieved, adding another IANB does not help much with pulpal anesthesia.

## When supplemental anesthesia is needed

Because the buccal infiltration of 1.8 mL of 4% articaine with 1:100,000 epinephrine has a limited success rate (42% for the first molars and 48% for the second molars)[8] following an IANB, it is best to proceed to an intraosseous injection using 1.8 mL of 3% mepivacaine distal to the first molar or mesial to the second molar. This recommendation is not based on the cardiovascular risks associated with a vasoconstrictor-containing anesthetic solution but rather clinical research that shows that 3% mepivacaine is reasonably effective and does not increase heart rate.[9,10] That is, a few patients may overreact to the heart rate increase with epinephrine-containing solutions, making treatment difficult or time-consuming because the patient has to be calmed before endodontic treatment can begin. However, many endodontists also use 2% lidocaine with 1:100,000 epinephrine for intraosseous anesthesia. Each clinician may want to experiment to see which anesthetic solution (3% mepivacaine or 2% lidocaine with 1:100,000 epinephrine) works best in his or her hands.

An infiltration of 1.8 mL of 4% articaine with 1:100,000 epinephrine is given over the site of the proposed intraosseous injection to help decrease the pain of the injection. Wait a few minutes and administer the intraosseous injection.

Retest the tooth with cold refrigerant. If the patient does not respond, proceed with treatment. Apply rubber dam and slowly begin the access preparation. Inform the patient that the procedure will be discontinued if pain is experienced. If pain occurs in dentin, remove the rubber dam and administer another cartridge of 3% mepivacaine or 2% lidocaine with 1:100,000 epinephrine intraosseously; this should be successful.[11] This regimen should work the majority of the time in anesthetizing molars. The clinician should ensure that there is lip numbness with the initial IANB and that anesthetic solution is being deposited into cancellous bone with the intraosseous injection.

If further pain is experienced in dentin, administer nitrous oxide. Because nitrous oxide has analgesic effects and relieves anxiety, it is effective when other supplemental techniques have failed. Naturally, nitrous oxide could be administered at the start of the appointment.

If initial pain occurs when the pulp is entered, remove the rubber dam and administer another cartridge of 3% mepivacaine or 2% lidocaine with 1:100,000 epinephrine intraosseously. If further pain is experienced, give an intrapulpal injection.

Occasionally, we have observed that when the pulp is initially exposed, the patient will experience pain, but the intrapulpal injection elicits no pain response from the patient. We feel that perhaps some change in intrapulpal pressure occurs when the pulp is entered and results in this initial pain. However, it is difficult to explain why no subsequent pain occurs upon the intrapulpal injection.

Anesthesia should be effective with the supplemental intraosseous injection for approximately 30 minutes with 3% mepivacaine[10] and 60 minutes with 2% lidocaine with 1:100,000 epinephrine.[12,13] If

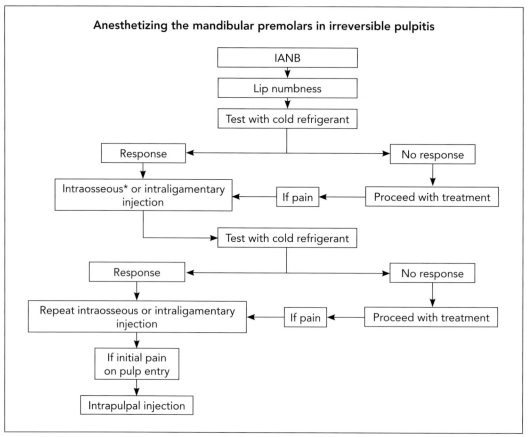

**Anesthetizing the mandibular premolars in irreversible pulpitis**

IANB
↓
Lip numbness
↓
Test with cold refrigerant

Response ← → No response

Intraosseous* or intraligamentary injection ← If pain ← Proceed with treatment

Test with cold refrigerant

Response ← → No response

Repeat intraosseous or intraligamentary injection ← If pain ← Proceed with treatment

If initial pain on pulp entry

Intrapulpal injection

**Fig 7-2** Algorithm for anesthetizing the mandibular first and second premolars in irreversible pulpitis. *Before an intraosseous injection, provide a buccal infiltration of 4% articaine with epinephrine.

the patient feels pain during the later stages of the appointment, repeat the intraosseous injection. Remember, it might also be possible that the IANB is wearing off. Another IANB may help if the in-traosseous injection does not seem to be working.

### Alternative choice for supplemental anesthesia

Although not as efficacious as intraosseous anesthesia, intraligamentary anesthesia can be given on the mesial and distal aspect of the tooth using 2% lidocaine with 1:100,000 epinephrine. Retest with cold refrigerant. If the patient does not respond, proceed with treatment. If the patient responds to cold, repeat the intraligamentary injection. The first intraligamentary injection may be successful from 63% to 74% of the time[14–16]; reinjection increases success to 92% to 96%.[14,15] Remember, the intralig-amentary injection may only be effective for 10 to 20 minutes. Therefore, it may need to be repeated.

## First and second premolars

An algorithm for anesthetizing the first and second premolars in irreversible pulpitis is presented in Fig 7-2. Administer topical anesthetic for at least 1 minute. Slowly administer an IANB using a two-cartridge volume of 2% lidocaine with 1:100,000 epinephrine. A slow injection (at least 60 seconds) will be less painful.[1] As an alternative, a two-stage injection technique may be used.[2] The use of the CompuDent

CCLAD system will also reduce the pain of injection.[3-7] Wait 10 minutes. Check for lip numbness. If not present, wait a few minutes. If no lip numbness occurs, perform another IANB or Gow-Gates injection. Once the lip is numb (soft tissue anesthesia is required in the mandible for success of the supplemental injections), test the tooth with cold refrigerant. If the patient feels the cold, add supplemental anesthesia. You could wait a few additional minutes and then retest the tooth with cold refrigerant because some patients have slow onset of pulpal anesthesia. If the patient has no response to cold, proceed with treatment. If the patient feels pain, add supplemental anesthesia.

## When supplemental anesthesia is needed

An infiltration of 4% articaine with 1:100,000 epinephrine is given over the site of the proposed intraosseous injection to help decrease the pain of the injection. Wait a few minutes and administer a supplemental intraosseous injection using 1.8 mL of 3% mepivacaine or 1.8 mL of 2% lidocaine with 1:100,000 epinephrine. Retest the tooth with cold. If the patient does not respond, proceed with treatment. Apply rubber dam and slowly begin the access preparation. Inform the patient that the procedure will be discontinued if pain is experienced. If initial pain occurs in dentin, remove the rubber dam and readminister the supplemental intraosseous injection using 1.8 mL of 3% mepivacaine or 1.8 mL of 2% lidocaine with 1:100,000 epinephrine. This regimen should work the majority of the time in anesthetizing premolars.

If further pain is experienced in dentin, administer nitrous oxide. Because nitrous oxide has analgesic effects and relieves anxiety, it is effective when other supplemental techniques have failed. Naturally, nitrous oxide could be administered at the start of the appointment.

If the initial pain occurs when the pulp is entered, remove the rubber dam and administer a cartridge of 3% mepivacaine or 2% lidocaine with 1:100,000 epinephrine intraosseously. If further pain is experienced, give an intrapulpal injection.

For supplemental intraosseous injections, anesthesia should be effective for around 30 minutes with 3% mepivacaine[10] and 60 minutes with 2% lidocaine with 1:100,000 epinephrine.[12,13] If the patient feels pain during the appointment, repeat the intraosseous injection. Remember, it might also be possible that the IANB is wearing off. Another IANB may help if the intraosseous injection does not seem to be working.

### Alternative choice for supplemental anesthesia

Although not as efficacious as intraosseous anesthesia, intraligamentary anesthesia can be given on the mesial and distal aspect of the tooth using 2% lidocaine with 1:100,000 epinephrine. Retest with cold refrigerant. If the patient does not respond, proceed with treatment. If the patient responds to cold, repeat the intraligamentary injection.

## Canine and lateral and central incisors

An algorithm for anesthetizing the canine, lateral incisor, and central incisor in irreversible pulpitis is presented in Fig 7-3.

Administer topical anesthetic for at least 1 minute. Slowly administer an IANB using a two-cartridge volume of 2% lidocaine with 1:100,000 epinephrine. A slow injection (at least 60 seconds) will be less painful.[1] As an alternative, a two-stage injection technique may be used.[2] The use of the CompuDent CCLAD system will also reduce the pain of injection.[3-7] Wait 15 to 20 minutes because onset of pulpal anesthesia is longer for the anterior teeth than the posterior teeth. Check for lip numbness. If not present, wait a few minutes. If no lip numbness occurs, perform another IANB or Gow-Gates injection. Once the lip is numb (soft tissue anesthesia is required in the mandible for success of the supplemental injections), add a labial infiltration of 1.8 mL of 4% articaine with 1:100,000 epinephrine. Test the tooth with cold refrigerant. If the patient responds to cold, add a lingual infiltration of 1.8 mL

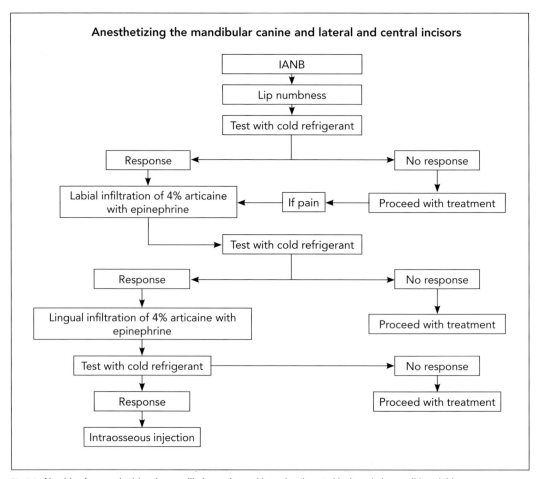

**Fig 7-3** Algorithm for anesthetizing the mandibular canine and lateral and central incisors in irreversible pulpitis.

of 4% articaine with 1:100,000 epinephrine. This regimen should work the majority of the time in anesthetizing the anterior teeth. If it fails, add supplemental intraosseous anesthesia.

### When supplemental intraosseous anesthesia is needed

Because intraligamentary anesthesia is not successful in anterior teeth,[17] intraosseous anesthesia is indicated. Administer an intraosseous injection with 1.8 mL of 3% mepivacaine or 2% lidocaine with 1:100,000 epinephrine distal to the anterior tooth to be anesthetized. Retest the tooth with cold refrigerant. If the patient does not respond, proceed with treatment. If the patient responds to cold, repeat the intraosseous injection.

Pulpal anesthesia should be effective for approximately 30 minutes with a labial infiltration of 1.8 mL of 4% articaine with 1:100,000 epinephrine. For intraosseous anesthesia, anesthesia should be effective for around 30 minutes with 3% mepivacaine[10] and 60 minutes with 2% lidocaine with 1:100,000 epinephrine.[12,13] If the patient feels pain during the later stages of the appointment, repeat the infiltration of 4% articaine with 1:100,000 epinephrine or repeat the intraosseous injection. Remember, it might also be possible that the IANB is wearing off. Another IANB may help if the intraosseous injection does not seem to be working.

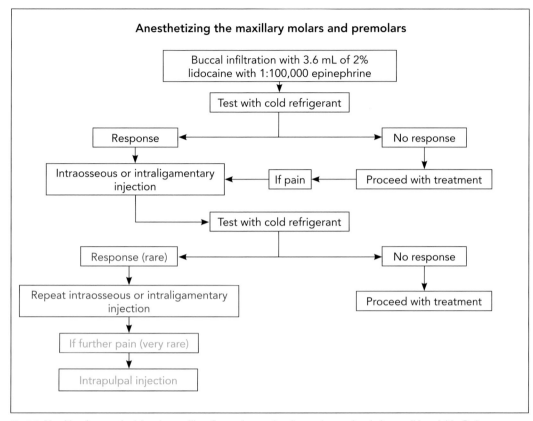

**Anesthetizing the maxillary molars and premolars**

Buccal infiltration with 3.6 mL of 2% lidocaine with 1:100,000 epinephrine

Test with cold refrigerant

Response → No response

Intraosseous or intraligamentary injection ← If pain ← Proceed with treatment

Test with cold refrigerant

Response (rare) → No response

Repeat intraosseous or intraligamentary injection → Proceed with treatment

If further pain (very rare)

Intrapulpal injection

**Fig 7-4** Algorithm for anesthetizing the maxillary first and second molars and premolars in irreversible pulpitis. Red, rare; green, very rare.

# Maxillary Anesthesia

## Molars and premolars

An algorithm for anesthetizing molars and premolars in irreversible pulpitis is presented in Fig 7-4.

Administer topical anesthetic for at least 1 minute. Slowly administer an infiltration using a cartridge of 2% lidocaine with 1:100,000 epinephrine. A slow injection (at least 60 seconds) will be less painful. As an alternative, a two-stage injection technique may be used.[2] The use of the CompuDent CCLAD system will also reduce the pain of injection.[3-7] Add another cartridge of 2% lidocaine with 1:100,000 epinephrine (total volume of 3.6 mL). The 3.6-mL volume helps to prolong the duration of anesthesia.[18] If lingual soft tissue anesthesia is needed, administer 2% lidocaine with 1:100,000 epinephrine to the palatal tissue. The CompuDent CCLAD system will reduce the pain of a palatal injection.[19,20] Wait 5 minutes, and then test the tooth with cold refrigerant. If there is no response from the patient, proceed with treatment. If the patient responds to cold, you could wait an additional 3 to 5 minutes and retest. If the patient is still responsive to cold, administer supplemental anesthesia.

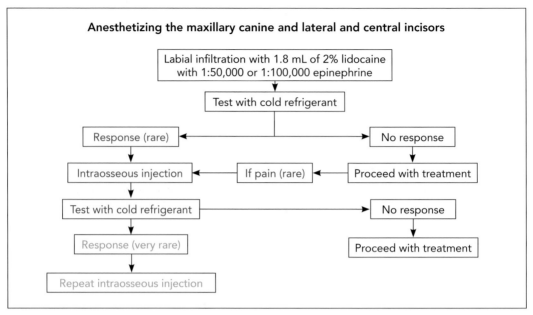

**Fig 7-5** Algorithm for anesthetizing the maxillary canine and lateral and central incisors in irreversible pulpitis. Red, rare; green, very rare.

## *When supplemental anesthesia is needed*

In some patients, infiltration anesthesia is not completely effective; therefore, the intraosseous injection is indicated. Administer an intraosseous injection with 1.8 mL of 3% mepivacaine or 2% lidocaine with 1:100,000 epinephrine on the distal of the tooth to be anesthetized, unless the tooth is a second molar, in which case use a mesial intraosseous injection. This regimen should work the majority of the time in anesthetizing the posterior teeth.

Duration of infiltration anesthesia in the maxilla is not as long as in the mandible. Therefore, if pain is experienced during the later stages of instrumentation or obturation, an additional infiltration injection is necessary. Occasionally, pain is experienced with the palatal canal of molars. Infiltration of 0.5 mL of anesthetic solution over the palatal apex enhances anesthesia[21] and may prove helpful.

### Alternative choice for supplemental anesthesia

Although not as efficacious as intraosseous anesthesia, intraligamentary anesthesia can be given on the mesial and distal aspect of the tooth using 2% lidocaine with 1:100,000 epinephrine. Retest with cold refrigerant. If the patient does not respond, proceed with treatment. If there is a response to cold, repeat the intraligamentary injection.

## Canine and lateral and central incisors

An algorithm for anesthetizing the canine, lateral incisor, and central incisor in irreversible pulpitis is presented in Fig 7-5.

Administer topical anesthetic for at least 1 minute. Slowly administer an infiltration using a cartridge of 2% lidocaine with 1:50,000 or 1:100,000 epinephrine. The higher concentration of epinephrine (1:50,000) will provide a more effective duration.[22] A slow injection (at least 60 seconds) will be less painful. As an alternative, a two-stage injection technique may be used.[2] The use of the CompuDent CCLAD system will also reduce the pain of injection.[3–7] If lingual soft tissue anesthesia is needed for a rubber dam clamp, administer 2% lidocaine with 1:100,000 epinephrine to the palatal tissue. The CompuDent CCLAD system will reduce the pain of a palatal injection.[19,20] Wait 5 minutes, and then test the tooth with cold refrigerant. If the patient does not respond, proceed with treatment. This regimen should work the majority of the time in anesthetizing the anterior teeth. If the patient responds to cold, you can wait an additional 3 to 5 minutes and retest. If the patient still responds to cold, administer supplemental anesthesia.

### When supplemental anesthesia is needed

Although supplemental anesthesia is rarely necessary, when given, the intraosseous injection should be successful. Because intraligamentary anesthesia is very painful in anterior teeth, has a success rate of only 39% in asymptomatic teeth, and provides only a 10-minute duration of anesthesia,[17] intraosseous anesthesia is the best choice. In some patients, infiltration anesthesia is not completely effective and intraosseous anesthesia is very helpful. Use 1.8 mL of 3% mepivacaine or 2% lidocaine with 1:100,000 epinephrine.

It is important to realize that anesthesia starts to decline after an initial infiltration in anterior teeth. If the patient experiences pain during the later stages of instrumentation or obturation, an additional 1.8 mL of 2% lidocaine with 1:100,000 or 1:50,000 epinephrine can be given. The additional infiltration will prolong anesthesia.[23] If the intraosseous injection is given, there may be a need for an additional intraosseous injection using 1.8 mL of anesthetic solution because the intraosseous injection will not provide 60 minutes of anesthesia in the maxilla.

# Other Considerations for Endodontic Anesthesia

## Symptomatic teeth with total pulpal necrosis and apical pathosis

When patients present with symptomatic teeth, and examination reveals total pulpal necrosis and periapical radiolucencies, this is an indication of pain in the periapical tissue. Because these teeth may be painful to manipulation and movement during treatment, extra care must be taken.

After giving topical anesthetic, administer the conventional injections: IANB and long buccal injection for mandibular teeth. For maxillary teeth with no swelling, administer anesthesia with conventional infiltrations. If soft tissue swelling (ie, cellulitis or abscess) is present, infiltrate on either side of the swelling or administer a block—either a second division nerve block, posterior superior alveolar (PSA) nerve block, or infraorbital nerve block depending on the tooth involved. These injections will provide some degree of bone and soft tissue anesthesia. After achieving signs of anesthesia, place rubber dam and *slowly* begin the access. Usually, the pulp chamber can be entered without discomfort, if the tooth is not torqued excessively. Hand and rotary file placement and debridement can be performed without much pain if instruments are finessed.

Occasionally, the conventional injections do not provide profound anesthesia, particularly in maxillary teeth. Do not use intraosseous injections, intraligamentary injections, or intrapulpal injections. While effective for teeth presenting with irreversible pulpitis, these injections would likely be very painful and ineffective for symptomatic necrotic teeth with apical pathosis. Rather, explain to the patient that he or she does not have profound anesthesia due to the inflammation in the bone surrounding the tooth and use gentle file manipulation.

## Asymptomatic teeth with total pulpal necrosis and apical pathosis

Patients presenting with asymptomatic teeth with pulpal necrosis are the easiest to anesthetize; patient comfort is usually attained without difficulty. Although it may be tempting to proceed without anesthesia, pain may be experienced during instrumentation if anesthesia is not administered.

After giving topical anesthetic, administer the conventional injections: IANB and long buccal injection for mandibular molars and infiltration injections in maxillary teeth. Proceed with access and file placement. Usually, the patient is comfortable. On rare occasions, there may be some discomfort during canal preparation requiring an intraosseous or intraligamentary injection. Do not inject intrapulpally because bacteria and debris may be forced from the canal into the periapical tissue. In the maxilla, an additional infiltration may be necessary if anesthesia begins to wear off.

## Incision and drainage

We should always attempt to achieve some level of anesthesia before performing an incision and drainage procedure. Patients will tolerate the procedure better if there is a degree of anesthesia. In the mandible, a conventional IANB injection and long buccal injection (for molars) are administered. In the maxilla, infiltrate 1.8 mL of 2% lidocaine with 1:100,000 epinephrine on either side of the labial or buccal swelling. Because we are mostly concerned with soft tissue anesthesia, the following injections may be used: a PSA nerve block for molars, a second division nerve block for molars and premolars, and an infraorbital injection in anterior teeth. For palatal swellings, infiltrate 0.5 mL of 2% lidocaine with 1:100,000 epinephrine over the greater palatine foramen for molars and premolars or the nasopalatine foramen for anterior teeth. However, do not use these injections if swelling is present over the foramen. Infiltrate on either side of the swelling. The use of the CompuDent CCLAD system will reduce the pain of palatal injections.[19,20] Because profound anesthesia is usually difficult to achieve, this should be explained to the patient.

### *Why not inject the swelling?*
The traditional belief is that injecting directly into a swelling is contraindicated. The reasons given were the possible spread of infection and that the anesthetic solutions would be affected by the lower pH and would be rendered less effective. However, a basic science investigation found that local anesthetics may be successful in inflamed tissue, which is acidified.[24] Regardless, the basic reasons we do not inject swellings is that it is very painful and it is relatively ineffective. The area of a cellulitis has an increased blood supply. Injecting into this area causes the anesthetic to be carried away into the systemic circulation rather than effectively numbing the area locally. Therefore, the anesthetic effect is diminished when we inject swellings.

## Periapical surgery

It must be remembered that anesthesia is required for both soft tissue and bone. In the mandible, the IANB and long buccal injections are reasonably effective. Additional infiltration injections in the vestibule are useful to achieve vasoconstriction, particularly in the anterior mandible. In the maxilla, infiltration injections are generally effective. Usually larger volumes are necessary to provide anesthesia over the surgical field. That is, for maxillary anterior teeth, a cartridge of 2% lidocaine with 1:50,000 epinephrine can be given over the tooth requiring an apicoectomy, and a cartridge of 2% lidocaine with 1:100,000 epinephrine is given over each adjacent tooth. Gutmann and coauthors[25] reported that higher concentrations of vasoconstrictors can be used during surgical procedures. In the premolars and molars, a cartridge of 2% lidocaine with 1:100,000 epinephrine can be given over the tooth requiring an apicoectomy, and a cartridge of 2% lidocaine with 1:100,000 epinephrine is given over each adjacent tooth. Palatal anesthesia is also required. After anesthetizing the palatal tissue initially, a cartridge of 2% lidocaine with 1:100,000 epinephrine is given over the apex of the tooth.

If the surgical area is inflamed or the patient is apprehensive, anesthesia may not be totally successful. After the flap is reflected, if anesthesia is inadequate, attempts to enhance or regain anesthesia through additional infiltrations or injecting the sensitive area are not particularly effective. Yamazaki and coauthors[26] found that the effectiveness of surgical anesthesia is decreased by half when compared with anesthesia for nonsurgical procedures. This occurs because when reflecting a flap and

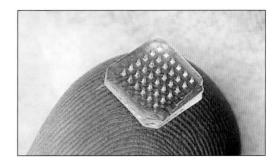

**Fig 7-6** Microneedles may be used in the future to deliver topical or local anesthetics across mucosal surfaces painlessly. (Courtesy of Jeong-Woo Lee, Georgia Tech.)

opening into bone, the anesthetic solution is diluted by bleeding and is removed by irrigation.[26] Ogawa and coauthors[27] reported similar findings experimentally.

We have found anecdotally that when surgical anesthesia during the latter part of the surgery is inadequate, giving a palatal infiltration over the surgical site is helpful in the maxilla. Additional consideration could be given to PSA nerve block or high tuberosity second division nerve block for molars and infraorbital nerve block for premolars. In the mandible, repeating the IANB sometimes helps to restore surgical anesthesia.

As a prophylactic measure, an intraosseous injection may be administered at the site after routine injections and before the surgery. This may enhance depth of anesthesia and may provide better hemostasis. Baker and coauthors[28] found that either infiltration or intraosseous anesthesia resulted in significantly less osseous bleeding than the use of no anesthesia. However, they did not study the combination of infiltration and intraosseous anesthesia for osseous bleeding. Further studies are needed to determine the anesthetic effects and amount of bleeding using the combination injections.

Use of a long-acting anesthetic has been advocated for surgery.[29,30] In the mandible, this is reasonably effective. In the maxilla, long-acting agents have a shorter duration of anesthesia and decreased epinephrine concentrations, which result in more bleeding during surgery.[31,32] For infiltration anesthesia for apicoectomy, Meechan and Blair[33] found that long-acting local anesthetics gave soft tissue anesthesia for twice as long as lidocaine with epinephrine without a significant reduction in the pain experience or in the timing of self-prescribed analgesia. Therefore, the use of long-acting agents with epinephrine offers no advantage over lidocaine with epinephrine when administered as a maxillary infiltration for apical surgery.

After periapical surgery, administration of a long-acting anesthetic has been suggested.[34] However, postsurgical pain is usually not severe and can be managed by nonprescription analgesics.[33,35–39] Morin and coauthors[40] found that women reported postsurgical pain from implant placement as more intense than what men reported, but men were more disturbed than women by low levels of pain that lasted several days.

# Future Directions

Research continues in the development of new or improved anesthetics. Capsaicin and transient receptor potential vanilloid-1 (TRPV-1) agonist and antagonists may in the future be used in the clinical management of pain associated with inflammation.[41–43]

Considerable ongoing research, therefore, is directed at the development of new local anesthetic formulations that allow clinicians to better treat patients in pain.

New modes of delivery of drugs are also being studied. Microneedles are a new technology to enhance delivery of drugs.[44,45] Gupta et al[46] demonstrated that microneedle-based lidocaine injection was as rapid and as effective as hypodermic syringe injection in inducing local anesthesia of the forearm and dorsum of the hand while resulting in less pain during injection. Perhaps microneedles could deliver topical or local anesthetics across mucosal surfaces painlessly (Fig 7-6).

# References

1. Kanaa M, Meechan J, Corbett I, Whitworth J. Speed of injection influences efficacy of inferior alveolar nerve blocks: A double-blind randomized controlled trial in volunteers. J Endod 2006;32:919–923.
2. Nusstein J, Steinkruger G, Reader A, Beck M, Weaver J. The effects of a 2-stage injection technique on inferior alveolar nerve block injection pain. Anesth Prog 2006;53:126–130.
3. Palm AM, Kirkegaard U, Poulsen S. The Wand versus traditional injection for mandibular nerve block in children and adolescents: Perceived pain and time of onset. Pediatr Dent 2004;26;481–484.
4. Oztas N, Ulusu T, Bodur H, Dougan C. The Wand in pulp therapy: An alternative to inferior alveolar nerve block. Quintessence Int 2005;36:559–564.
5. Sumer M, Misir F, Koyuturk AE. Comparison of the Wand with a conventional technique. Oral Surg Oral Med Oral Pathol Oral Radiol Endod 2006;101:106–109.
6. Yesilyurt C, Bulut G, Taşdemir T. Pain perception during inferior alveolar injection administered with the Wand or conventional syringe. Br Dent J 2008;205:258–259.
7. Yenisey M. Comparison of the pain levels of computer-controlled and conventional anesthesia techniques in prosthodontics treatment. J Appl Oral Sci 2009;17:414–420.
8. Fowler S, Drum M, Reader A, Beck M. Anesthetic success of an inferior alveolar nerve block and supplemental articaine buccal infiltration for molars and premolars in patients with symptomatic irreversible pulpitis. J Endod 2016;42:390–392.
9. Replogle K, Reader A, Nist R, Beck M, Weaver J, Meyers WJ. Cardiovascular effects of intraosseous injections of 2 percent lidocaine with 1:100,000 epinephrine and 3 percent mepivacaine. J Am Dent Assoc 1999;130:649–657.
10. Gallatin E, Stabile P, Reader A, Nist R, Beck M. Anesthetic efficacy and heart rate effects of the intraosseous injection of 3% mepivacaine after an inferior alveolar nerve block. Oral Surg Oral Med Oral Pathol Oral Radiol Endod 2000;89:83–87.
11. Reisman D, Reader A, Nist R, Beck M, Weaver J. Anesthetic efficacy of the supplemental intraosseous injection of 3% mepivacaine in irreversible pulpitis. Oral Surg Oral Med Oral Pathol Oral Radiol Endod 1997;84:676–682.
12. Dunbar D, Reader A, Nist R, Beck M, Meyers WJ. Anesthetic efficacy of the intraosseous injection after an inferior alveolar nerve block. J Endod 1996;22:481–486.
13. Guglielmo A, Reader A, Nist R, Beck M, Weaver J. Anesthetic efficacy and heart rate effects of the supplemental intraosseous injection of 2% mepivacaine with 1:20,000 levonordefrin. Oral Surg Oral Med Oral Pathol Oral Radiol Endod 1999;87:284–293.
14. Walton RE, Abbott BJ. Periodontal ligament injection: A clinical evaluation. J Am Dent Assoc 1981;103:571–575.
15. Cohen H, Cha B, Spangberg L. Endodontic anesthesia in mandibular molars: A clinical study. J Endod 1993;19:370–373.
16. Nusstein J, Claffey E, Reader A, Beck M, Weaver J. Anesthetic effectiveness of the supplemental intraligamentary injection, administered with a computer-controlled local anesthetic delivery system, in patients with irreversible pulpitis. J Endod 2005;31:354–358.
17. White JJ, Reader A, Beck M, Meyers WJ. The periodontal ligament injection: A comparison of the efficacy in human maxillary and mandibular teeth. J Endod 1988;14:508–514.
18. Mikesell A, Drum M, Reader A, Beck M. Anesthetic efficacy of 1.8 mL and 3.6 mL of 2% lidocaine with 1:100,000 epinephrine for maxillary infiltrations. J Endod 2008;34:121–125.
19. Primosch RE, Brooks R. Influence of anesthetic flow rate delivered by the Wand local anesthetic system on pain response to palatal injections. Am J Dent 2002;15:15–20.
20. Nusstein J, Lee S, Reader A, Beck M, Weaver J. Injection pain and postinjection pain of the anterior middle superior alveolar injection administered with the Wand or conventional syringe. Oral Surg Oral Med Oral Pathol Endod 2004;98:124–131.
21. Guglielmo A, Drum M, Reader A, Nusstein J. Anesthetic efficacy of a combination palatal and buccal infiltration of the maxillary first molar. J Endod 2011;37:460–462.
22. Mason R, Drum M, Reader A, Nusstein, Beck M. A prospective, randomized, double-blind comparison of 2% lidocaine with 1:100,000 and 1:50,000 epinephrine and 3% mepivacaine for maxillary infiltrations. J Endod 2009;35:1173–1177.
23. Scott J, Drum M, Reader A, Nusstein J, Beck M. The efficacy of a repeated infiltration in prolonging duration of pulpal anesthesia in maxillary lateral incisors. J Am Dent Assoc 2009;140:318–324.
24. Tsuschiya H, Mizogami M, Ueno T, Takakura K. Interaction of local anaesthetics with lipid membranes under inflammatory conditions. Inflammopharmacology 2007;15:164–170.
25. Gutmann JL, Frazier LW, Baron B. Plasma catecholamine and haemodynamic responses to surgical endodontic anaesthetic protocols. Int Endod J 1996;29:37–42.
26. Yamazaki S, Seino H, Ozawa S, Ito H, Kawaai H. Elevation of a periosteal flap with irrigation of the bone for minor oral surgery reduces the duration of action of infiltration anesthesia. Anesth Prog 2006;53:8–12.
27. Ogawa S, Watanabe M, Kawaai H, Tada H, Yamazaki S. Lidocaine concentration in mandibular bone after subperiosteal infiltration anesthesia decreases with elevation of periosteal flap and irrigation with saline. Anesth Prog 2014;61(2):53–62.
28. Baker TF, Torabinejad M, Schwartz SF, Wolf D. Effect of intraosseous anesthesia on control of hemostasis in pigs. J Endod 2009;35:1543–1545.
29. Davis W, Oakley J, Smith E. Comparison of the effectiveness of etidocaine and lidocaine as local anesthetic agents during oral surgery. Anesth Prog 1984;31:159–164.
30. Rosenquist J, Rosenquist K, Lee P. Comparison between lidocaine and bupivacaine as local anesthetics with diflunisal for postoperative pain control after lower third molar surgery. Anesth Prog 1988;35:1–4.

31. Gross R, McCartney M, Reader A, Beck M. A prospective, randomized, double-blind comparison of bupivacaine and lidocaine for maxillary infiltrations. J Endod 2007;33:1021–1024.

32. Crout RJ, Koraido G, Moore PA. A clinical trial of long-acting local anesthetics for periodontal surgery. Anesth Prog 1990;37:194–198.

33. Meechan JG, Blair GS. The effect of two different local anaesthetic solutions on pain experience following apicectomy. Br Dent J 1993;175:410–413.

34. Malamed S. Handbook of Local Anesthesia, ed 5. St Louis: Mosby, 2004.

35. Chong BS, Pitt Ford TR. Postoperative pain after root-end resection and filling. Oral Surg Oral Med Oral Pathol Oral Radiol Endod 2005;100:762–766.

36. Iqbal MK, Kratchman SI, Guess GM, Karabucak B, Kim S. Microscopic periradicular surgery: Perioperative predictors for postoperative clinical outcomes and quality of life assessment. J Endod 2007;33:239–244.

37. Penarrocha M, Garcia B, Marti E, Balaguer J. Pain and inflammation after periapical surgery in 60 patients. J Oral Maxillofac Surg 2006;64:429–433.

38. García B, Penarrocha M, Martí E, Gay-Escodad C, von Arx T. Pain and swelling after periapical surgery related to oral hygiene and smoking. Oral Surg Oral Med Oral Pathol Oral Radiol Endod 2007;104:271–276.

39. Tsesis I, Fuss Z, Lin S, Tilinger G, Peled M. Analysis of postoperative symptoms following surgical endodontic treatment. Quintessence Int 2003;34:756–760.

40. Morin C, Lund JP, Villarroel T, Clokie CM, Feine JS. Differences between the sexes in post-surgical pain. Pain 2000;85:79–85.

41. Knotkova H, Pappagallo M, Szallasi A. Capsaicin (TRPV1 agonist) therapy for pain relief: Farewell or revival? Clin J Pain 2008;24:142–154.

42. Kissin I. Vanilloid-induced conduction analgesia: Selective, dose-dependent, long-lasting, with a low level of potential neurotoxicity. Anesth Analg 2008;107:271–281.

43. Gerner P, Binshtok AM, Wang CF, et al. Capsaicin combined with local anesthetics preferentially prolongs sensory/nociceptive block in rat sciatic nerve. Anesthesiology 2008;109:872–878.

44. Al-Qallaf B, Das DB. Optimizing microneedle arrays to increase skin permeability for transdermal drug delivery. Ann N Y Acad Sci 2009;1161:83–84.

45. Wu Y, Qiu Y, Zhang S, Qin G, Gao Y. Microneedle-based drug delivery: Studies on delivery parameters and biocompatibility. Biomed Microdevices 2008;10:601–610.

46. Gupta J, Denson DD, Felner EI, Prausnitz MR. Rapid local anesthesia in humans using minimally invasive microneedles. Clin J Pain 2012;28:129–135.

# Index

Page numbers followed by "f" denote figures; those followed by "t" denote tables.